Progress
in Drug
Research

Vol. 53

Edited by Ernst Jucker, Basel

Board of Advisors
Joseph M. Colacino
Pushkar N. Kaul
Vera M. Kolb
J. Mark Treherne
Q. May Wang

Authors
Jacob Szmuszkovicz
Satya P. Gupta
Bijoy Kundu, Sanjay K. Khare and
Shiva K. Rastogi
Paul Spence
Mary S. Barnette

Springer Basel AG

Editor

Dr. E. Jucker
Steinweg 28
CH-4107 Ettingen
Switzerland
e-mail: jucker.pdr@bluewin.ch

Visit our PDR homepage: http://www.birkhauser/books/biosc/pdr

© 1999 Springer Basel AG
Originally published by Birkhäuser Verlag in 1999
Softcover reprint of the hardcover 1999
Printed on acid-free paper produced from chlorine-free pulp. TCF ∞
Cover design and layout: Gröflin Graphic Design, Basel

ISBN 978-3-0348-9749-5   ISBN 978-3-0348-8735-9 (eBook)
DOI 10.1007/978-3-0348-8735-9

9 8 7 6 5 4 3 2 1

Contents

Foreword by the Editor

Volume 53 of *Progress in Drug Research* contains five review articles and the various indexes which facilitate the use of monograph and also help to establish PDR as an encyclopedic source of information in the complex and fast growing field of drug research.The first article in this volume is devoted to κ-agonists, an important group of compounds which are being tested as agents with diuretic, analgesic and neuroprotective properties.The remaining contributions deal with quantitative structure-activity relationships of various classes of antihypertensive agents, with combinatorial chemistry as a powerful tool for accelerating the drug discovery process, with the complete characterisation of an organism's gene expression leading to optimisation of the search for new drugs. The last contribution reviews the role of phosphodiesterase inhibitors in the developments of novel therapies for asthma and chronic obstructive pulmonary disease.

All of these reviews contain extensive bibliographies, thus enabling the interested reader to have easy access to the original literature.

In the 40 years of PDR's existence, drug research has undergone drastic changes; the original purpose of this series of monographs, however, remained unchanged: dissemination of information about the actual trends and crucial points of drug research. The Editor is anxious to maintain the high standard of these monographs and is grateful to the contributing authors for their willingness to undertake the hard work of writing comprehensive review articles for the benefit of all involved with drug research.

In ending this foreword, I would like to thank the authors for their contributions, the Members of the Board of Advisors for their advice and the reviewers for their help in improving these monographs. Last but not least, I am grateful to Birkhäuser Publishers, and in particular to Ruedi Jappert, Janine Kern, Bernd Luchner, Eduard Mazenauer, Claus Puhlmann and Gregor Messmer, with whom I have a cooperative relationship that is harmonious and rewarding. My very special thanks go to Mr. Hans-Peter Thür, the CEO of Birkhäuser Publishers. Over many years I did and still do enjoy Mr. Thür's constant support and encouragement to continue with the editorship of PDR.

Basel, September 1999   Dr. E. Jucker

Progress in Drug Research, Vol. 53 (E. Jucker, Ed.)
©1999 Birkhäuser Verlag, Basel (Switzerland)

U-50,488 and the κ receptor Part II*: 1991–1998

By Jacob Szmuszkovicz

Department of Chemistry and Bio-
chemistry, University of Notre
Dame, Notre Dame, IN 46556-5670,
USA

*Part I was published in vol. 52
of this series.

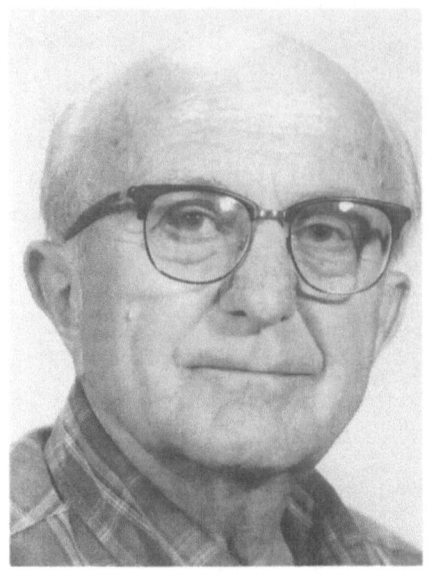

Jacob Szmuszkovicz

was born in Lódz, Poland. He received a B.Sc. degree at the American University of Beirut and a Ph.D. degree at the Hebrew University and the Weizmann Institute. After postdoctoral appointments at Harvard University, the University of Wisconsin and Columbia, he joined the Upjohn Company. He retired from Upjohn as a distinguished scientist and joined the Department of Chemistry and Biochemistry at the University of Notre Dame.

Summary

This review, Part II, follows an earlier article, Part I, published in volume 52 of this series. Part II is a discussion of centrally and peripherally acting κ agonists which can be considered analogs of U-50,488. Included also are three classes of κ agonists which fall outside of the scope of the general structure of U-50,488. These are benzodiazepines, phenothiazines and diazobicyclononanones. The discussion also covers other pertinent topics including labelled ligands and sigma receptor.

Contents

Jacob Szmuszkovicz

Keywords

Analgesics, κ agonists, U-50,488, κ receptor, sigma receptor, centrally acting analgesics, peripherally acting analgesics, dysphoria.

Glossary of abbreviations

SC, subcutaneous; NMDA, N-methyl-D-aspartate; nM, nanomolar; IC_{50}, inhibitory concentration$_{50}$; LVD, rabbit vas deferens essay; DUP, DuPont; U, Upjohn; ICI, Imperial Chemical Industries; RP, Rhone-Poulenc; i.v., intravenous; i.p., intraperitoneal; icv, intracerebroventricular; EMD, E. Merck Darmstadt; MAC, mouse abdominal constriction test.

1 Introduction

1.1 General remarks

This review is a sequel to the article published in volume 52 of this series which was entitled "U-50,488 and the κ receptor: A personalized account covering the period 1973 to 1990". The reader is encouraged to peruse the abovementioned Part I of this series as background for Part II. Several concise reviews on this subject have appeared during 1981 to 1998 [1–8]. A comprehensive review of the chemistry of 1,2-diamines has recently been published [9]. Part II of this review does not include morphine and peptide related κ agonists.

1.2 Therapeutic potential of κ agonists

The main therapeutic potential for centrally acting κ agonists (see section 2) is the treatment of severe to moderate pain. This class of drugs possesses several advantages over mu agonists. κ agonists do not cause respiratory depression, constipation and physical dependence liability. Centrally acting κ agonists also have neuroprotective effects and may be useful for the treatment of stroke [10]. They produce water diuresis and have an antitussive effect (for references see [6]); they also have potential as agents for hypertension [11, 12].

4

Another major interest in κ agonists relates to their potential as peripherally acting analgesics (see section 6), useful for the treatment of inflammatory conditions.

1.3   Ongoing basic research

Basic research on κ receptor related science is progressing. Some of the areas of interest include the relationship between μ and κ receptor [13, 14], κ receptor subtypes (see section 9), interaction with the cholinergic system [15–19] site-directed mutagenesis studies [20, 21] studies with knockout mice [22], immunomodulation [23], renal function [24], cocaine addiction [25], anticonvulsant effects possibly involving glycine/NMDA receptor complex [26], feeding and neuroendocrine regulation [27].

1.4   The cocaine-procaine and the morphine-U-50,488 events

During a lecture in 1977 [28], Dr. Harris Isbell summarized the search for a non-addicting analgesic organized by the Committee on Drug Addiction and Narcotics in 1929. The committee was strongly influenced by the finding that procaine, a synthetic drug, did not have the euphoric properties of cocaine and took the place of cocaine as a local anesthetic in medical practice (Fig. 1).

Morphine has served as a template for several generations of medicinal chemists. Modifications of the morphine molecule produced a vast range of compounds with the mild propoxyphene at one end, potent drugs like methadone in the middle and, finally, extremely potent drugs such as etorphine (Immobilon) and sufentanil at the other end. Despite a wide variation in structures, the pharmacology of these morphine related compounds is similar. Thus, Isbell concluded in 1977 that the discovery of the perfect analgesic had not been realized yet.

Today, the cocaine-procaine experience may be compared to the morphine-U-50,488 development. A major step towards the goal of finding a non-addicting strong analgesic has been accomplished by the Upjohn discovery of U-50,488 [29]. Hopefully, in the near future the dysphoric side-effects of U-50,488 series will be better understood and resolved and, thus, pave the way for the κ agonist to become a pain remedy.

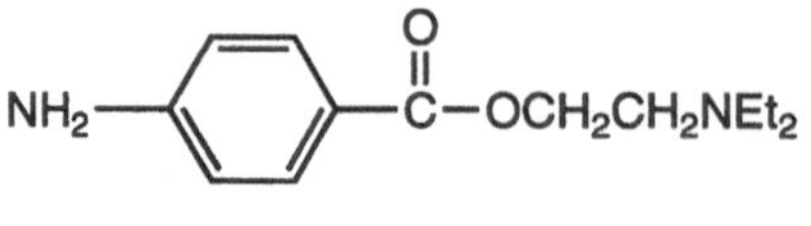

Fig. 1
Structures of procaine and cocaine.

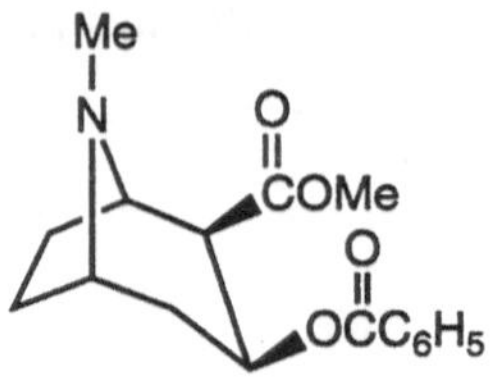

2 Centrally acting U-50,488 analogs

2.1 Glaxo piperidine and piperazine analogs

The Glaxo scientists concentrated their efforts on U-50,488 analogs in which one nitrogen is either part of the piperdine ring (Fig. 25) [30, 31] or piperazine ring (Fig. 26) [32]. This effort produced some very active κ agonists. In the piperidine series (Fig. 2) the 3-oxopyrrolidinyl compound A and the ketal compound B were most active. In the piperazine series (Fig. 3) the carbomethoxy pyrrolidine compound A is most active and the activity resided in (R)-enantiomer. The above compounds displayed high selectivity for the κ opioid receptors over both μ and δ receptors. They were also potent antinociceptive agents as determined by the mouse acetylcholine-induced abdominal constriction test (sc).

Compoundd GR 89696 (Fig. 3) was found to be neuroprotective in both global and cerebral ischaemia animal models [10].

GR 89696 was found to an agonist at κ-2 receptor and antagonist at κ-1 receptors in the guinea pig hippocampus. κ-2 receptors may represent an important route to the regulation of NMDA receptor function in certain neuropathologies [33].

The Adolor group reported orally on the analog of GR 89696 with improved peripheral selectivity but no details were published [34].

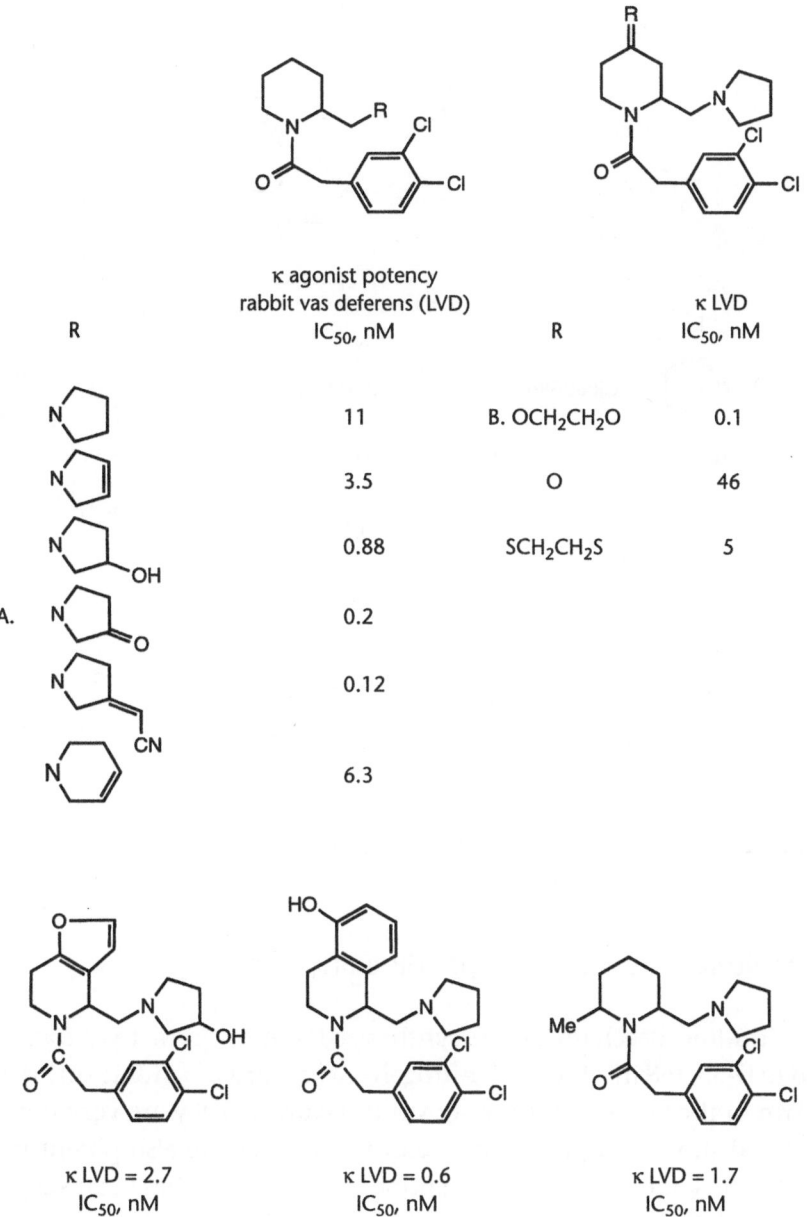

R	κ agonist potency rabbit vas deferens (LVD) IC$_{50}$, nM	R	κ LVD IC$_{50}$, nM
A.	11	B. OCH$_2$CH$_2$O	0.1
	3.5	O	46
	0.88	SCH$_2$CH$_2$S	5
	0.2		
	0.12		
	6.3		

κ LVD = 2.7 IC$_{50}$, nM

κ LVD = 0.6 IC$_{50}$, nM

κ LVD = 1.7 IC$_{50}$, nM

Fig. 2
Glaxo analogs of U-50,488 in which one nitrogen is part of a piperidine ring.

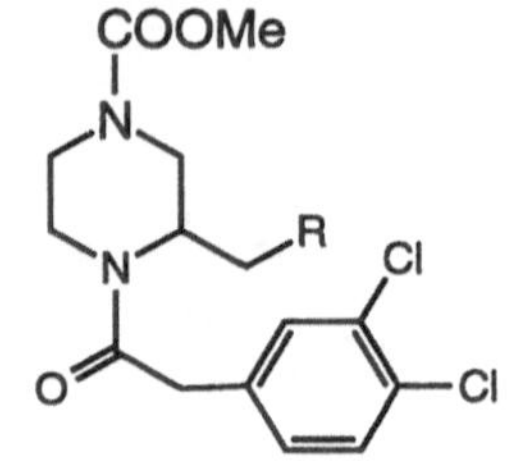

	R		κ agonist potency rabbit vas deferens (LVD) IC_{50}, nM
A. (±)	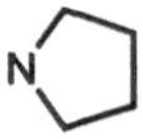	GR 89696	0.041
(R)	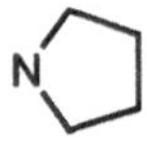	GR 103545	0.018
	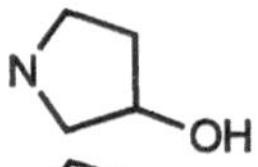		0.34
	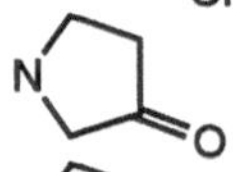		0.34
	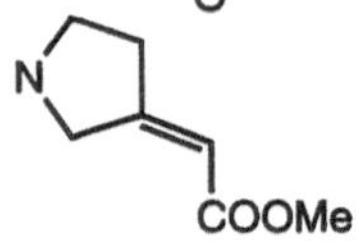		0.28

Fig. 3
Glaxo analogs of U-50,488 in which one nitrogen is part of a piperazine ring.

2.2 SmithKline Beecham piperidine analogs

The SmithKline Beecham group synthesized some very active κ agonists related to U-50,488 in which one nitrogen is a part of a piperidine ring (Fig. 4) [35]. Two of the compounds are shown in Figure 4. They are very potent κ ligands and show very good mu/κ selevitivity. They are also potent in the mouse tail flick model of antinociception. Compound B has been subjected to clinical trial as a κ selective analgesic.

Compound C (Fig. 4) was described in a patent [36]. No opioid receptor binding data was reported but in standard rodent analgesic assays potent activity was observed after sc injection (mouse writhing $ED_{50} = 0.005$ mg/kg).

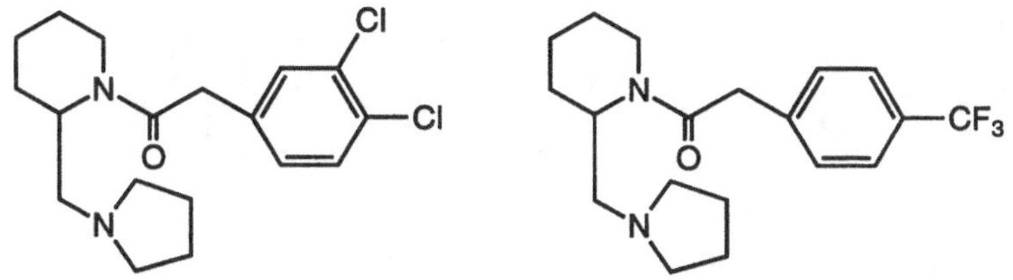

	receptor binding affinity Ki, nM			mouse tail flick
	κ	μ	μ/κ	ED$_{50}$, mg/kg sc
A.	0.24	1560	6500	50
B.	0.57	2340	4100	110

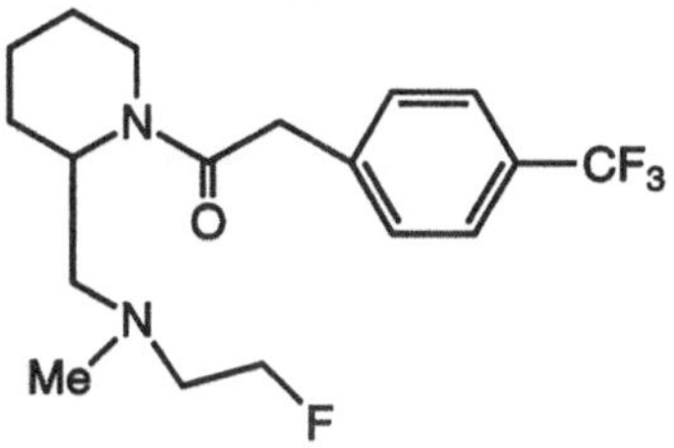

Fig. 4
SmithKline Beecham analogs of U-50,488 in which one nitrogen is part of a piperidine ring.

The SmithKline Beecham group described a series of U-50,488 analogs in which one nitrogen is part of a tetrahydroisoquinoline ring (Fig. 5) [37, 38]. The general trend of the receptor binding profile in this series tends to be morphine-like; namely, the compounds exhibit affinity to κ as well as to μ and δ receptors. The presence of the fused aromatic ring has caused an increase in μ affinity. This increase is particularly striking in the case of the 5-hydroxy compound E when compared to the unsubstituted compound D. The authors ascribe it to the presence of the phenolic ring, mimicking the tyramine moiety, as in the alkaloid agonists of the morphine series. The best mu/κ ratio is exhibited by compound D which does not have substituents on either ring of the tetrahydroisoquinoline moiety.

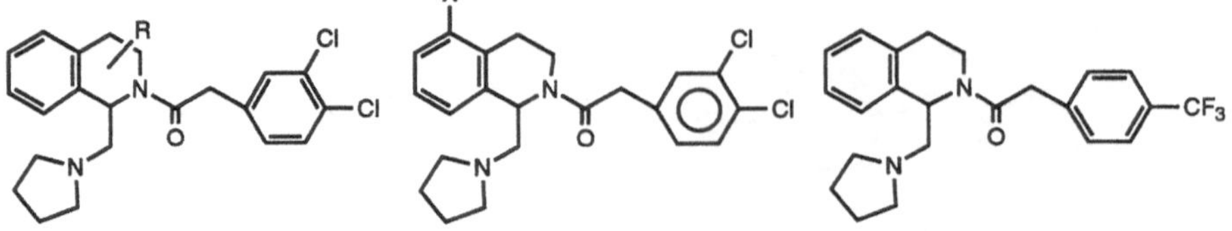

A, B, C   D, E   F

receptor binding affinity
Ki, nM

	all are (−)	κ	μ	δ	μ/κ
A	R = 3-Me cis	0.43	11.1	43.6	26
B	R = 4-Me trans	0.6	56.5	158	94
C	R = 4.4-Me$_2$	2.3	239	1010	104
D	X = H	0.2	30.2	113	151
E	X = OH	0.09	0.49	7.09	5.4
F		0.24	10.7	149	44

Fig. 5
SmithKline Beecham analogs of U-50,488 in which one nitrogen is part of a tetrahydroisoquinoline ring.

The above group has extended the above SAR to include two compounds in which one nitrogen is part of a thienopiperidine ring (Fig. 6) [38]. Compound A showed the best mu/κ ratio of the compounds shown in Figures 5 and 6.

The SmithKline Beecham group described U-50,488 analogs in which one nitrogen is part of a piperidine ring and the aromatic ring is extended to tetraline and tetralone. Four of these are shown in Figure 7 [39].

Overall this series showed lack of correlation between κ binding affinity and antinociceptive potency *in vivo* as shown in Figure 7.

The most interesting compound C showed moderate κ affinity (Ki = 47 nM), negligible affinity for mu, delta and sigma receptors (Ki > 1000 nM), *in vivo* subcutaneous antinociceptive activity, reduced propensity to cause sedation and diuresis and, finally, it displayed lesser propensity to aversive side-effects.

A paper also appeared from this group [40] describing the receptor binding and antinociceptive activity of racemates and enantiomers of a large number of compounds in the series discussed above.

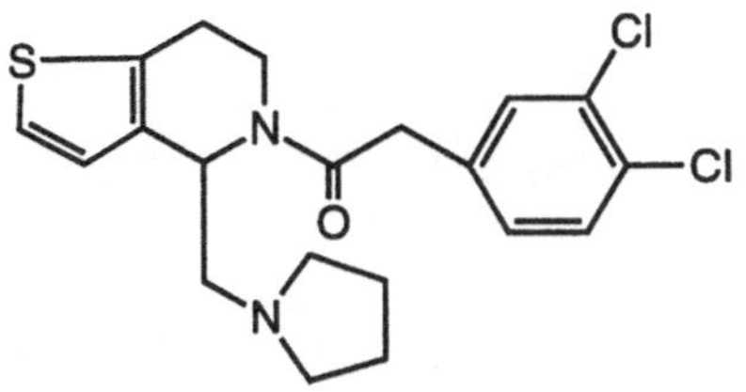

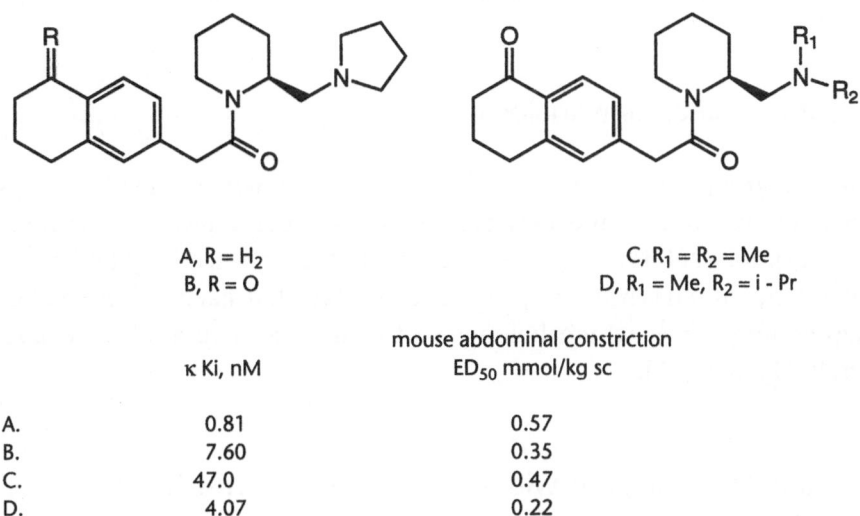

	binding affinity Ki, nM			
	κ	μ	δ	μ/κ
A	0.22	47.2	153	215
B	0.46	47	362	102

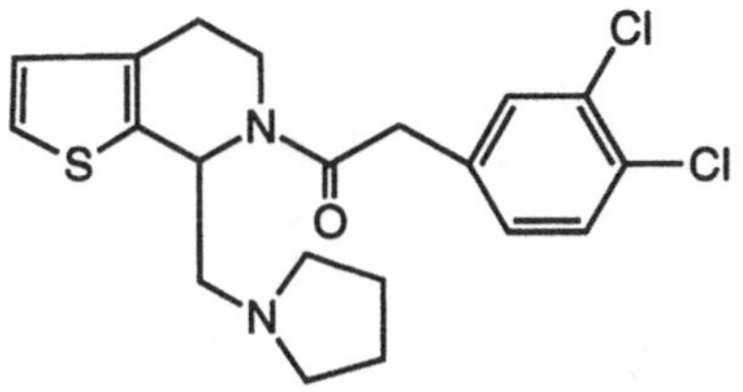

Fig. 6
SmithKline Beecham analogs of U-50,488 in which one nitrogen is part of a thienopiperidine ring.

A, R = H₂
B, R = O

C, R₁ = R₂ = Me
D, R₁ = Me, R₂ = i - Pr

	κ Ki, nM	mouse abdominal constriction ED₅₀ mmol/kg sc
A.	0.81	0.57
B.	7.60	0.35
C.	47.0	0.47
D.	4.07	0.22

Fig. 7
SmithKline Beecham analogs of U-50,488 in which one nitrogen is part of a piperidine ring.

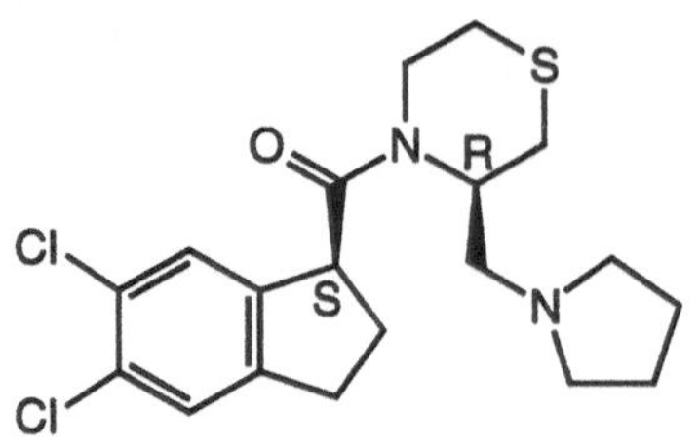

R-84760

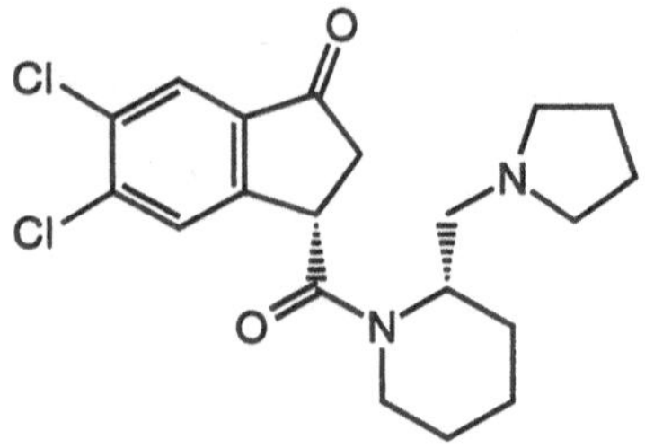

A.

IC_{50}, nM
$\kappa = 0.9$
$\mu = 230$

	κ	μ	δ	μ/κ
		IC_{50}, nM		
R-84760	0.436	297	1030	681
U-50,488	7.59	571	10.400	75.2

Fig. 8
Sankyo analogs of U-50,488 in which one nitrogen is part of a six-membered ring and the amide side-chain has restricted rotation.

2.3 Sankyo piperidine analogs

The Sankyo group synthesized analogs of U-50,488 in which one nitrogen is part of a six-membered ring and the amidic side chain has restricted rotation (Fig. 8) [41]. R-84760 is a κ agonist with high affinity, selectivity and functional potency and has been subjected to extensive pharmacology. An earlier Sankyo compound A, which belongs to the same structural class, is also shown in Figure 8 [42].

2.4 Parke-Davis analogs with conformationally restricted aromatic rings

In elaboration of the earlier leads PD 117302 and PD 129290 (CI-977, enadoline) (Fig. 9, compound A and B) [43] Parke-Davis scientists found that com-

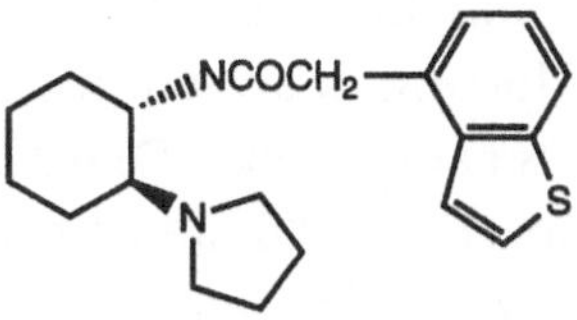

A. (PD 117302)

κ Ki = 3.7 nM
μ:κ = 110

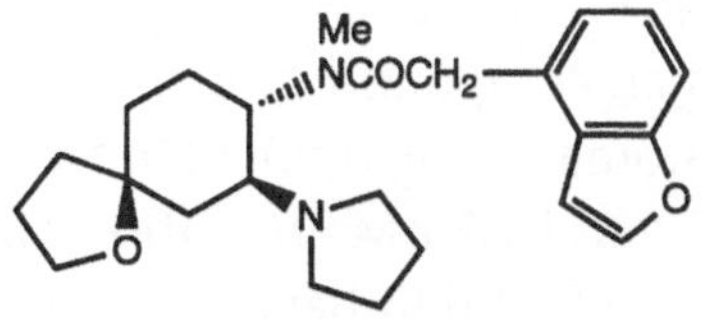

B. (PD 129290)
Cl-977 enadoline

κ Ki = 0.83 nM
μ:κ = 1520

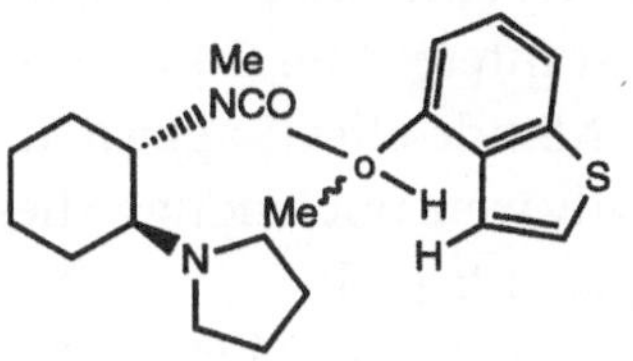

C.
1:1 mixture of two diastereosiomers

κ Ki = 172 nM
μ Ki = 2460
μ:κ = 14

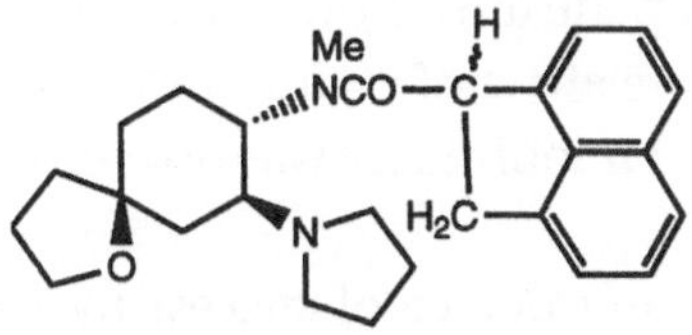

D.
diastereosiomer I: κ Ki = 0.37
                       μ Ki = 244
                       μ:κ = 659

diastereosiomer II: κ Ki = 1.2
                       μ Ki = 273
                       μ:κ = 227

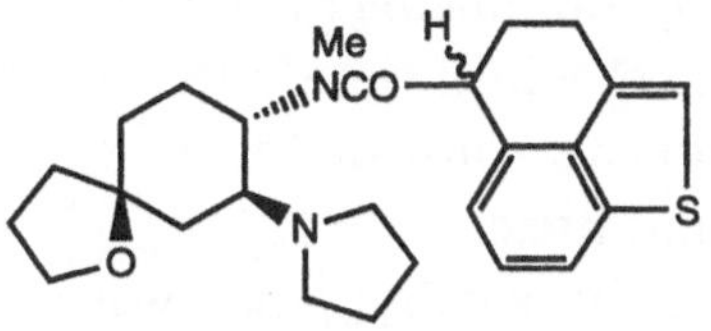

E.
diastereosiomer I: κ Ki = 4.65
                       μ Ki = 507
                       μ:κ = 109

diastereosiomer II: κ Ki = 11.1
                       μ Ki = 62
                       μ:κ = 5.6

Fig. 9
Parke-Davis compounds with conformationally restricted aromatic rings.

pound C, which has a methyl group in the side chain, had much lower affinity than compound A (Ki 172 vs 3.7 nM). Introduction of acenaphthene as the aromatic ring resulted in two diastereoisomers I and II (Fig. 9D) with κ Ki = 0.37 and 1.2 nM; μ/κ ratio = 659 and 227, respectively. Diastereoisomer I was also found to have high selectivity with respect to the δ receptor, δ Ki = 578 nM, δ/κ ratio = 1562. The corresponding naphthalene analogue showed κ Ki = 3.35 nM. Finally, the dihydronaphthothiophene derivatives were prepared (Fig. 9, E). Diastereoisomer I was found to have higher κ receptor affinity and higher mu/κ selectivity than diastereoisomer II (κ Ki = 4.65, 11.1 and μ/κ ratio = 109, 5.6, respectively).

Of the class of compounds summarized in Figure 9, compound B (enadoline) appears to be the most interesting. Clinical trials with enadoline have been reported. Although CNS side-effects appeared at high doses, dysphoria and psychotomimetic activity were not amongst them. Enadoline is currently in clinical trials in stroke patients [44].

The Parke-Davis group designed some highly lipophilic compounds based on the rationale that this may lead to peripherally selective agents (Fig. 10) [45]. Compound A, in which a benzhydryl group replaced the eastern methylene group bearing the aromatic ring of U-50,488, had poor activity as a κ agonist. When the two phenyl groups of the benzhydryl substituent were constrained into a planar configuration, the resulting fluorene derivative (compound B) was active. The planarity of this molecule was further modified by introducing the 1,2-diphenylcyclopropene unit shown in compounds C and D, which were both active. The sedative effect of compound D (in the rotarod test) provided evidence that increased lipophilicity was not sufficient to limit its access to CNS.

The benzhydryl group was used with greater degree of success by the E. Merck group in EMD 61753 (asimadoline) shown in Figure 27. For a discussion of this benzhydryl group in relation to hydrophobic collapse see Section 6.1.

2.5 DuPont-Merck benzologs of U-50,488

The DuPont-Merck group [46, 47] elaborated further on their earlier benzolog lead (Compound A in Fig. 11; see also Fig. 12 in part I) which arose from the combination of the structural features of U-50,488 and 2-aminotetralin. The aminotetralin is present in compound B (Fig. 11), which has been reported

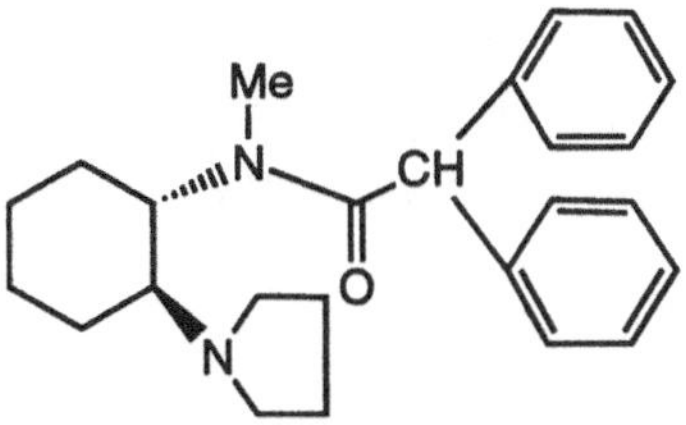

A.
κ EC$_{50}$ (LVD) > 10 μM

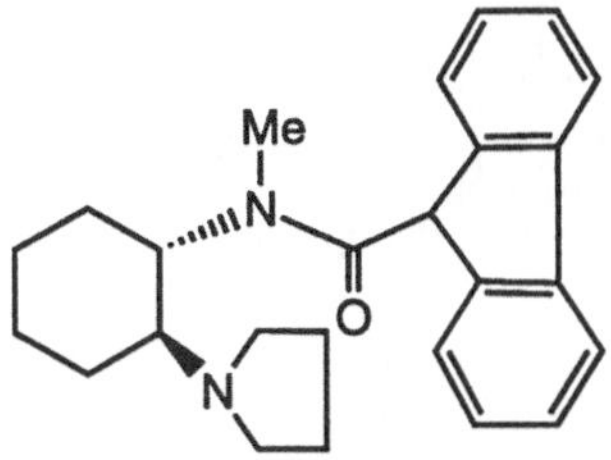

B.
κ EC$_{50}$ (LVD) > 22 nM

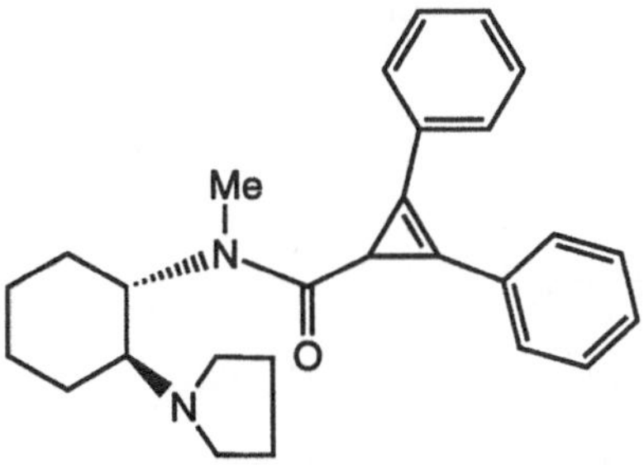

C.
κ EC$_{50}$ (LVD) = 32 nM

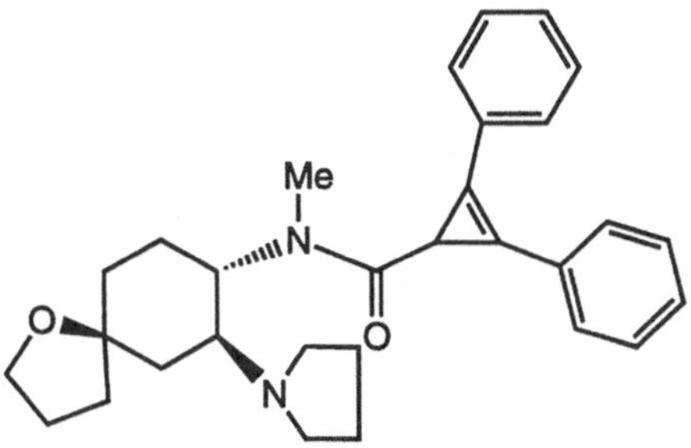

D.
κ EC$_{50}$ (LVD) = 9.6 nM
log P = 4.39
rotarod (mouse) ED$_{50}$ = 0.6 mg/kg

Fig. 10
Parke-Davis lipophilic κ agonists rigid benzhydryl analogs. (LVD = rabbit vas deferens assay)

to be a potent analgesic [46], and is also a part of ethylketocyclazocine frame-work. DuP 747 emerged as the most interesting candidate as a result of an extensive SAR study [47]. The benzolog feature has been included in the analysis of the north-west region of U-50,488 (and section 2.11 of this review).

2.6 Hoechst Marion Roussel benzologs with cyclopentane rings

Niravoline (RU-51599) is a Hoechst Marion Roussel compound (Fig. 12) [49, 49a]. It belongs to the structural class of benzologs of U-50,488 in which the

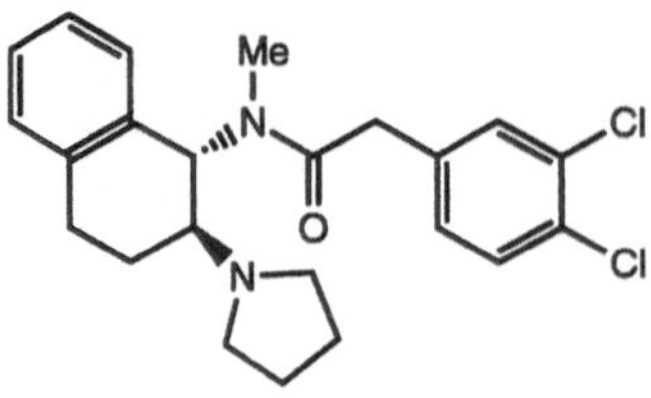

Jacob Szmuszkovicz

A

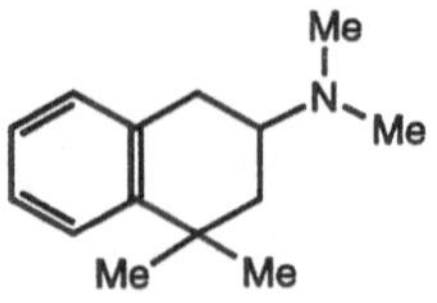

B

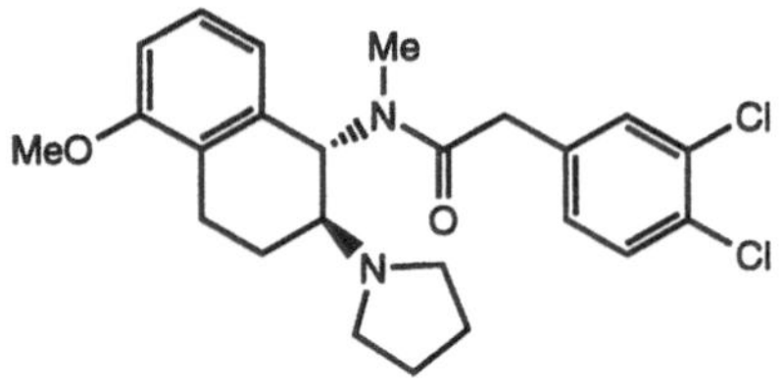

DuP 747

Opiod receptor binding

Compound	κ Ki, nM	μ Ki, nM	δ Ki, nM	σ Ki, nM
A	10	545	10,000	10,000
A [48]	5.2	> 1000	–	–
DuP 747	6	304	2,090	5,160
U-50,488	15	825	21,000	696

Fig. 11
Benzologs of U-50,488: DuP 747

cyclohexane ring was replaced by cyclopentane. Mu agonists, such as morphine and methadone, in addition to a plethora of effects, also cause antidiuresis in hydrated animals and humans. κ agonists induce diuresis by inhibiting the release of vasopressin (antidiuretic hormone). Niravoline has marked diuretic activity in animals and humans with low analgesic potency in animals. It may have potential as a diuretic agent.

2.7 Open chain analogs

In continuation of their study of the open chain analogs of U-50,488 ([50] and also Fig. 9 in Part I) ICI scientists identified three interesting κ agonists

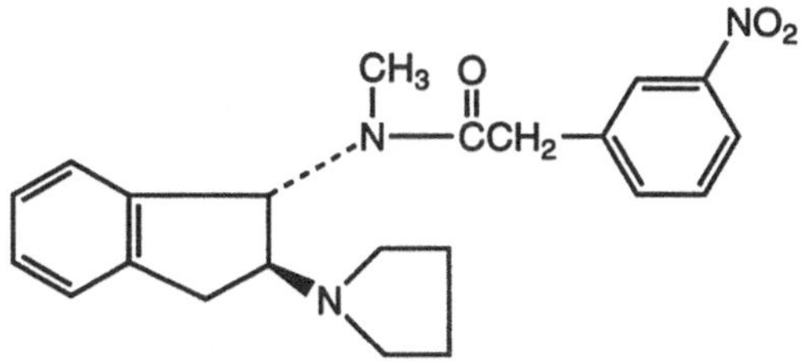

Niravoline (Ru 51599)

κ IC$_{50}$ = 1.83 nM
μ IC$_{50}$ = 1141 nM

Fig. 12
Analgesic and diuretic activity of niravoline.
In dogs, niravoline induced a dose-dependent increase in urine output reaching 161,341 and 321% of the initial value at 0.025, 0.05 and 0.1 mg/kg i.v. respectively. Analgesic activity in mice using acetic acid-induced writhing was absent up to 1 mg/kg i.v., and significant at 3 mg/kg. Similar dose range was observed in the hot plate test.

shown as A, B and C in Figure 13. They were also very active as analgesics *in vivo* s.c. in mice, and produced marked sedation in mice s.c. [52].

Some very interesting results were obtained by Rensselaer-Rochester group in the open chain U-50,488 analog bearing a meta aminophenyl group on the ethylene side chain [51] (Fig. 14). This represents an extension of the ICI series [52]. The (S)-(+) isomers were two orders of magnitude more potent than the corresponding (R)-(–) isomers for binding to the μ, δ and κ receptors. Both A compounds had very high affinity for the κ receptor. In both cases the Ki values for the acetamides were very similar to those of the corresponding amines indicating, perhaps, that only one donor hydrogen on the amine is required for bonding.

Novel hydroxamic acid derivatives of open-chain analogs of U-50,488 (for example, the compound shown in Fig. 15) represent a modification of the previously reported ICI leads and were reported by Pfizer in a patent as κ receptor agonists [53].

17

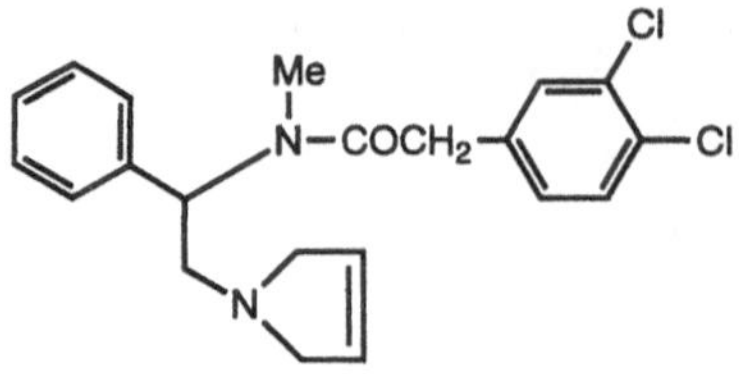

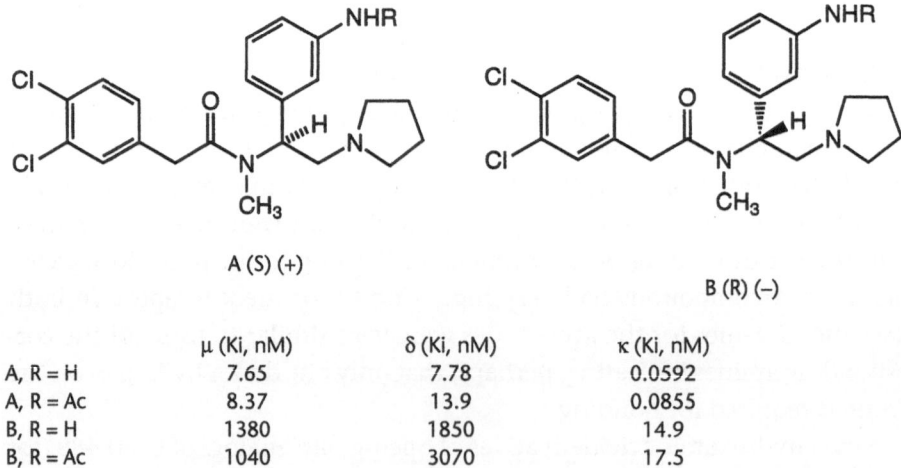

A.
κ IC$_{50}$ = 10.8 nM

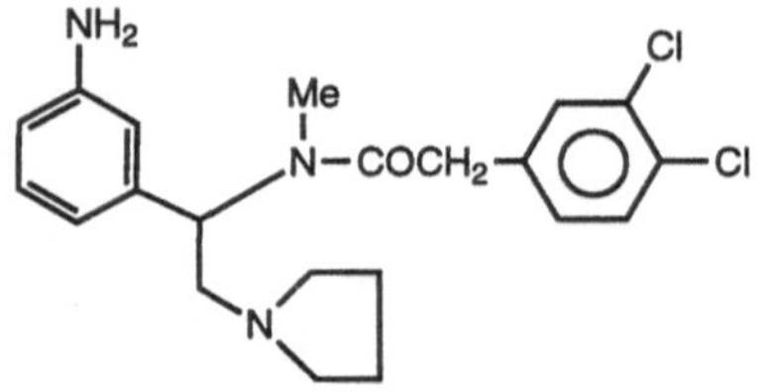

B.
κ IC$_{50}$ = 14.3 nM

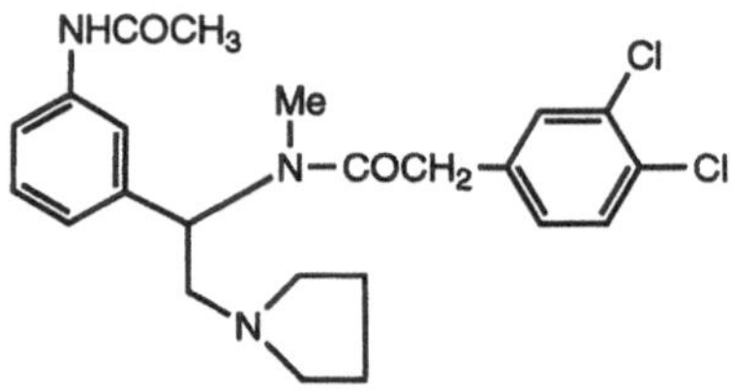

C.
κ IC$_{50}$ = 5.5 nM

Fig. 13
ICI open chain analogs of U-50,488.

A (S) (+)

B (R) (−)

	μ (Ki, nM)	δ (Ki, nM)	κ (Ki, nM)
A, R = H	7.65	7.78	0.0592
A, R = Ac	8.37	13.9	0.0855
B, R = H	1380	1850	14.9
B, R = Ac	1040	3070	17.5

Fig. 14
Open chain analogs of U-50,488 containing a meta aminophenyl group.

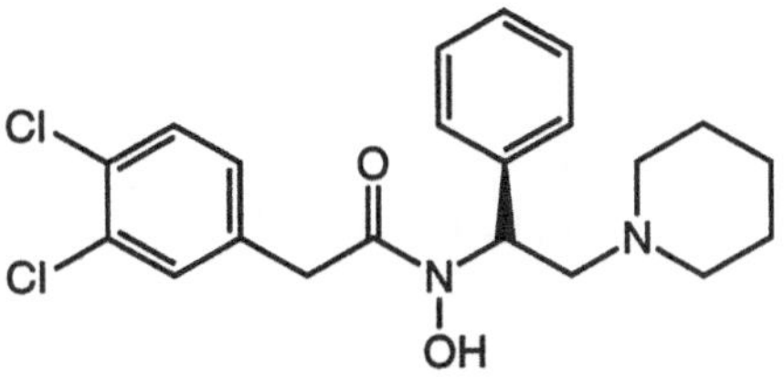

Fig. 15
Pfizer hydroxamic acid derivative.

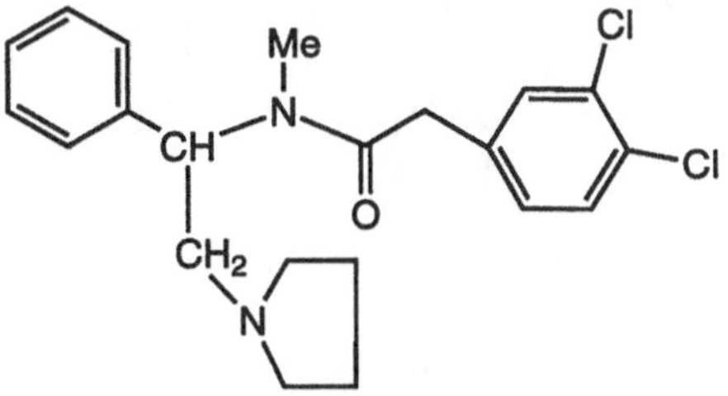

ICI 199,441

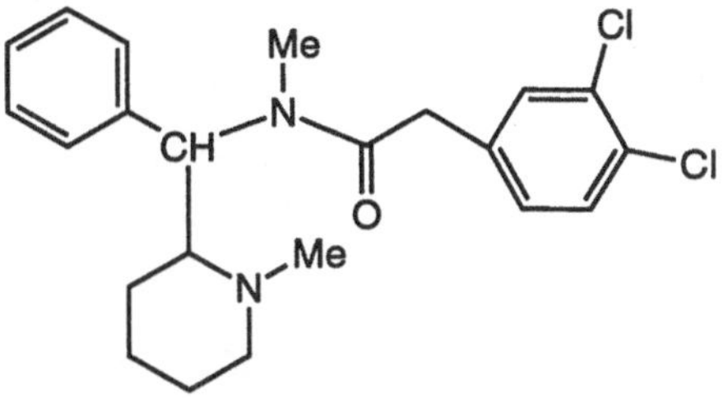

A. Mouse phenylquinone writhing

Ki, nM	ED$_{50}$ mg/kg
κ = 7	sc = 1.7
μ = 270	po = 10

Fig. 16
DuPont Merck semi-open chain compound.

2.8 DuPont Merck semi-open chain compounds

An interesting analog was published by the DuPont Merck group (Fig. 16, compound A) [54] which represents a hybrid of an open chain analog such as ICI 199441 (Fig. 16 and also section 2.7), and an analog in which the basic nitrogen is incorporated in a piperidine ring (see Fig. 15).

2.9 Spiro analogs related to U-62,066 (spiradoline)

In the category of spiro derivatives of U-62,066 (spiradoline) the National Taiwan University-DuPont Merck group described ketal and spiro-α-methyl-

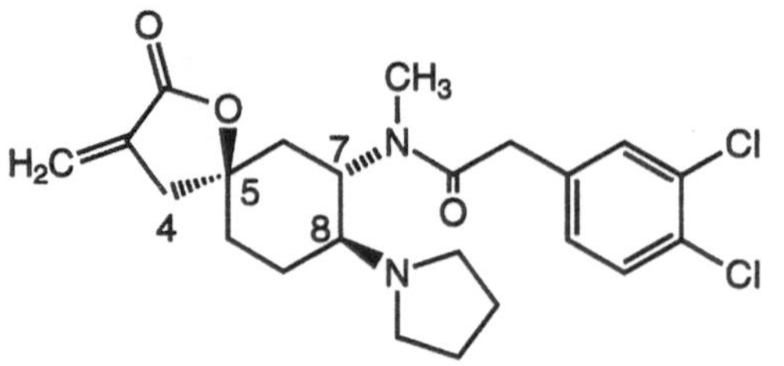

A.
κ Ki = 109 nM
μ:κ = 29

κ Ki = 1100 nM
μ:κ = 2.4

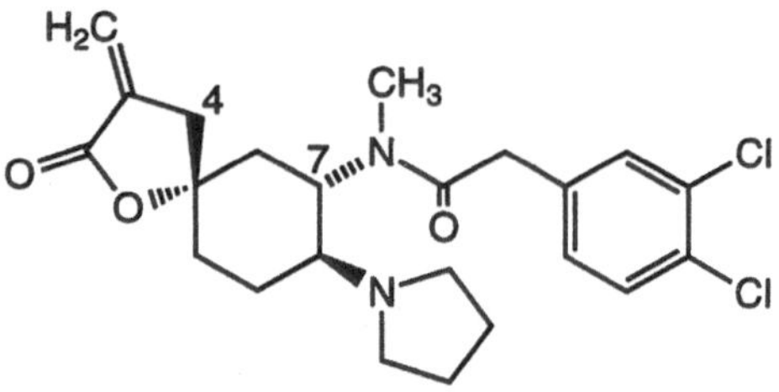

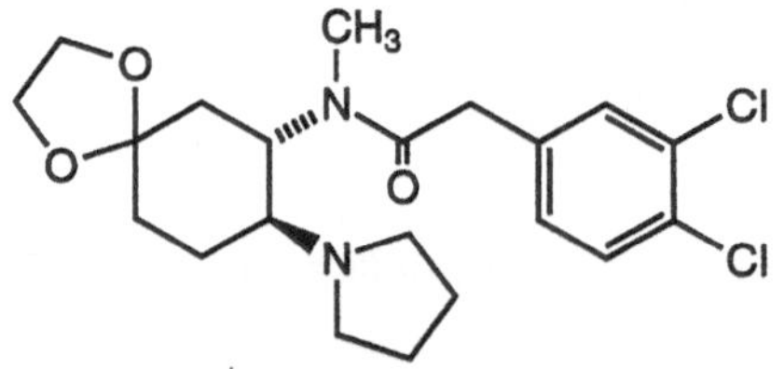

κ Ki = 94 nM
μ:κ = 55

B.
κ Ki = 1.5 nM
μ:κ = 468

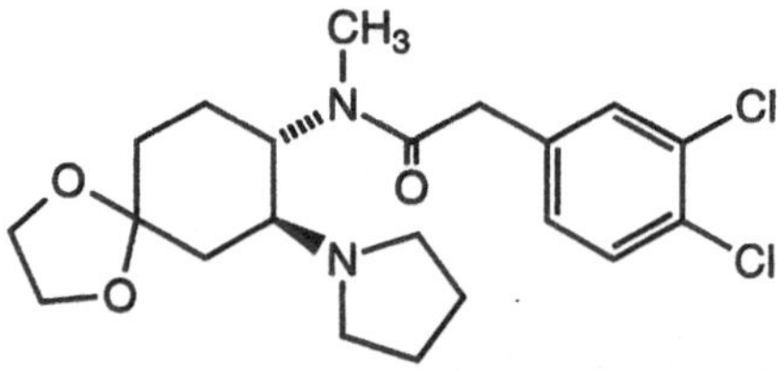

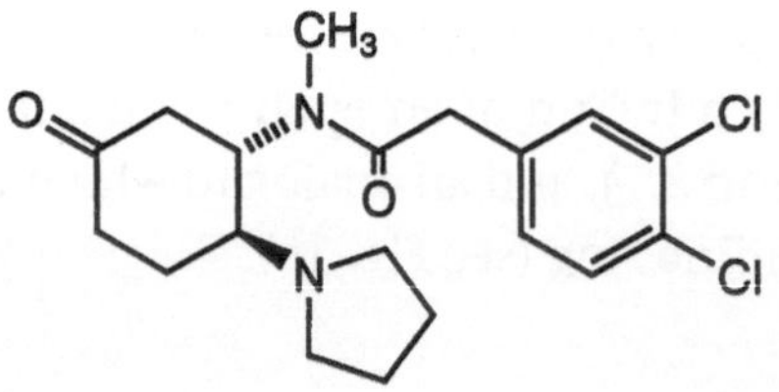

κ Ki = 78 nM
μ:κ = 166

Fig. 17
National Taiwan University-DuPont Merck compounds: Ketone and spiro derivatives of U-50,488 involving the cyclohexane ring.

ene-γ butyrolactone compounds (Fig. 17) [55] (see also [56]). The ketal (meta to pyrrolidine) compound B, which is an oxygen analog of U-62,066, showed the best affinity and selectivity toward the κ receptor in this series. The butyrolactone compound A was an irreversible (wash-resistant) ligand at the κ receptor but showed only moderate affinity and selectivity.

2.10 Rigidified lactam and spiro side chain analogs of U-50,488

In the rigidified lactam side-chain analog of U-50,488 [57] (Fig. 18) compound A showed good κ affinity about in the range of U-50,488, but the selectivity was inferior. In this series affinity is the function of the orientation of the phenyl ring and the presence of 3,4-dichloro substitution.

Considerable loss of affinity occurred with spiro substitution on the side chain of U-50,488 as shown in Fig. 19 [58].

2.11 The northwest region of U-50,488

The northwest region of U-50,488 has been subjected to some scrutiny which is summarized in Figure 20 [59] and references therein]. This group of five active κ agonists represents different degrees of unsaturation including a double bond in the cyclohexane ring, a phenyl substituent and an adjacent benzene ring. Modeling studies, inclusive of U-50,488, determined the size and shape of the hydrophobic pocket of the κ receptor with which the northwest part of the ligand interacts.

2.12 Examples of substitution in the cyclohexane ring of U-50,488 which eliminates κ activity

As shown in Figure 21, the structures of analogs of U-50,488 are without significant κ agonist activity. This group includes the phenalene A [60], the aza analog B [61] and three compounds (C, D, E) with an additional pyrrolidine substituent on the cyclohexane ring [62].

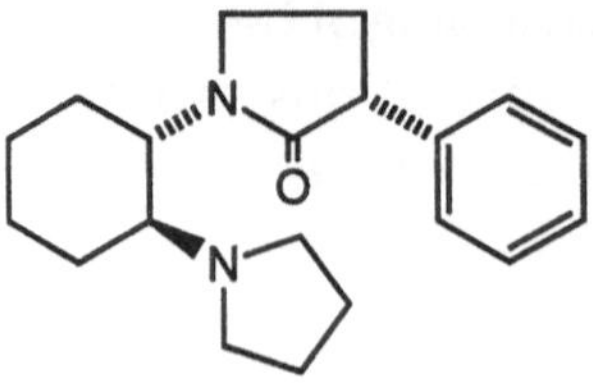

κ Ki = 416 nM
μ:κ = > 24

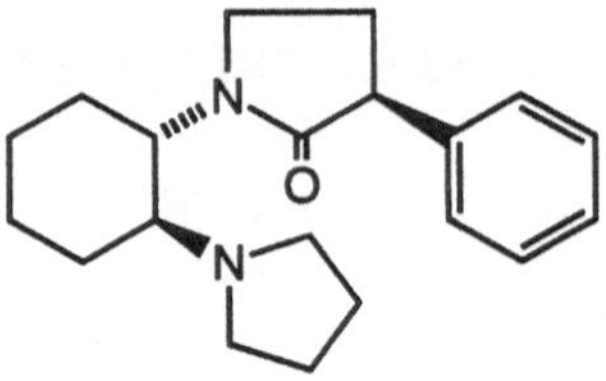

κ Ki = 672 nM
μ:κ = 13

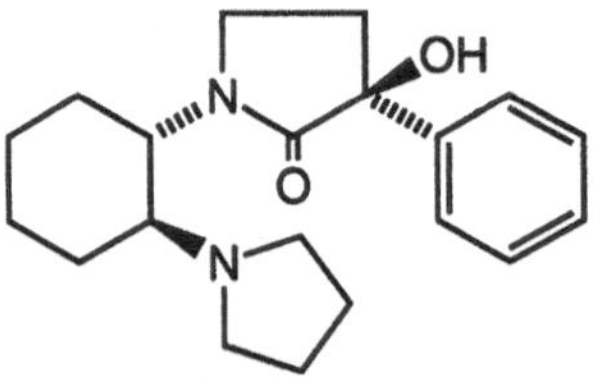

κ Ki = 382 nM
μ:κ = > 26

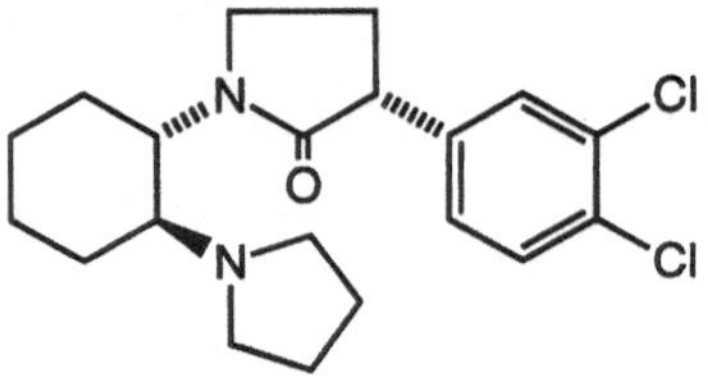

κ Ki = 10 nM
μ:κ = 23

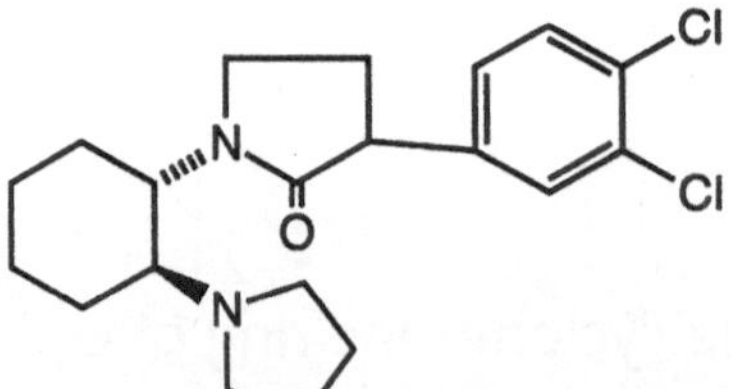

κ Ki = 92 nM
μ:κ = 9.4

Fig. 18
Rigidified lactam side-chain analogs of U-50,488.

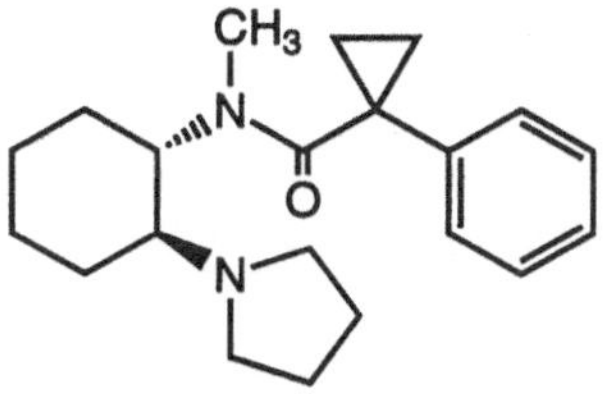

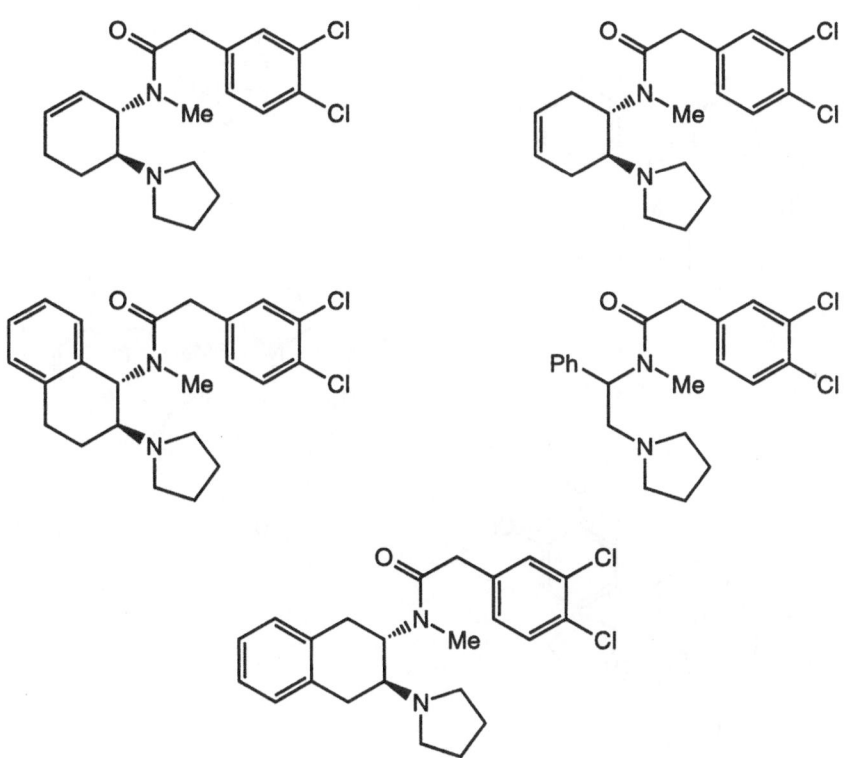

κ Ki = 14,400 nM
μ:κ = 0.13

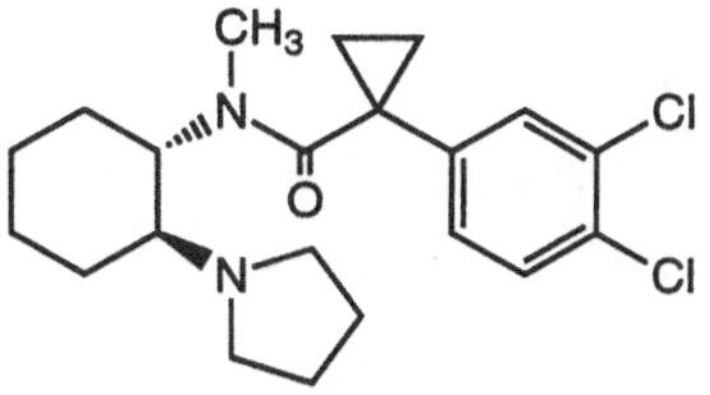

κ Ki = 9730 nM
μ:κ = 0.14

Fig. 19
Spiro derivatives involving the side-chain of U-50,488.

Fig. 20
Compatibility of bulk and unsaturation with κ agonist activity in the northwest region of U-50,488.
All the above compounds are active κ agonists.

23

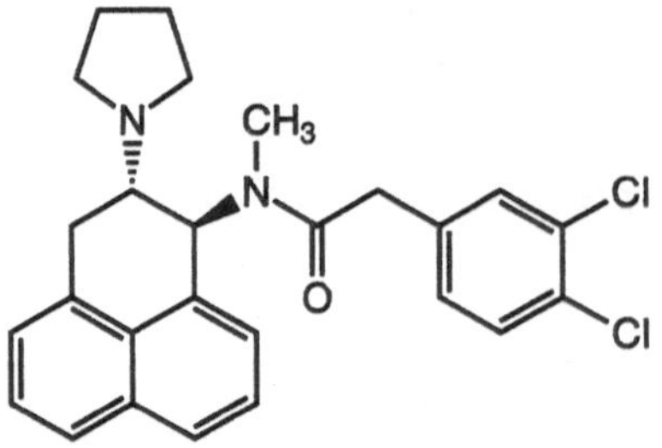

A.

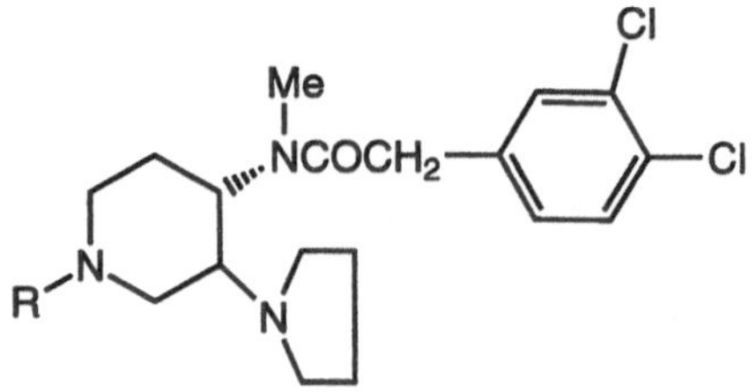

B.
R = H
R = CH₂Ph
R = Cbz

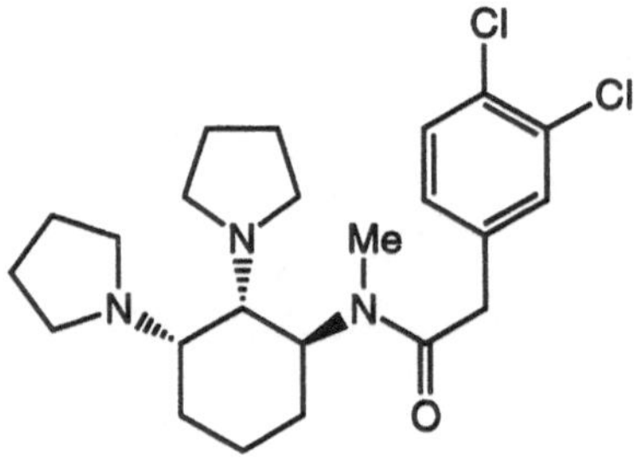

C.

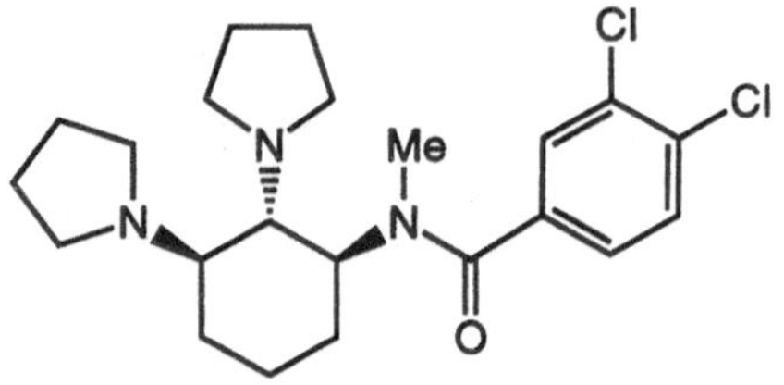

D.

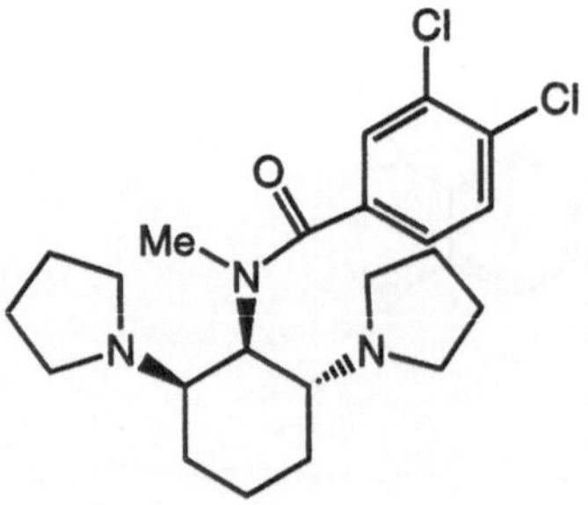

E.

Fig. 21
Analogs of U-50,488 without significant κ agonist activity.

3   Other centrally acting κ agonists

3.1   SmithKline Beecham ligands incorporating the benzodiazepine moiety in the 1,3-diaminobenzamide series

In an extension of the κ agonist lead tifluadom, SmithKline Beecham scientists have synthesized several anologs (Fig. 22) [63] which do not contain the N-C-C-N (sp^2) feature which is present in 1,2-diamine κ agonists. Instead they incorporated the N-C-C-C-N (sp^2) feature. In particular the 2-thienyl derivative A (Fig. 22) showed comparable κ 1 receptor potency to tifluadom but higher selectivity for the κ vs the μ receptor. All these compounds were devoid of significant affinity for both CCK-A and CCK-B receptors. It is of interest to note that when the deschloro compounds (A, B, C) were converted to chloro derivatives in position 7 of the benzodiazepine ring (Compounds D, E, F), marked loss of affinity to the κ-1 receptor and the μ receptor occurred.

3.2   Rhone-Poulenc phenothiazine ligands with the 1,2-diaminoamide or surrogate amide motif

Rhone-Poulenc scientists have described two analogs of their earlier 1,2-diamine phenothiazine RP-60180 (apadoline) (Fig. 23) [64]. Compound RP-61127 incorporates an imidazoline as an amide mimic and shifts the μ/κ ratio in favor of the μ receptor. This effect becomes even more pronounced when the amide of apadoline is replaced by an amidine substituent in compound A.

3.3   Diazobicyclononanone class

It is refreshing to be exposed in the area of opiates to a structure which does not resemble morphine or 4-phenylpiperidine.

The first representatives of a new structural class of κ agonists have been prepared. The 3,7-diazobicyclo[3.3.1]nonan-9-one HZ2 shown in Figure 24 displays an impressive separation of κ and μ affinities. In contrast to the corresponding compound, in which the methyl group on nitrogen-3 is replaced

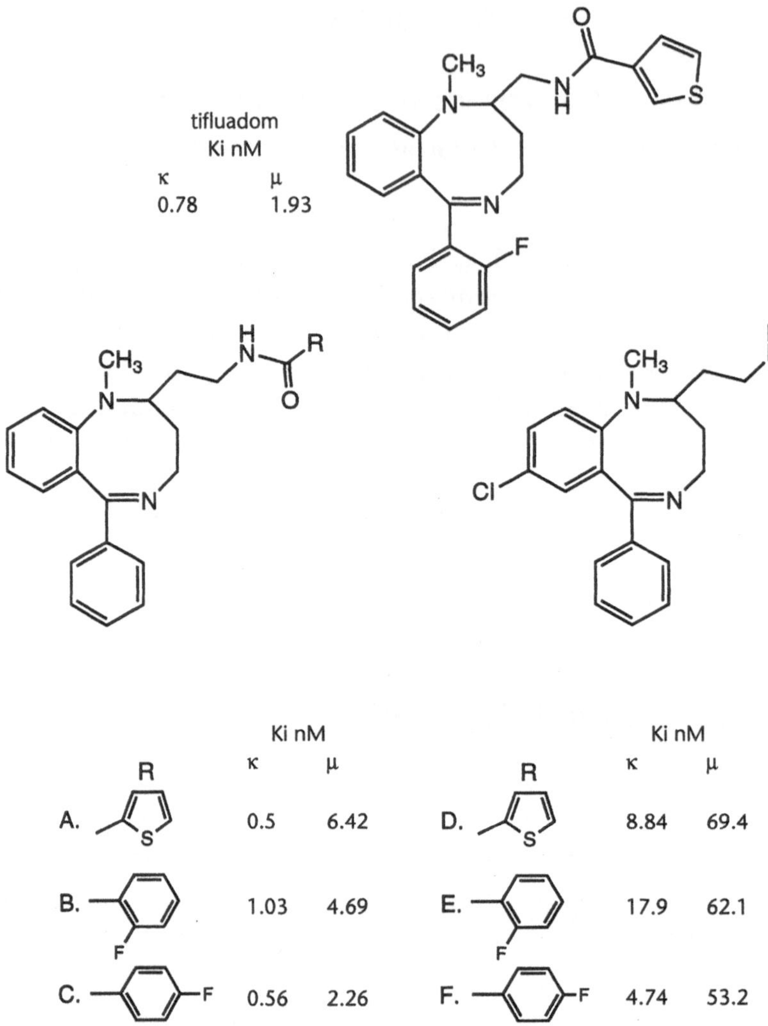

tifluadom
Ki nM

κ	μ
0.78	1.93

Fig. 22
Ligands incorporating the benzodiazepine moiety.

	R	Ki nM κ	μ		R	Ki nM κ	μ
A.	thiophene	0.5	6.42	D.	thiophene	8.84	69.4
B.	2-F-phenyl	1.03	4.69	E.	2-F-phenyl	17.9	62.1
C.	4-F-phenyl	0.56	2.26	F.	4-F-phenyl	4.74	53.2

by hydrogen, HZ2 showed high oral bioavailability in different animal species [65–67]. Consistent with the expected profile for a κ receptor agonist, HZ2 produced sedation and diuresis. The dose-dependent emesis, also seen in the antinociceptive dose range, is not typical of a κ receptor mediated effect and may be related to the complex template of this compound.

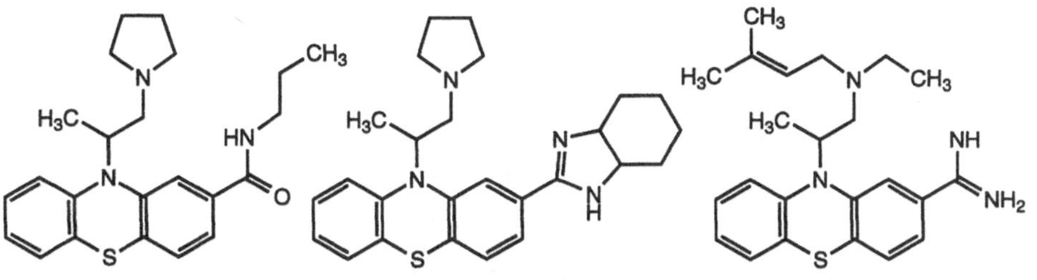

Apadoline RP-60180	RP-61127	A.
IC$_{50}$ nM	IC$_{50}$ nM	IC$_{50}$ nM
κ = 3	κ = 0.37	κ = 11
μ = 215	μ = 6.3	μ = 0.01

In vivo analgesic results for apadoline compared to morphine (ED$_{50}$ s.c. mg/kg)

	PBQ writhing (mouse)	hot plate (mouse)	tail flick (mouse)	tail flick (rat)	paw pressure (rat)
apadoline	0.08	> 30	0.8	> 20	1
morphine	0.04	7.5	2.4	2.5	0.3

Fig. 23
Rhône-Poulenc phenothiazine derivatives.

The authors have carried out some molecular modeling studies and concluded that the essential feature responsible for the opioid character of this compound is the aryl-propyl-amine element distributed along the N7-C6-C5-C4-aryl bonds (Fig. 24). Minimization of compound HZ2 against ketazocine produced a good fit.

This new template should be promising in developing new active κ-1 ligands. It is hoped that this structure will be elaborated on in order to achieve a fully economical template devoid of unnecessary and, possibly, deleterious groups. At the present time the necessity for the presence of both pyridine rings and both carbomethoxy groups (remindful of hypotensive dihydropyridines) is subject to question. The possible significance of the transannular N–C = 0 interactions should also be investigated. Once the SAR of the molecule is elucidated and the structure (perhaps) simplified, it is possible that the emetic effect will be eliminated.

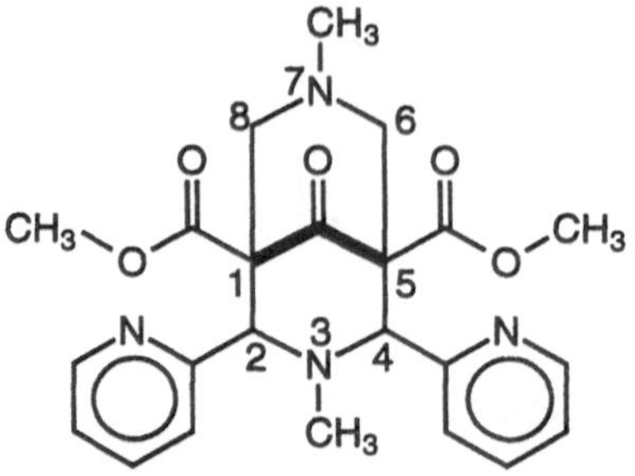

HZ2

κ Ki = 15 nM
μ Ki = > 1000 nM

	mouse (mg/kg)			rat (mg/kg)		
	i.v.	i.p.	p.o.	i.v.	i.p.	p.o.
LD$_{50}$ range (approx.)	26.1–31.6	464–681	464–681	31.6–46.4	464–681	464–681

Fig. 24
Structure of Grünenthal-University of Bonn-Hungarian Academy of Sciences 3,7-diazabicyclo [3.3.1] nonan-9-one compound HZ2.

4   Modeling and computational studies

Some modeling and computational methodology experiments in the U-50,488 series have been described [32, 35, 50, 59, 67–71, 71a].

In one of these studies the Parke-Davis group reported an interesting molecular modeling study [69] in which five known κ agonists were selected as representatives of various chemical series. These are shown in Figure 25 as A, B, C, D and E. Based on this model fewer then ten compounds were synthesized and tested. Those synthetic compounds belonged to three structural series, namely pyrrolidine-1,2,-diamino-amide,1,2-diamino-macrocyclic-amide and arylamine series. Representative compounds of these three series are shown in Figure 25 as F, G and H with the corresponding biological data. The most interesting compound is the aryloxy amine compound H with κ Ki = 160 nM and μ/κ ratio > 60. Since four of the five κ agonists

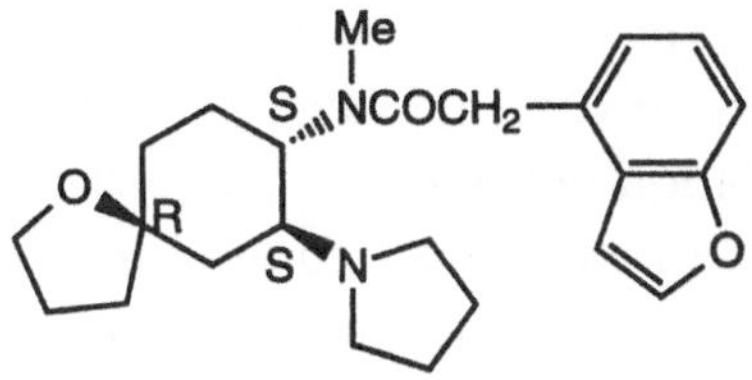

A.

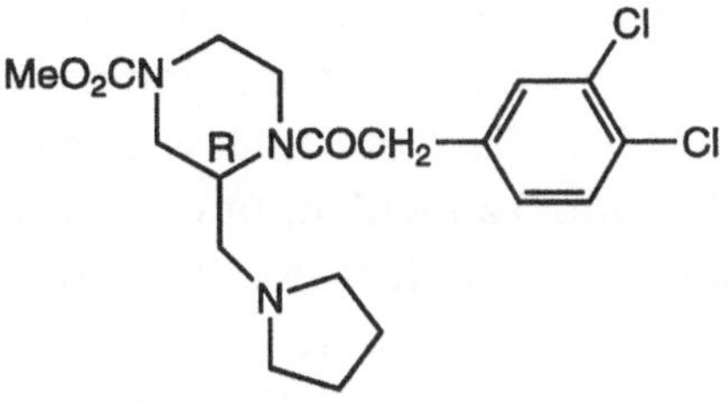

B.

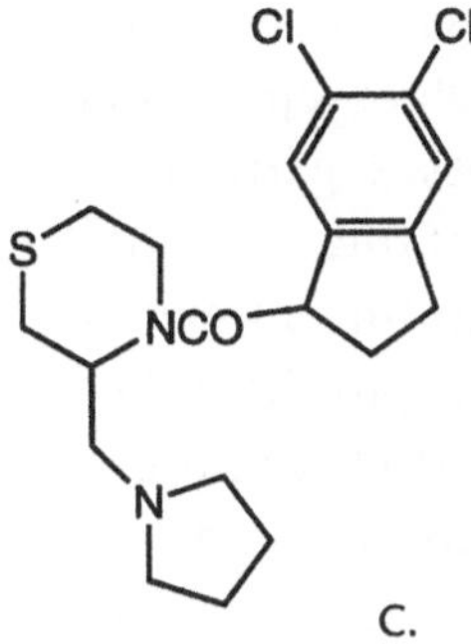

C.

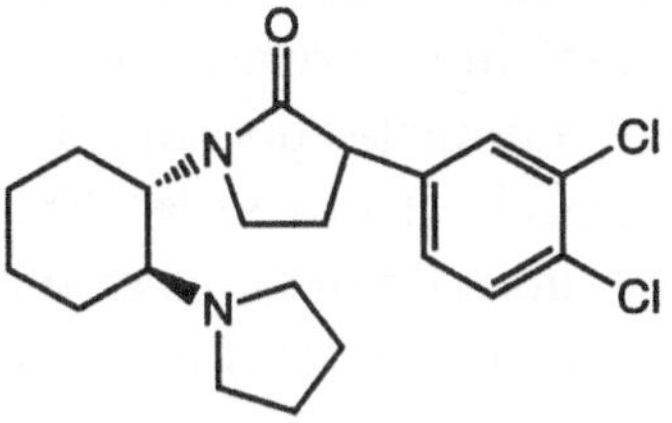

D.

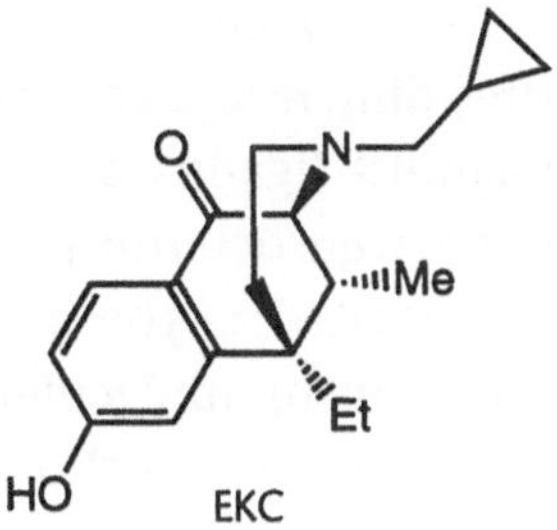

EKC

E.

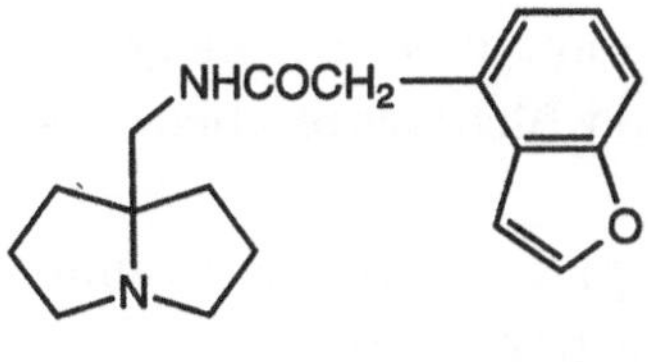

F.

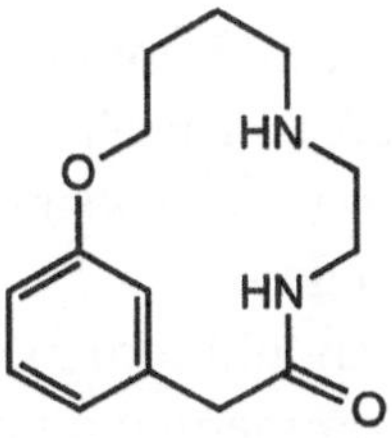

G.

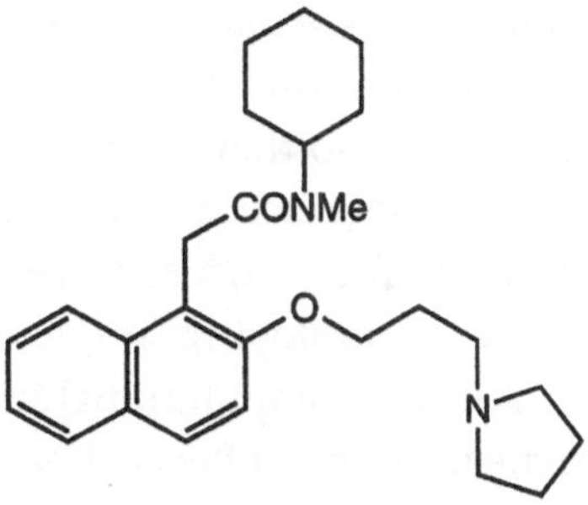

H.

		receptor affinity Ki, nM	
	F.	G.	H.
κ	940	> 10,000	160
μ	3350	> 10,000	> 10,000
μ:κ	3.5		> 60

Fig. 25
Parke-Davis modeling study.

used as models for this study were 1,2-diaminobenzoamides it is possible to provide a distant correlation between the structure of compound H and U-50,488 series. Nevertheless, compound H represents an interesting non-1,2-diamino lead which, hopefully, will be elaborated upon. But unless a different approach is used in choosing some of the model compounds, it is likely that the future outcome of this experiment will be a compound similar in structure to U-50,488. The future modeling could, for example, include compound H along with a hypotensive and cognition enhancing templates.

In an extensive study [71a] the Minnesota group has investigated the three-dimensional structure, dynamics and bonding models of representative κ agonist ligands of the 1,2-diamino-arylacetamide class. Ligand binding modes were determined using automated docking of two of these ligands and extrapolated to the other ligands of this series. The binding modes were refined using molecular dynamics simulations of the receptor-ligand complexes. The results show that a salt bridge is formed between the amino proton of the ligands and the carboxylate group of Asp^{138} in TM3. Additional ligand contacts with κ specific residues were also noted which may partly explain the κ selectivity in the series. Significantly, little evidence was found to link the 1,2-diaminoarylacetamide class of ligands with the opiate based ligands. It is interesting to note that U-50,488 was designed by the author of this review so that the structure would not be superimposable on the morphine model (see section 2 in part I). The above elaborate Minnesota group study confirms, in a very elegant way, the conclusion which was reached originally by employing simple modeling.

A future computational study should address the problems of how to eliminate dysphoric effects already commented on in sections 8 and 11.

5   Degradation product of U-62,066 (spiradoline)

A novel degradation product of spiradoline was obtained in aqueous solution stored at 80°C in the course of heat strain stability studies. The structure of the degradation product B was proved by spectroscopy and synthesis (Fig. 26) [72]. Compound B was synthesized in two steps: spiradoline was hydrolyzed with acid to give the diamine A; oxidation of A with mercuric acetate afforded B in 30% yield.

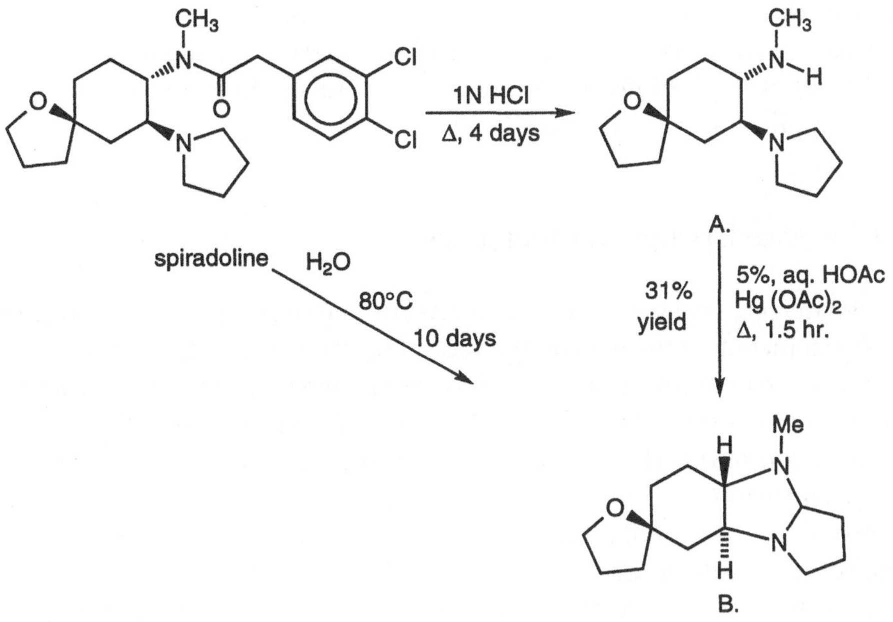

Fig. 26
Degradation product of spiradoline.

The degradation was promoted by bubbling air or oxygen into the solution or by adding α,α'-azobisisobutyronitrile for radical initiation. It was suppressed by bubbling nitrogen. The mechanism is considered to involve an oxidation by the oxygen radical.

6   Peripherally acting U-50,488 analogs

The interest in κ agonists as potentially useful centrally acting analgesics has been extended to their potential as peripherally acting analgesics. The presence of κ receptors in the peripheral terminals of primary afferent neurons points the way to the development of new drugs to treat inflammatory conditions [6]. A turtle stimulates for this research has been provided by the demonstration that U-50,488 and U-69,593 are potent peripheral analgesics [73–75].

The quaternization method used to produce peripheral selectivity with μ agonists was less successful when applied to κ agonist in the U-50,488 class and led to a reduction in κ receptor affinity of 200 times and more [7].

The following sections describe some successful methodology used to produce peripheral κ agonists in the U-50,488 class of compounds.

6.1   E. Merck peripheral analgesics

The E. Merck group has developed a class of diarylacetamide derivatives of U-50,488 including the benzhydryl motif [76]. The benzhydryl group is present in some lipophilic drugs devoid of central effects such as non-sedating antihistaminics (for references see [76]). As is shown in Figure 27, some of the members of this class showed good κ affinity and opioid receptor selectivity. Furthermore, compound EMD61753 (asimadoline) shows a profile similar to that of antiinflammatory drugs rather than centrally acting opiates (such as morphine or ICI 197067, see Fig. 27) in the formalin test in mice.

An extensive pharmacological profile of EMD61753 has been carried out [77] and has further shown that it is orally effective with limited ability to cause centrally mediated sedation, putative aversion, diuresis and antinociception. This compound has potential as a peripherally acting analgesic in which pain of inflammatory origin may be alleviated without causing undesirable central side-effects.

The four enantiomers of each of the peripherally selective κ agonists EMD 60400 and EMD 61753 were synthesized and their affinity for the κ receptor determined [78]. The results are shown in Figure 28.

The benzhydryl group present in EMD 61753 (Figs. 27 and 28) deserves a comment. This structural feature is present in a large number of biologically active compounds and as benzodiazepines and tricyclic CNS drugs. It has been proposed [79, 80] as a motif that resists hydrophobic collapse in aqueous media by preventing the formation of inactive collapsed conformation due to stacking of multiple aromatic groups upon each other.

As extensive biochemical and pharmacological study of the central and peripheral actions of ICI 60400 was performed by the E. Merck group (Fig. 29) [81]. ICI 197067 and ICI 20448 were tested for comparison: the first is a centrally acting κ agonist and the second has been described as having limited access to the CNS (see Fig. 10 in part I). EM 60400 showed high affinity

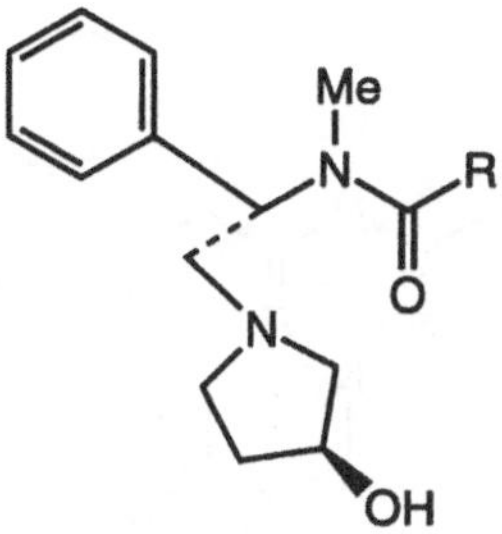

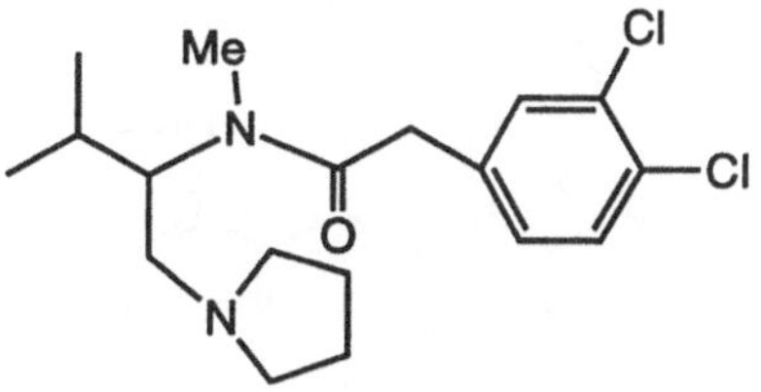

ICI 197067

| | κ Ki, nM* | mouse formalin test ID$_{50}$ mg/kg sc | |
		early phase	late phase
R = —CH(Ph)(Ph) EM 61,753, asimadoline	2	ICI 197067 0.04	0.02
R = —CH(Ph)(isopropyl)	3	morphine 1.7	3.4
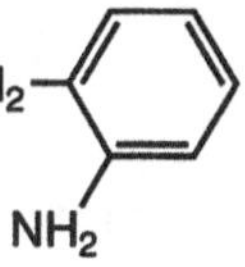 R = —CH₂-C₆H₄-NH₂ EMD 60400	1	EMD61753 > 2	0.24
A. R 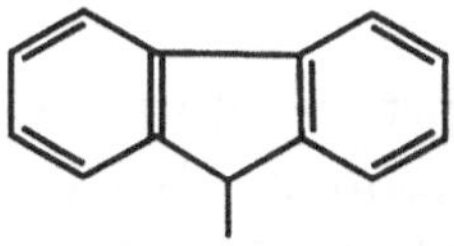 = (fluorene)	6		
R = (dihydroanthracene)	4		
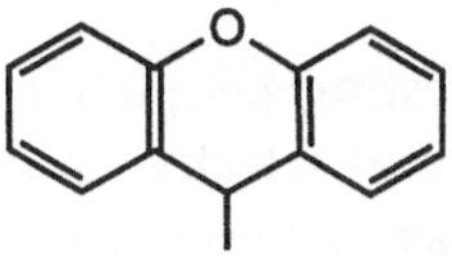 R = (xanthene)	4		

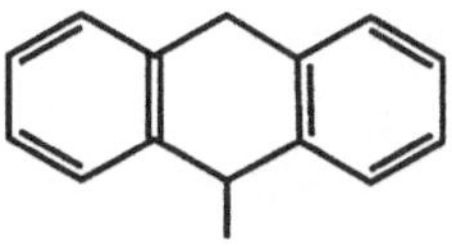

* All the CH-substituted compounds shown here possess Ki ≥ 100 nM for the μ and δ receptors. Only compound A showed μ Ki = 40 nM and δ Ki = 60 nM.

Fig. 27
E. Merck peripheral κ agonists.

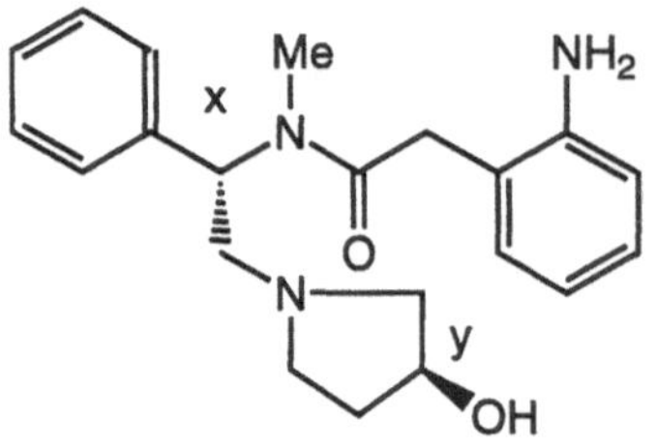

EMD 60400 (S, S)

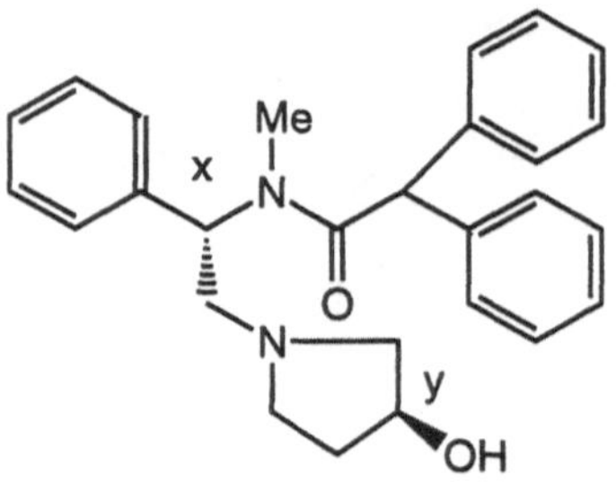

EMD 61753 (S, S)
Asimadoline

| Configuration | | κ affinity | |
| chiral | chiral | IC$_{50}$ nM | |
center x	center y	EMD 60400 (series)	EMD 61753 (series)
S	S	2.8	5.6
S	R	42.3	190
R	S	41.7	267
R	R	>10,000	>10,000

Fig. 28
The configuration and κ receptor binding affinity of the four enantiomers of E. Merck EMD 60400 and EMD 61753.

and selectivity for the κ receptor with a degree of peripheral activity. The three compounds have different tendencies to elicit centrally mediated sedative and putative aversion (ICI 19 7067 > EMD 60400 > ICI 20448) which corresponds to their ability to cross the blood brain barrier.

6.2 Minnesota group peripheral analgesics

The Minnesota group synthesized some interesting peripheral κ agonist based on the amino derivative of the potent and selective κ agonist ICI 199441 (Fig. 9, part I). This amino derivative was converted to α-conjugate of L-aspartic acid (Compound A), its D-diastereoisomer (Compound B) and the β-conjugate to L-aspartic acid (Compound C) (Fig. 30) [82]. In addition to retaining κ receptor affinity and selectivity the aspartate conjugates A, B and C were found to be less effective than the parent compound ICI 199441 in producing CNS-mediated opioid antinociception after peripheral admin-

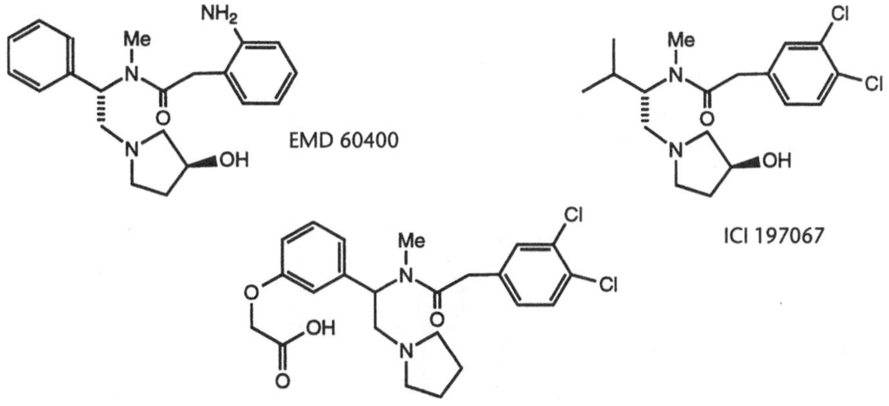

EMD 60400

ICI 197067

ICI 204448

	Receptor binding affinity IC$_{50}$, nM			Mouse formalin ID$_{50}$ mg/kg sc	
	κ	μ	δ	early phase	late phase
EMD 60400	2.8	500	333	0.44	0.47
ICI 197067	1.5	100	1200	0.04	0.02
ICI 20448	13.0	233	167	18.9	12.6

Fig. 29
EMD 60400, an E. Merck κ agonist. Comparison with ICI 197067 and ICI 20448.

istration and may be useful as peripherally acting opioid agonists. Another potential application is the treatment of gastrointestional mobility disorders (for references see [82]).

6.3 Glaxo piperazine peripheral analgesics

The Glaxo piperazine series (see Fig. 3) was also modified to produce hydrophilic derivatives as peripherally selective κ agonists (Fig. 31) [83]. The model lipophilic compound, GR 103545 (see Fig. 3) had a measured log D = 3.14. Lipophilicity was reduced by two modifications, namely replacing the N-carbomethoxy group with the non polar acetyl group and the introduction of a 3-hydroxy group in the pyrrolidine ring. Selected substituents were

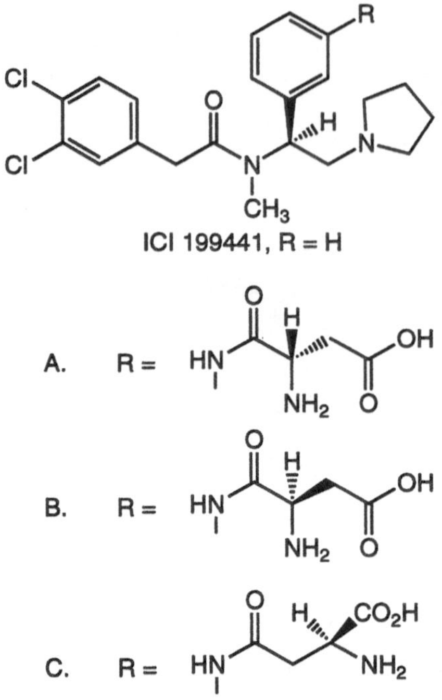

Jacob Szmuszkovicz

ICI 199441, R = H

A.   R =

B.   R =

C.   R =

	Receptor binding affinity Ki, nM			Antinociceptive potencies in mice (writhing) ED$_{50}$, nmole/kg		
	κ	μ	δ	i.c.v.	i.v.	i.v./i.c.v.
ICI 199441	–	–	–	11.8	16.5	1.4
A	0.34	462	1072	6.8	105	15.7
B	1.20	280	573	46	2015	43.6
C	–	–	–	11	628	56.5

Fig. 30
The Minnesota peripheral κ agonists.

then incorporated into the aromatic ring to produce a range of log D's. The most interesting compound was the sulphone followed by GR 94839 (Fig. 31) [76]. The sulphone was almost 3000 times more potent upon intra-cerebroventricular (i.c.v.) as compared to subcutaneous (s.c.) administration. GR 103545 was almost equipotent when administered by the peripheral or central routes as above. Thus, the sulphone shows significant peripheral selectivity *in vivo* and was compared to ICI 204448 (see also Fig. 10 in Part I).

36

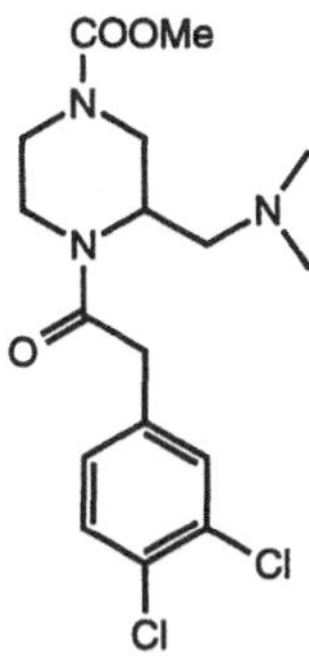

GR 103545

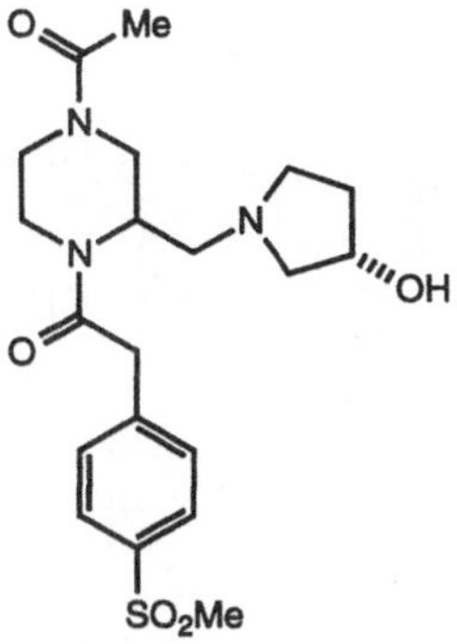

sulphone

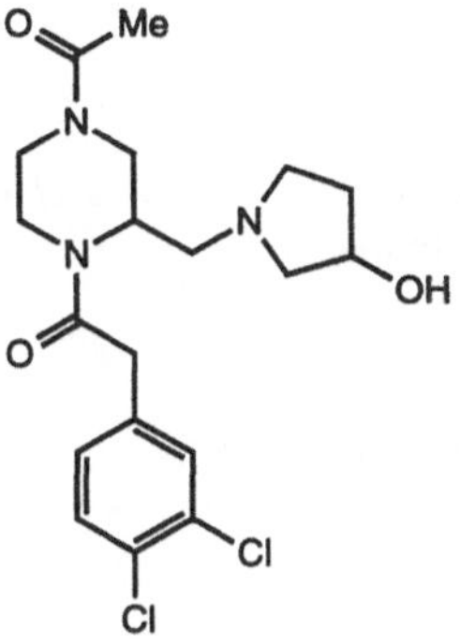

GR 94839

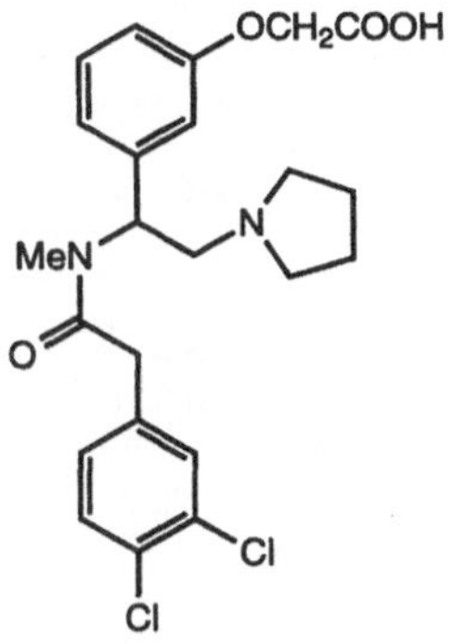

ICI 204448

| | measured Log D | LVD IC$_{50}$, nM | Mouse ACh-induced abdominal constriction ED$_{50}$, mg/kg | | |
			s.c.	i.c.v.	s.c./i.c.v
GR 103545	3.1	0.02	0.0003	0.0002	1.5
Sulphone	<0.5	0.9	2.21	0.0008	2762
ICI 204448	0.3	7.4	4.4	0.13	34
GR 94839	-	1.4	1.9	0.008	238

Fig. 31
Glaxo sulphone, a peripherally selective agonist.

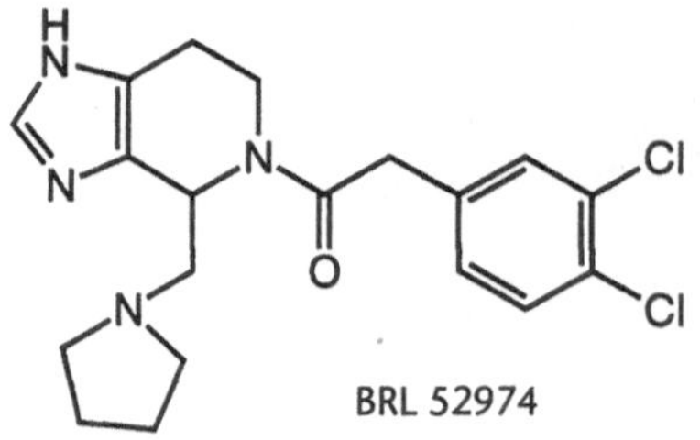

BRL 52974

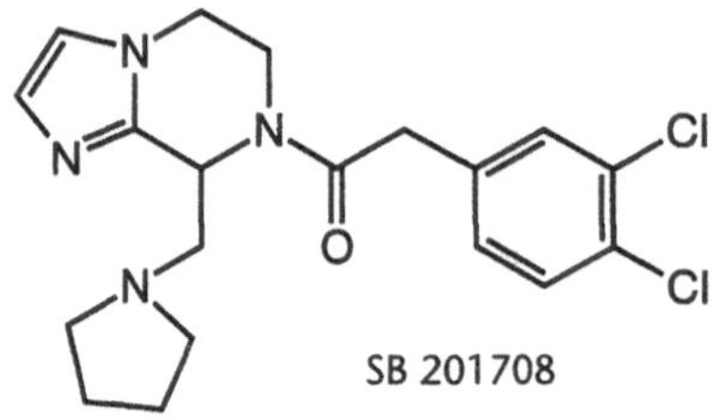

SB 201708

	κ binding Ki, nM	MAC* s.c.	MAC i.c.v. ED$_{50}$, mg/kg	MAC s.c./i.c.v.
BRL 52974	0.19	43.5	0.15	290
SB 201708	0.23	0.051	-	-

*MAC = mouse abdominal constriction test, following administration by the subcutaneous (s.c.) route and intracerebroventricular (i.c.v.) routes.

Fig. 32
SmithKline Beecham imidazopiperidines.

6.4   SmithKline Beecham imidazopiperidine peripheral analgesics

The SmithKline Beecham group described imidazopiperidines shown in Figure 32 [6]. BRL 52974 contains a hydrogen bonding NH group which results in increased hydrophilicity over the closely related BRL 201708. This is expressed in the MAC test results which correlate brain penetration with central and/or peripheral antinociceptive activity. Limited access of BRL 52974 to the brain was also shown by an *ex vivo* binding model. The compound was not detected in brain homogenates up to 4 h past sc dosing. These results confirm the inability of BRL 52974 to cross the blood brain barrier after single systemic administration.

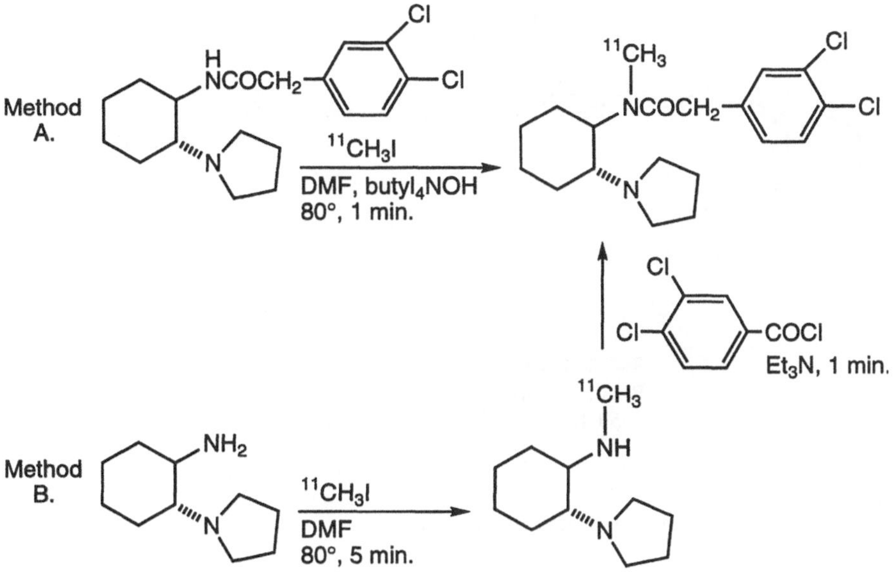

Fig. 33
Two synthesis of N-(¹¹C-methyl)-U-50,488.

7 Labelled ligands

7.1 Radiochemical synthesis

The radiochemical synthesis of ^{11}C-methyl-U-50,488 has been accomplished [84] in one step by direct methylation with ^{11}C-methyliodide (Fig. 33: Method A) in 22 min, or in two steps (Fig. 33: Method B) in 27 min. The labeled compound will be useful for the study of κ subtype receptors using position emission tomography.

[18]F fluoroalkylated derivatives of U-50,488 have also been considered [85] and the corresponding ^{19}F analogs were prepared. Fluoroalkylation proved detrimental to ligand affinity and therefore, the fluoroethyl and the fluoro-propyl analogs shown in Figure 21 are not suitable for PET studies. In the course of this synthesis the authors have first attempted direct alkylation of the amide (N-normethyl U-50,488). These unsuccessful attempts have been

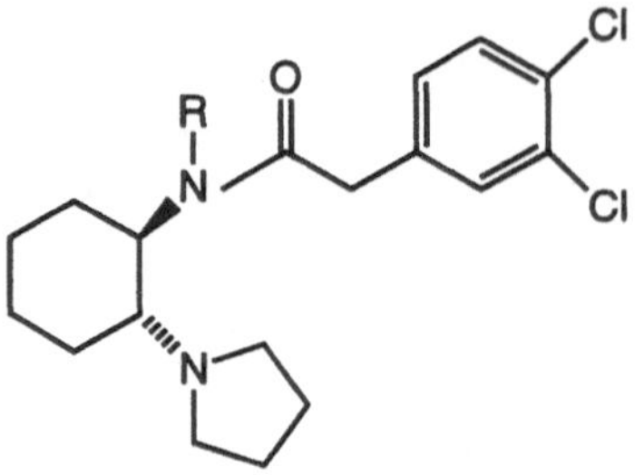

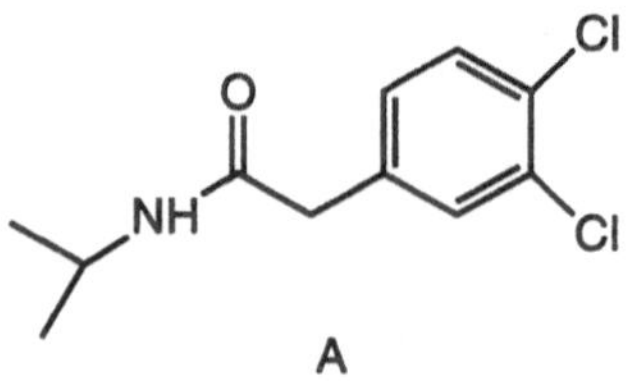

	κ Ki, nM
R = CH$_2$CH$_2$F	440
R = CH$_2$CH$_2$CH$_2$F	870
U-50,488	8.5

Fig. 34
Fluoroalkyl derivatives of U-50,488 and compound A.

encountered in the literature before. The alternative synthesis, in which trans-1-pyrrolidino-2-aminocyclohexane precursor was alkylated and then acylated, was fruitful. Time constraints make it unlikely that it could be adapted for synthesis of the corresponding ^{18}F-labeled compounds. The authors provide an interesting analysis of the unsuccessful alkylation experiments, as well as results of model study with compound A (structure shown in Fig. 34).

It is known that in the SAR of U-50,488 activity is optimal in the case of the methyl group on the amidic nitrogen. The presence of the fluorines in the cases above further extends this SAR.

7.2   Fluorescence labelled ligand

A fluorescein isothiocyanate-conjugated arylacetamide (FITC-AA, for clarity the letters composing the acronym are underlined) based on ICI [52] open chain U-50,488 analog, is shown in Figure 35 [86, 51]. This compound displayed high affinity for the κ receptor and was used in indirect immunofluorescence experiments to specifically stain κ receptors on lymphoytes. Racemic FITC-AA has been used to label κ receptors expressed on a mouse

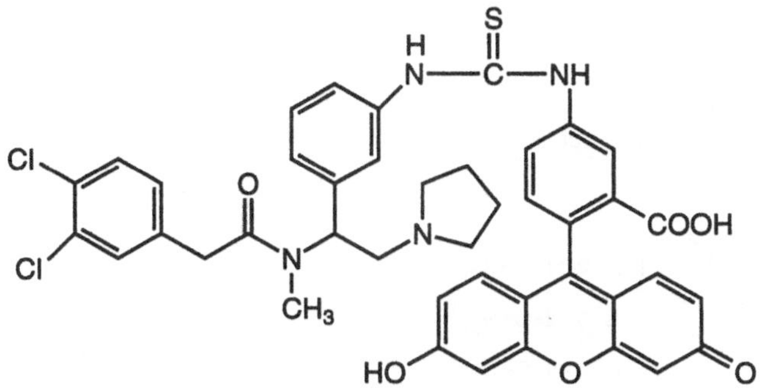

FITC – AA

Ki nM for FITC – AA

	μ	δ	κ
Racemic	176	1.84	8.2
(S) (+)	98	0.898	1.4
(R) (–)	1190	85.7	139

Fig. 35
Structure of FITC – AA used for identification of κ receptors in the immune system by indirect immuno-fluorescence.

thymoma and on mouse thymocytes [86]. The (S) isomer was two orders of magnitude more potent than the (R) isomer in binding to μ, δ and κ sites. Unlike the starting material NH_2 compound and its acetyl derivative [51] the (S)-FITC-AA showed less site selectivity, likely due to the presence of fluorescein in the ligand.

7.3 Electrophilic affinity ligands

The University of Washington group developed selective electrophilic affinity ligands based on the structure of the ICI κ agonist ICI-199,441 (Fig. 36) as potential affinity probes for the characterization of κ receptors [87]. The isothiocyanate group was chosen as the electrophilic functionality since it does not readily react with water, but does with amino acid thiol groups. The isothiocyanate group has been used previously for this purpose to modify U-50,488 (see Fig. 15 in part I). The ligand shown in Figure 36 exhibited affinity in the range of ICI-199,441 and U-69,593 with C and D lagging behind.

41

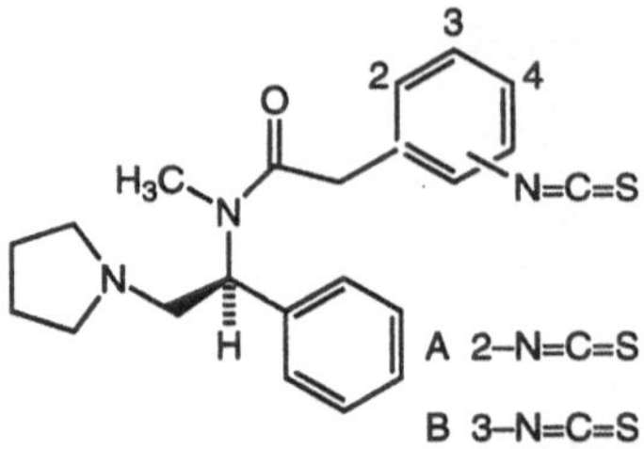

A 2–N=C=S

B 3–N=C=S

C 4–N=C=S

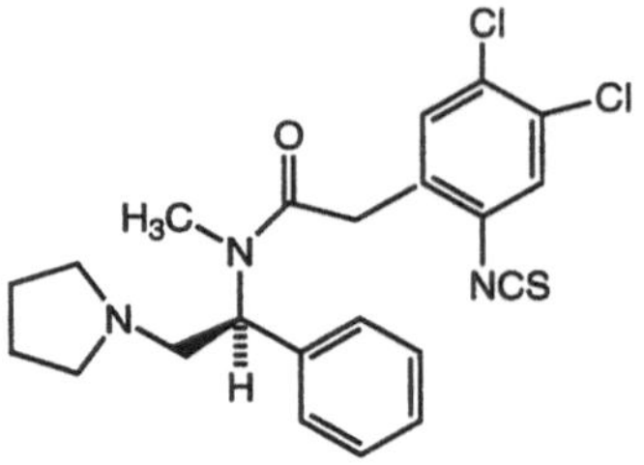

D

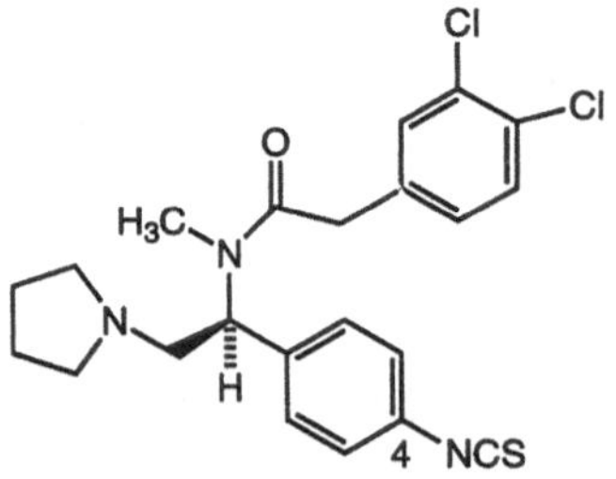

E

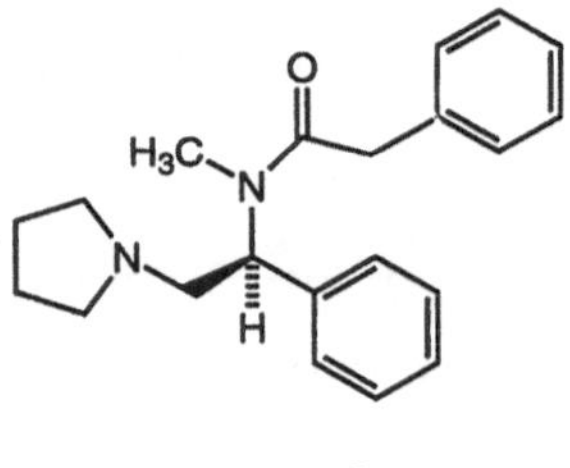

F

	κ IC_{50}, nM
ICI-199,441	1.5
A	2.3
B	3.3
C	14
D	9.5
E	1.8
F	1.4
U-69,593	2.1

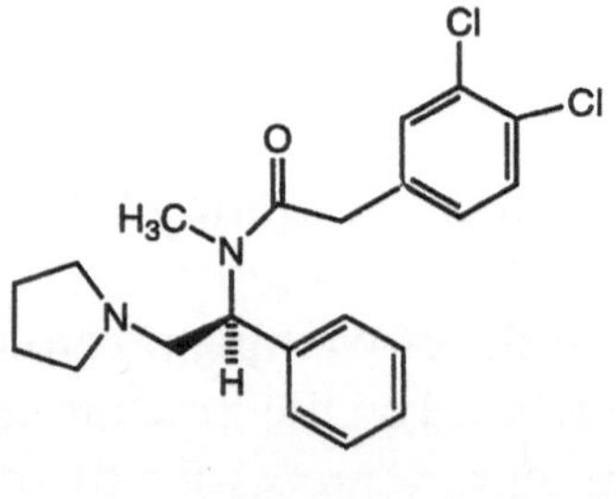

ICI 199,441

Fig. 36
κ receptor affinity labels employing –N=C=S.

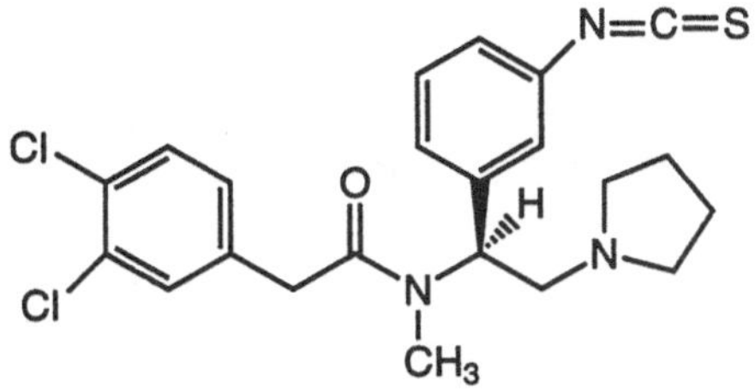

DIPPA

κ IC$_{50}$, nM = 2.21

Fig. 37
Additional κ receptor affinity label employing –N=C=S.

All the ligands showed good selectivity for the κ receptors as compared to μ and δ.

The Minnesota group [88] developed a closely related labeled ligand (Fig. 37) also derived from ICI-199,441 (Fig. 36), namely DIPPA or 2-(3,4-dichlorophenyl)-N-methyl-N-[(1S)-1-(3-isothiocyanatophenyl)-2-(1-pyrrolidinyl)ethyl]acetamide (the acronymous identified by the underlined letters). DIPPA was selective to the κ receptor as compared to μ and δ; in the mouse-flick assay DIPPA (0.53 μmol/Kg sc) was found to be an antagonist selective for the κ receptor, and thus constitutes the first example of an aryl-acetamide label with κ antagonist activity *in vivo*. The parent compound, ICI-199,441, was found to have no antagonist activity within the same time period (48 h). It appears that the isothiocyanate group is responsible for the antagonist activity of DIPPA as a consequence of covalent binding to the κ receptor.

For another irreversible ligand in the U-50,488 class, containing the spiro-α-methylene-γ-butyrolactone moiety, see Figure 17 [55].

8   U-50,488 template and the sigma receptor

No κ agonist related to U-50,488 has yet achieved therapeutic application primarily because of the dysphoric side effect. Perhaps it is not too surprising considering the close relationship between the structure of U-50,488 and the corresponding cis compound (Fig. 38) which is a sigma receptor ligand [89].

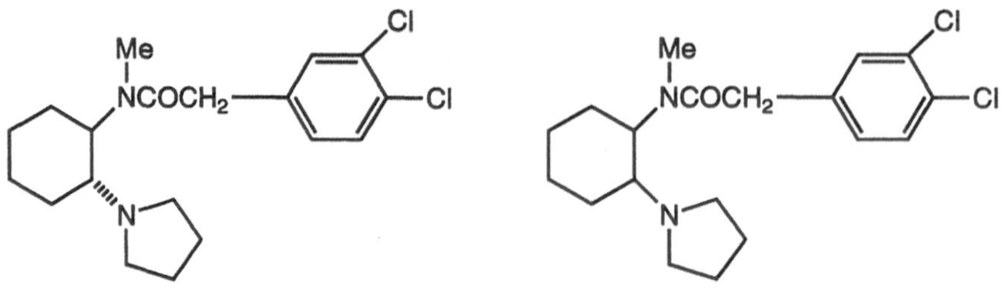

Fig. 38
Structure of U-50,488 (trans) and the cis isomer A.

However, it should be possible to design a compound in which the conformational overlap between U-50,488 template (trans) and the corresponding cis template is either reduced or preferably eliminated. This approach may produce a compound which does not produce dysphoria.

The sigma-1 receptor has been sequenced and cloned. The discovery of other members of the sigma receptor family and the evidence of the role they play in cholesterol biosynthesis has provided interesting targets for drug development. For a summary and references see [90].

Figure 39 summarizes part of a large amount of work done by the NIH group on the SAR of U-50,488 agonist class with respect to sigma affinity (for references see Fig. 39). The structures of all the agonists have been modified by elimination of the amide carbonyl group to produce potent σ ligands. For example, U-50,488 exhibited weak affinity for σ receptors labeled by ^{3}H-(+)-3-PPP. Change in stereochemistry of U-50,488 from trans to cis produced an almost total loss of affinity for κ receptor and a large increase in affinity for σ receptor. Thus, 1S,2R-(–)-cis diastereoisomer (Fig. 38, Compound A) had a Ki of 81 nM for σ receptor and negligible affinity for κ receptor. Conversion of the carbonyl group to a methylene produced is compound B, cis (–), with a Ki of 1.3 nM for σ receptor. Further simplification of U-50,488 to structure C produced a highly active and selective sigma ligand.

Many of the κ agonists described in this review have been simplified to produce potent sigma ligands and are also shown in Figure 39. Thus, the SAR of compound C shows considerable conformational freedom and suggests

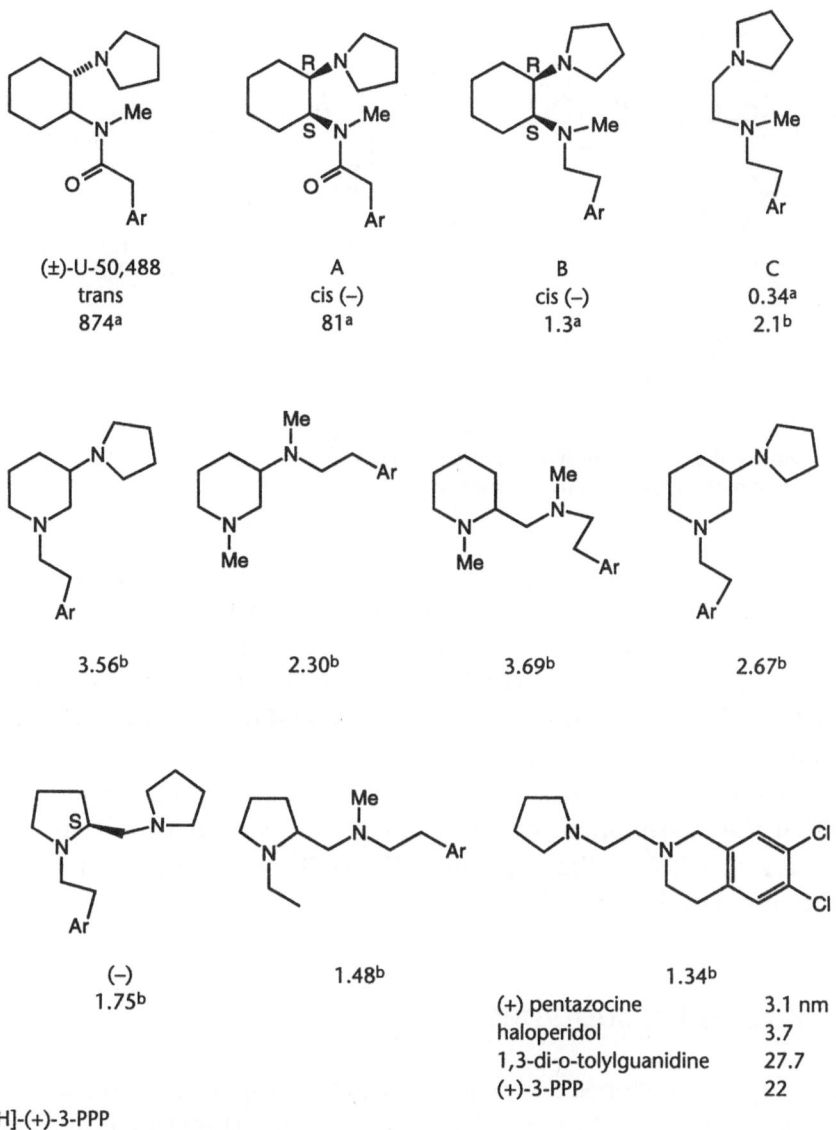

(±)-U-50,488	A	B	C
trans	cis (–)	cis (–)	0.34[a]
874[a]	81[a]	1.3[a]	2.1[b]

3.56[b]   2.30[b]   3.69[b]   2.67[b]

(–)   1.48[b]   1.34[b]
1.75[b]

(+) pentazocine	3.1 nm
haloperidol	3.7
1,3-di-o-tolylguanidine	27.7
(+)-3-PPP	22

[a] [³H]-(+)-3-PPP
[b] Standard: [³H]-(+)-pentazocine
Ar = 3,4-dichlorophenyl. Numbers represent Ki in nM.
Adapted from [89, 91–95]

Fig. 39
NIH group results: sigma binding affinities.

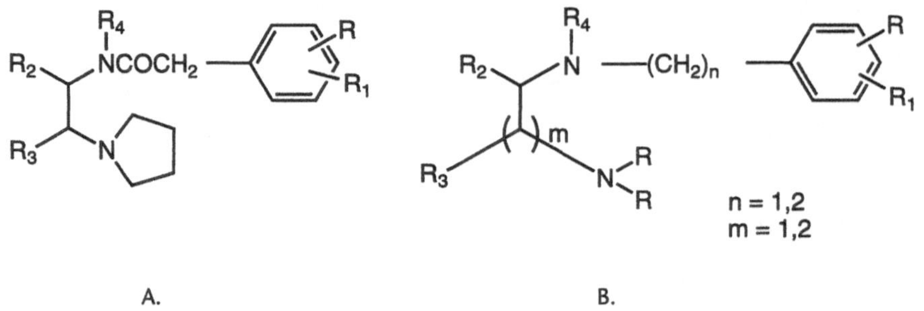

Fig. 40
A. The template of U-50,488 which has survived modifications.
B. The present status of the σ template related to A.

that the σ receptor is not subject to the strict steric requirements which have been shown in the case of U-50,488 analogs with respect to the κ receptor.

The template of U-50,488 which has survived modifications and retained κ activity is shown in Figure 40 as structure A, and the present status of the σ template related to A is shown as structure B.

Further research is required to modify the template of U-50,488 in such a way that the "dysphoric" conformation, which is shared by U-50,488 in structure A (Fig. 38), is eliminated from U-50,488 in order to produce a compound devoid of dysphoric effects.

9   κ receptor subtypes

The κ receptor was cloned and sequenced and corresponds to κ-1 subtype. It has high affinity for dynorphin A (1–17), U-50,488, U-60,593, ethylketocyclazocine, bremazocine and tifluadom. These ligands also bind to κ-2-subtype with the exception of U-69,593 which selectively binds to the κ-1 with high affinity. There are no selective ligands for the κ-2 yet. A third site, κ-3 has been proposed which demonstrates high affinity to naloxone benzoylhydrazone but none to U-50,488 [27, 96, 96a, 97]. Evidence has been provided for the existence of four κ receptor subtypes [98–100].

10 Developmental states of κ agonists

The clinical testing of several κ agonists has been discontinued due to dose limiting dysphoria, but clinical interest continues with several others. The developmental status of κ agonists has been summarized recently [101]. Clinical investigation of the following compounds continues: Apadoline (RP 60180, Rhone-Poulenc, Fig. 23), Asimadoline (EMD 61743, E. Merck, Fig. 27), TRK 820 (TORAY, structure unpublished) [102], DuP747 (DuPont Merck, Fig. 11), Enadoline (CI-977, Park-Davis, Fig. 9).

11 Final comments

In the biology area future directions are pointing towards the development of a selective κ agonist with diuretic properties and low analgesic activity (see Fig. 12); a selective κ agonist as neuroprotective agent; and a peripherally acting analgesic. The existence of multiple κ binding sites is awaiting confirmation by cloning studies and may pave the way to the development of a centrally acting analgesic devoid of undesirable side-effects.

In the chemistry area some of the most novel development in this field include the 1,3-diamines in the benzodiazepine series (Section 3.1), and the diazobicyclononanone series (Section 3.3).

The 1,2-diaminobenzamide template deserves refinement. First, we need analogs which will not share conformational overlap with the σ ligands (see Section 8). Secondly, we need to introduce structural modifications in order to render the ligands more specific for the different κ receptor subtypes.

References

1   D.C. Rees, in: G.P. Ellis and D.K. Luscombe (eds): Progress in Medicinal Chemistry, Vol. 29, Elsevier Science Publishers, B. V. 1992, 109–139.

2   D.I.C. Scopes: Drugs of the Future *18*, 933 (1993).

3   A.F. Casy, in: The Steric Factor in Medicinal Chemistry, Dissymmetric Probes of Pharmacological Receptors, Plenum Press, New York and London 1993, 531–548.

4   D.I.C. Scopes: Exp. Opin. Invest. Drugs *3*, 369 (1994).

5   A. Barber and R. Gottschlich: Exp. Opin. Invest. Drugs *6*, 1351 (1997).

6   G. Ghardina, G.D. Clarke, M. Grugni, M. Sbacchi and V. Vecchietti: H. Farmaco *50*, 405 (1995).

7   A. Barber and R. Gottschlich: Med. Res. Rev. *12*, 525 (1992).

8   A. Herz, in: L.F. Tseng (ed): The Pharmacology of Opioid Peptides, Harwood Academic Publishers 1995, 287.

9   D. Lucet, T. Le Gall and C. Mioskowski: Angew Chem. Int. Ed. *37*, 2580 (1998).

10   P.J. Birch, H. Rogers, A.G. Hayes, N. Hayward, M.B. Tyers, D.I.C. Scopes, A. Naylor and D.B. Judd: Br. J. Pharmacol. *103*, 1819 (1991).

11   Q.J. Zhai and A.J. Ingenito: J. Cardiovasc. Pharmacol. *31*, 806 (1998).

12   M.M. McConnaughey, Q.Z. Zhai and A.J. Ingenito: J. Pharm. Pharmacol. *50*, 1121 (1998).

13   Z.Z. Pan, S.A. Tershner and H.L. Fields: Nature *389*, 382 (1997).

14   Z.Z. Pan: TiPS *19*, 94 (1998).

15   T.J. Feuerstein and W. Seeger: Pharmacol. Ther. *74*, 333 (1997).

16   M. Hiramatsu, H. Murasawa, T. Nabeshima and T. Kameyama: J. Pharmacol. Exp. Therap. *284*, 858 (1998).

17   M. Hiramatsu, T. Hyodo and T. Kameyama: Neurosci. Letts. *236*, 45 (1997).

18   M. Ukai, N. Shinkai and T. Kameyama: Eur. J. Pharmacol. *281*, 173 (1995).

19   M. Hirokami, H. Togashi, M. Matsumoto, M. Yoshioka and H. Saito: Eur. J. Pharmacol. *253*, 9 (1994).

20   A.D. Blake, G. Bot and T. Reisine: Chem. & Biol. *3*, 967 (1996).

21   T.G. Metzger and D.M. Ferguson: FEBS Letts. *375*, 1 (1995).

22   S.R. Childers: Cur. Biol. *7*, R695 (1997).

23   D.D. Taub, T.K. Eisenstein, E.B. Geller, M.W. Adler and T.J. Rogers: Proc. Natl. Acad. Sci. USA *88*, 360 (1991).

24   D.R. Kapusta: Clin. & Experim. Pharmacol. and Physiol. *22*, 891 (1995).

25   R. Spangler, A. Ho, Y. Zhou, C.E. Maggos, V. Yuferov and M.J. Kreek: Mol. Brain Res. *38*, 71 (1996).

26   G. De Sarro, G.R. Trimarchi, S. Sinopoli, Y. Masuda and A. De Sarro: Gen. Pharmac. *24*, 439 (1993).

27   B.N. Dhawan, F. Cesselin, R. Raghubir, T. Reisine, P.B. Bradley, P.S. Portoghese and M. Hamon: Pharmacol. Rev. *48*, 567 (1996).

28   H. Isbell: Clin. Pharmacol. Therap. *22*, 377 1977.

29   J. Szmuszkovicz and P.F. VonVoigtlander: J. Med. Chem. *25*, 1125 (1982).

30   D.I.C. Scopes, N.F. Hayes, D.E. Bays, D. Belton, J. Brain, D.S. Brown, D.B. Judd, A.B. McElroy, C.A. Meerholz, A. Naylor et al.: J. Med. Chem. *35*, 490 (1992).

31   A.G. Hayes, P.J. Birch, N.J. Hayward, M.J. Sheehan, H. Rogers, M.B. Tyers, D.B. Judd, D.I.C. Scopes and A. Naylor: Br. J. Pharmacol. *101*, 944 (1990).

32   A. Naylor, D.B. Judd, J.E. Lloyd, D.I.C. Scopes, A.G. Hayes and P.J. Birch: J. Med. Chem. *36*, 2075 (1993).

33   R.M. Caudle, A.J. Mannes, M.J. Iadarola: J. Pharmacol. Exp. Therap. *283*, 1342 (1997).

34   Y. Zhang, I. Cassel, L. Cortes-Burgos, J. Daubert, R. DeHaven, D. DeHaven-Hudkins, F. Gaul, S. Gottshall, S. Greiner, M. Koblish et al.: Am. Chem. Soc. Nat. Meeting, Boston, MA Medi. 297 (1998).

35   V. Vecchietti, A. Giordani, G. Giardina, R. Colle and G.D. Clarke: J. Med. Chem. *34*, 397 (1991).

36   Zambeletti patent WO9117981 (1991).

37   V. Vecchietti, G.D. Clarke, R. Colle, G. Dondio, G. Giardina, G. Petrone and M. Sbacchi: J. Med. Chem. *35*, 2970 (1992).

38   V. Vecchietti, G.D. Clarke, R. Colle, G. Giardina, G. Petrone and M. Sbacchi: J. Med. Chem. *34*, 2624 (1991).

39   G. Giardina, G.D. Clarke, G. Dondio, G. Petrone, M. Sbacchi and V. Vecchietti: J. Med. Chem. *37*, 3482 (1994).

40   R. Colle, G.D. Clarke, G. Dondio, G. Giardina, G. Petrone, M. Sbacchi and V. Vecchietti: Chirality *4*, 8 (1992).

41   K. Fujibayashi, K. Kubota and K. Saito: Eur. J. Pharmacol. *343*, 171 (1998).

42   Sankyo patent EP356247; JP90149560.

43   P.R. Halfpenny, D.C. Horwell, J. Hughes, C. Humblet, J.C. Hunter, D. Neuhaus and D.C. Rees: J. Med. Chem. *34*, 190 (1991).

44   F.C. Tortella, J. Rose, L. Robles, J.E. Moreton, J. Hughes and J.C. Hunter: J. Pharmacol. Exp. Therap. *282*, 286 (1997).

45   V. Sabin, D.C. Horwell, A.T. McKnight and P. Broqua: Bioorg. & Med. Chem. Letts. *7*, 291 (1997).

46   P. Rajagopalan, R.M. Scribner, P. Pennev, W.K. Schmidt, S.W. Tam, G.F. Steinfels and L. Cook: Bioorg. & Med. Chem. Letts. *2*, 715 (1992).

47   P. Rajagopalan, R.M. Scribner, P. Pennev, P.L. Mattei, H.S. Kezar, C.Y. Cheng, R.S. Cheeseman, V.R. Ganti, A.L. Johnson, M.A. Wuonola et al.: Bioorg. & Med. Chem. Letts. *2*, 721 (1992).

48   J.P. Freeman, E.T. Michalson, S.V. D'Andrea, L. Baczynskyj, P.F. VonVoigtlander, R.A. Lahti, M.W. Smith, C.F. Lawson, T.A. Scahill, S.A. Mizsak et al.: J. Med. Chem. *34*, 1891 (1991).

49   G. Hamon, F. Clémence, M. Fortin, O. Le Martret, S. Jouquey, J.C. Vincent, F. Petit and D.G. Bichet: Brit. J. Pharmacol. *114*, 310P (1995).

49a   I. Bemana and S. Nagao: J. Neurotrauma *15*, 117 (1998).

50   G.F. Costello, R. James, J.S. Shaw, A.M. Slater and N.C.J. Stutchbury: J. Med. Chem. *34*, 181 (1991).

51   A.D. Pechulis, S. Archer, M.P. Wentland, A.M. Colasurdo and J.M. Bidlack: Bioorg. & Med. Chem. Letts. *7*, 2271 (1997).

52   J.J. Barlow, T.P. Blackburn, G.F. Costello, R. James, D.J. Le Count, B.G. Main, R.J. Pearce, K. Russell, and J.S. Shaw: J. Med. Chem. *34*, 3149 (1991).

53   Pfizer patent, EP-789021-A (1997).

54   DuPont Merck patent WO9212128 (1992).

55   C.-Y. Cheng, S.-C. Wu, L.-W. Hsin and S.W. Tam: J. Med. Chem. *35*, 2243 (1992).

56   M.W. Mc Millan and J. Szmuszkovicz, U.S. patent 4,360,531 (1982), also describe the ketals.

57   C.-Y. Cheng, H.-Y. Lu, F.-M. Lee and S.W. Tam: J. Pharmac. Sci. *79*, 758 (1990).

58   C.-Y. Cheng, H.-Y. Lu and F.-M. Lee: Eur. J. Med. Chem. *26*, 125 (1991).

59   S. Zhao, J.P. Freeman, P.F. VonVoigtlander, W.J. Howe and J. Szmuszkovicz: Bioorg. & Med. Chem. Letts. *4*, 2139 (1994).

60   S. Zhao, J. P. Freeman, P. F. VonVoigtlander, M. W. Smith and J. Szmuszkovicz: Bioorg. & Med. Chem. Letts. *12*, 2641 (1993).

61   S.V. D'Andrea, E.T. Michalson, J.P. Freeman, C.G. Chidester and J. Szmuszkovicz: J. Org. Chem. *56*, 3133 (1991).

62   S. Zhao, J.P. Freeman, C.G. Chidester, P.F. VonVoigtlander, S.A. Mizsak and J. Szmuszkovicz: J. Org. Chem. *58*, 4043 (1993).

63   A. Cappelli, M. Anzini, S. Vomero, M.C. Menziani, P.G. De Benedetti, M. Sbacchi, G.D. Clarke and L. Mennuni: J. Med. Chem. *39*, 860 (1996).

64   C. Guyon, V. Fardin, A. Carruette, C. Garret, B. Plau, G. Taurand: AFMC International Medicinal Chemistry Symposium/AIMECS 1995.

65   W. Brandt, S. Drosihn, M. Haurand, U. Holzgrabe and C. Nachtsheim: Arch. Pharm. Pharm. Med. Chem. *329*, 311 (1996).

66   B. Kögel, T. Christoph, E. Friderichs, H.-H. Hennies, T. Matthiesen, J. Schneider and U. Holzgrabe: CNS Drug Reviews *4*, 54 (1998).

67   A. Borsodi, S. Benyhe, U. Holzgrabe, A. Märki and C. Nachtsheim: Reg. Pep *54*, 27 (1994).

68   C.J. De Ranter and C.L. Verlinde, in: B. Jensen, F.S. Jorgensen and H. Kofod (eds.): Frontiers in Drug Research, Munksgaard, Copenhagen 1990, 30–44.

69   M. Higginbottom, W. Nolan, J. O'Toole, G.S. Ratcliffe, D.C. Rees and E. Roberts: Bioorg. & Med. Chem. Letts. *5*, 841 (1993).

70   M. Froimowitz, C.M. DiMeglio and A. Makriyannis: J. Med. Chem. *35*, 3085 (1992).

71   A.P. Ijzerman: Rec. Trav. Chim Pays-Bas *112*, 169 (1993).

71a   G. Subramanian, M.G. Paterlini, D.L. Larson, P.S. Portoghese and D.M. Ferguson: J. Med. Chem. *41*, 4777 (1998).

72   M. Ogata, R. Shimizu and H. Abe: J. Pharmac. Sci. *82*, 91 (1993).

73   Y. Kolesnikov, S. Jain, R. Wilson and G.W. Pasternak: Eur. J. Pharmacol. *310*, 141 (1996).

74   G. Catheline, G. Guilbaud, V. Kayser: Eur. J. Pharmacol. *357*, 171 (1998).

75   Y. Kolesnikov, S. Jain, R. Wilson and G.W. Pasternak: Eur. J. Pharmacol. *310*, 141 (1996).

76.   H. Rogers, P.J. Birch, S.M. Harrison, E. Palmer, G.R. Manchee, D.B. Judd, A. Naylor, D.I.C. Scopes and A.G. Hayes: Br. J. Pharmacol. *106*, 783 (1992).

76   R. Gottschlich, K.A. Ackermann, A. Barber, G.D. Bartoszyk and H.E. Greiner: Bioorg. & Med. Chem. Letts. *4*, 677 (1994).

77   A. Barber, G.D. Bartoszyk, H.M. Bender, R. Gottschlich, H.E. Greiner, J. Harting, F. Mauler, K.-O. Minck, R.D. Murray and M. Simon: Br. J. Pharmacol. *113*, 1317 (1994).

78   R. Gottschlich, M. Krug, A. Barber and R.M. Devant: Chirality *6*, 685 (1994).

79   R.A. Wiley and D.H. Rich: Med. Res. Rev. *3*, 327 (1993).

80   D.H. Rich, in: B. Testa, E. Kyburz, W. Fuhrer and R. Giger (eds.): Perspectives in Medicinal Chemistry, VCH, New York 1993, 15.

81   A. Barber, G.D. Bartoszyk, H.E. Greiner, F. Mauler, R.D. Murray, C.A. Seyfried, M. Simon, R. Gottschlich, J. Harting and I. Lues: Br. J. Pharmacol. *111*, 843 (1994).

82   A.-C. Chang, A. Cowan, A.E. Takemori, and P.S. Portoghese: J. Med. Chem. *39*, 4478 (1996).

83   P.J. Birch, A.G. Hayes, M.R. Johnson, T.A. Lea, P.J. Murray, H. Rogers and D.I.C. Scopes: Bioorg. & Med. Chem. Letters. *2*, 1278 (1992).

84   G.D. Noble, R.F. Dannals, H.T. Ravert, A.A. Wilson and H.N. Wagner Jr.: J. Labelled Compounds and Radiopharmaceut. *31*, 81 (1992).

85   P.L. Chesis and M.J. Welch: Int. J. Radiat. Appl. Instrum. Part A. Appl. Radiat. Isot. *41*, 267 (1990).

86   D.M.P. Lawrence, W. El-Hamouly, S. Archer, J.F. Leary and J.M. Bidlack: Proc. Natl. Acad. Sci. USA *92*, 1062 (1995).

87   S.A. Weerawarna, R.D. Davis and W.L. Nelson: J. Med. Chem. *37*, 2856 (1994).

88   A.-C. Chang, A.E. Takemori and P.S. Portoghese: J. Med. Chem. *37*, 1547 (1994).

89   B.R. de Costa, K.C. Rice, W.D. Bowen, A. Thurkauf, R.B. Rothman, L. Band, A.E. Jacobson, L. Radesca, P.C. Contreras, N.M. Gray et al.: J. Med. Chem. *33*, 3100 (1990).

90   F.F. Moebius, J. Striessnig and H. Glossmann: TiPS *18*, 67 (1997).

91   B.R. de Costa, C. Dominguez, X.-S. He, W. Williams, L. Radesca and W. Bowen: J. Med. Chem. *35*, 4334 (1992).

92   B.R. de Costa, W.D. Bowen, S.B. Hellewell, C. George, R.B. Rothman, A.A. Reid, J.M. Walker, A.E. Jacobson and K.C. Rice: J. Med. Chem. *32*, 1996 (1989).

93   L. Radesca, W.D. Bowen, L. Di Paolo, and B.R. de Costa: J. Med. Chem. *34*, 3058 (1991).

94   B.R. de Costa, L. Radesca, L. Di Paolo and W.D. Bowen: J. Med. Chem. *35*, 38 (1992).

95   W.D. Bowen, J.M. Walker, B.R. de Costa, R. Wu, P.J. Tolentino, D. Finn, R.B. Rothman and K.C. Rice: J. Pharmacol. Exp. Therap. *262*, 32 (1992).

96   B. Nock, in: L.F. Tseng (ed.): The Pharmacology of Opioid Peptides, Harwood Academic Publishers, New York 1995, 29.

96a   M. Satoh and M. Minami: Pharmacol. Ther. *68*, 343 (1995).

97   S.P.H. Alexander and J.A. Peters, in: TIPS, Receptor and Ion Channel Nomenclature Supplement *58* (1998).

98   R.B. Rothman, V. Bykov, B.G. Xue, H. Xu, B.R. de Costa, A.E. Jacobson, K.C. Rice, J.E. Kleinman and L.S. Brady: Peptides *13*, 977 (1992).

99   R.B. Rothman, H. Xu, G.U. Char, A. Kim, B.R. de Costa, K.C. Rice and D.M. Zimmerman: Peptides *14*, 17 (1993).

100   Q. Ni, H. Xu, J.S. Partilla, B.R. de Costa, K.C. Rice and R.B. Rothman: Peptides *14*, 1279 (1993).

101   A. Barber, R. Gottschlich: Exp. Opin. Invest. Drugs *6*, 1351 (1997).

102   Scrip. no. *2002*, 25 (1995)

Progress in Drug Research, Vol. 53 (E. Jucker, Ed.)
© 1999 Birkhäuser Verlag, Basel (Switzerland)

Quantitative structure-activity relationships of antihypertensive agents

By Satya P. Gupta

Department of Chemistry, Birla Institute of Technology and Science, Pilani 333031, India

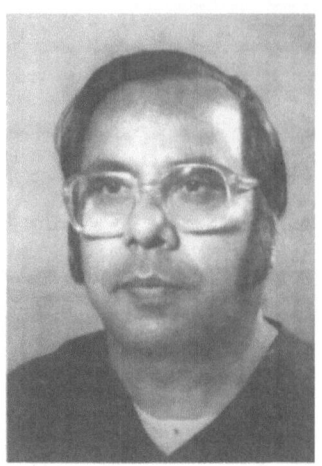

Satya P. Gupta

was born in in 1945 in Uttar Pradesh in India. He obtained his M.Sc. degree in physical chemistry in 1967 and D.Ph. degree in quantum chemistry in 1971, both from the University of Allahabad. He worked on the development of molecular orbital theory and proposed a new molecular orbital method called IOC-ω-technique (inclusion of overlap charges in ω-technique), which was then found very useful in dealing with the problems of conjugated systems. After his Ph.D. degree, Dr. Gupta moved to Tata Institute of Fundamental Research (TIFR), Bombay, where he worked on molecular biology and studied the structure and function of biomembranes. In 1973, he joined Birla Institute of Technology and Science (BITS), Pilani, where he is now a professor of chemistry and is working on theoretical aspects of drug design.

Summary

Quantitative structure-activity relationships of various classes of antihypertensive agents, e.g. sympatholytic agents, diuretics, direct or peripheral vasodilators, potassium channel activators, angiotensin-converting enzyme inhibitors, renin inhibitors and miscellaneous agents (platelet aggregation inhibitors) are reviewed. This review gives an overall picture of the mode of action of each class of drugs and points out their specific physicochemical and structural properties governing their action. For example, in the case of centrally acting drugs (sympatholytic agents) it has surfaced that the prime factors governing their activity are lipophilic and steric properties of the molecules, and at the receptor level a charge-transfer complex is formed between the molecule and the receptor. It is, however, observed that for peripherally acting sympatholytic agents the prime role is played by only lipophilicity. In the case of diuretics, the electronic characters of molecules are found to be more dominant than their lipophilic property, but for direct vasodilators and ACE inhibitors both electronic and lipophilic properties seem to be equally important. In renin or platelet aggregation inhibitors, the structural properties appear to be more important. However, the fundamental property that is overwhelmingly involved in the majority of antihypertensive agents appears to be the lipophilicity, suggesting that in most of the cases the hydrophobic interaction would play the major role in drug action.

Contents

Keywords

Antihypertensive agents, hypotensive agents, sympatholytic agents, diuretics, vasodilators, angiotensin-converting enzyme (ACE) inhibitors, renin inhibitors, carbonic anhydrase inhibitors, platelet aggregation inhibitors, potassium channel activators, clonidines, imidazolidines, arylquinolizines, central α-agonists, peripheral α-antagonists, sulfonamides

Glossary of abbreviations

ACE, angiotensin-converting enzyme; BP, blood pressure; Boc, $(CH_3)_3C-O-CO$; CA, carbonic anhydrase; Cys, cysteine; C_{100}, dose ($\mu mol/kg$) causing doubling of arterial blood pressure; D, distribution coefficient (octanol-phosphate buffer system); D_2^*, molar concentration of drug causing 50% of the maximal response and corrected for protonation; ED_{30}, effective dose of the drug ($\mu mol/kg$, corrected for protonation) causing 30% decrease in arterial blood pressure; E_{exc} (P), excitation energy of the protonated form of the molecule; $E_{HOMO}(P)$, energy of the highest occupied molecular orbital of the protonated form of the molecule; E_s, Taft's steric constant; F, inductive (field) electronic factor; IC_{50}, molar concentration of the drug leading to 50% inhibition of the binding of substrate to the receptor; K_a, dissociation constant of acid; MAC, mercaptoacetic acid; MED, minimum effective dose; P, partition coefficient (octanol-water system); Par, parachor; QSAR, quantitative structure-activity relationship; R, resonance electronic parameter; SHR, spontaneously hypertensive rat; π, hydrophobic constant; σ, Hammett's electronic constant; Δppm, chemical shift; V_w, van der Waals volume; $t_{1/2}$, time in minutes for half of the reaction; r, correlation coefficient; s, standard deviation; $F_{x,y}$, F-ratio between the variances of calculated and observed activities (x: number of independent variables; y = n–x–1)

1   Introduction

Hypertension is one of the cardiovascular diseases which is most common throughout the world. It is generally defined as an elevation of systolic and/or diastolic arterial blood pressure, which is 120/80 mm Hg in normal situation. A value of 140/90 mm is generally accepted as the upper limit of normotension. Hypertension with certain risk factors such as hypercholesterolemia, diabetes, smoking and a family history of vascular disease predisposes to arteriosclerosis and consequent cardiovascular morbidity and mortality. The treatment of hypertension leads to reduced risk of hypertensive renal failure, haemorrhagic stroke, myocardial infarction and cardiac failure.

In most cases, the cause of the hypertension can not be clearly defined. Such hypertension is termed as essential hypertension. In a few cases (5–15%), the hypertension is secondary to definable causes, such as renal artery stenosis, a pheochromocytoma, or an endocrine disorder. This type of hypertension is known as secondary hypertension. Although the exact etiology of essential hypertension is still not well known, the following factors are supposed to play causative roles.

1. *Neural factors*: Excessive sympathetic nerve discharge, probably triggered by stress or emotionality early in the development of hypertension, is thought to play a major role in the etiology of this disease. Increased sympathetic outflow from the brain promotes an increased cardiac output and elevated peripheral resistance. Noradrenaline is the principal nerve transmitter both centrally and peripherally, but abnormal serotonin, dopamine or adrenaline levels may also play a critical role in the etiology of hypertension.
2. *Electrolyte factors*: The main cause of elevated arterial blood pressure is supposed to be the inability of the kidney to excrete the adequate daily amount of salt and water [1, 2]. Abnormal retention of salt and water increases the blood volume, which increases the work load on the heart by increasing blood flow.
3. *Vasoconstriction*: It has been suggested that intermittent increases in cardiac output induce wall thickening [3]. This leads to vasoconstriction, offering resistance to blood flow.

4. *Hormonal factors*: The release of a hormone, called aldosterone, from the adrenal gland induces sodium and water retention, leading to an increase in the blood pressure by a volume mechanism [4, 5]. The main physiological stimulus for the release of this hormone is an octapeptide (Asp-Arg-Val-Tyr-Ile-His-Pro-Phe) called angiotensin II. The formation of angiotensin II from its precursor angiotensin I, a decapeptide (Asp-Arg-Val-Tyr-Ile-His-Pro-Phe-His-Leu), is mediated by an enzyme known as angiotensin-converting enzyme (ACE).

In addition to the above principal factors, the genetic factors are also supposed to be involved in hypertension [6]. Parents and siblings of individuals with essential hypertension are generally affected by the same condition.

2 Antihypertensive (hypotensive) agents

Based upon the above-mentioned etiological factors, the antihypertensive agents can be put into the following categories.

2.1 Sympatholytic agents

Sympatholytic agents produce their antihypertensive effects by inhibiting directly or indirectly the nerve discharge. They include centrally acting α-adrenergic stimulants (central α-agonists), peripherally acting α-adrenergic blocking agents (peripheral α-antagonists), adrenergic neuron blockers, β-adrenergic blocking agents (β-blockers), and ganglionic blocking agents.

2.2 Diuretics

Diuretics are the agents that increase the rate of urine formation and its excretion. This leads to the reduction of extracellular fluid volume and sodium ion concentration, which is associated with a decrease in cardiac output; and thus diuretics act as antihypertensive agents. Thiazides and related compounds comprise the most frequently used antihypertensive agents.

2.3   Direct or peripheral vasodilators

Direct or peripheral vasodilators act by inducing relaxation in vascular smooth muscles and consequently decreasing the peripheral resistance without any significant effect on sympathetic nervous system. Agents like diazoxide and sodium nitroprusside are treated as direct vasodilators.

2.4   Angiotensin-converting enzyme (ACE) and renin inhibitors

The angiotensin-converting enzyme (ACE) inhibitors inhibit the formation of angiotensin II from its precursor angiotensin I and thus prevent the release of aldosterone from the adrenal gland. The interference of the synthesis of angiotensin I can also lead ultimately to the inhibition of the release of aldosterone. Thus, the inhibitors of renin, the enzyme which mediates the synthesis of angiotensin I, can also be exploited as antihypertensive agents.

2.5   Miscellaneous

Hypertension has also been found to be associated with lowered level of cyclic adenosine-3',5'-monophosphate (cAMP). Therefore, inhibitors of cAMP phosphodiesterase, the enzyme that catalyzes the conversion of cAMP to adenosine-5'-monophosphate and is thus responsible, in part, for lowering the intracellular level of cAMP, can also act as antihypertensive agents. Similarly, inhibitors of several other enzyme systems, such as monoamine oxidase, tyrosine kinase and dopamine β-hydroxylase, which affect the noradrenaline pathway, were also explored for the development of hypertension therapy, but little success was achieved. Some platelet aggregation inhibitors were, however, found to be more promising as antihypertensive agents [7].

All the above categories of antihypertensive agents have different sites and mechanisms of action. Since essential hypertension is largely an asymptomatic condition, its treatment is largely dictated by the side-effects of the drugs. However, the sites and mechanisms by which the drugs lower the blood pressure greatly determine their usefulness as well as their side-effects. Therefore, the challenge for medicinal chemists and pharmacologists in developing antihypertensive agents is to identify the compounds with a site and mechanism of action unique to the control of blood pressure so as to avoid side-effects.

For in-depth studies on sites and mechanisms of drug actions, quantitative structure-activity relationships (QSARs) of drugs have been of great help. QSARs not only provide deeper insight into the mechanisms and sites of drug action but also rationalize the drug synthesis because of their predictive ability. Therefore, in succession to our efforts to present comprehensive reviews on QSARs of variety of drugs [8-16], a detailed review of QSARs of antihypertensive agents is presented.

3 QSAR results and discussion

3.1 Sympatholytic agents

Among the sympatholytic agents, the centrally acting α-agonists have been widely studied. Since the development of clonidine (**1**), an analogue of α-adrenergic naphthazole (**2**), as an effective antihypertensive agent, clonidine-like compounds have drawn considerable interest for the development of antihypertensive drugs. Clonidine elicits its potent central antihypertensive action through stimulation of α-receptors in the medulla.

1   **2**

The tendency of imidazolidine class of drugs (clonidine analogues) to accumulate in the brain, expressed as log (C_{brain}/C_{iv}), where C_{brain} refers to the rat-brain concentration of the drug (ng/g of brain tissue, wet weight) achieved at the moment of maximal decrease in the blood pressure following intravenous administration of a certain dose C_{iv} (µg/kg of body weight), was shown to have a high parabolic dependence on a distribution coefficient (D) measured in octanol-phosphate buffer system (Eq. 1) [17, 18]. However, the

$$\log (C_{brain}/C_{iv}) = 0.574 \log D - 0.133 (\log D)^2 - 0.094$$
$$n = 14, \ r = 0.987, \ s = 0.14, \ F_{2,11} = 211.83 \tag{1}$$

$$\log (1/ED_{30}{}^*) = 0.491(\pm 0.28) \log D - 0.253 (\pm 0.22) (\log D)^2 + 0.789$$
$$n = 27, \ r = 0.647, \ s = 0.79, \ F_{2,24} = 8.62 \tag{2}$$

$$\log (1/ED_{30}{}^*) = 0.105 \ (\pm 0.03) \ \Sigma Par - 0.00032 \ (\pm 0.00008) \ (\Sigma Par)^2$$
$$- 0.695 \ (\pm 0.17) \ \Delta pK_a{}^\circ + 5.333 \ (\pm 1.89) \ E_{HOMO} \ (P)$$
$$+ 6.752 \ (\pm 2.225) \ E_{exc} \ (P) + 2.494$$
$$n = 27, \ r = 0.952, \ s = 0.34, \ F_{5,21} = 40.34 \tag{3}$$

antihypertensive activity studied for a series of imidazolidines (3) in terms of $ED_{30}{}^*$, the dose of the drug (µmol/kg, corrected for protonation) causing 30% decrease in mean arterial blood pressure, was not found so well correlated with this distribution coefficient (Eq. 2) [19]. Rather, Timmermans et al. [19] found the antihypertensive activity to be significantly correlated with various other physicochemical and electronic parameters as shown in Eq. (3), where ΣPar refers to the parachor values of the substituents, $\Delta pK_a{}^\circ$ to the effect of substituents on the dissociation of the compound, and E_{HOMO} (P) and E_{exc} (P), the two quantum mechanical parameters, to the energy of the highest occupied molecular orbital and the excitation energy of the protonated form of the molecule, respectively. Parachor is defined as the product of molecular volume and the fourth root of surface tension. Since surface tension can be related to the overall lipophilic behaviour of the molecule, the parachor may be treated as variable containing lipophilic as well as steric properties. Thus, these two properties appear to be important in the activity. Further, the role of $\Delta pK_a{}^\circ$ can be ascribed to its profound influence on the lipophilicity. Thus, lipophilicity, or essentially the distribution coefficient, particularly of lipid-water phase, which is taken as a measure of lipophilicity (or hydrophobicity), seems to play a major role in antihypertensive activity. However, since $\Delta pK_a{}^\circ$ also reflects electronic effects, the drug-receptor inter-

3

action may be assumed to involve some electronic interaction. The dependence of the activity on E_{exc} and E_{HOMO} (an index of electron donor ability) together suggests that a charge-transfer phenomenon may occur between the drug and receptor molecules.

In all the above equations, n refers to the number of data points used to derive the equation, r is the correlation coefficient, s is the standard deviation, F is the F-ratio between the variances of calculated and observed activities, and the figures within parentheses are the 95% confidence intervals (such figures written without ± sign would refer to standard errors of the coefficients of variables).

Although Equation (3) exhibits a highly significant correlation, it does not provide any clear picture of the mode of drug action at the receptor level, as the *in vivo* effects involve kinetics other than mere receptor occupation. Equation (1) derived by Timmermans et al. [18] could be used to separate these two aspects and to calculate the brain concentration (nmol/g of brain tissue, wet weight) associated with a decrease in arterial blood pressure to 30% [19]. This new ED_{30}, referred to as $(ED_{30})_{cald}$, was considered a measure of the concentration of the drugs at the central α-adrenoceptor level, independent of the processes that ultimately provide this concentration in the receptor compartment, since these kinetic events are already accounted for by Equation (1). The $(ED_{30})_{cald}$, presumed to be a more suitable biological parameter, was then found to be correlated with a steric parameter rather than any parameter associated with lipophilic character of the molecule (Eq. 4) [19]. In Equation (4), ΣE_s stands for the Taft steric constants of the substituents. Also, in this equation, the presence, in place of ΔpK_a°, of ΣR, the parameter describing the electronic effects of substituents through resonance, suggests that the resonance effect of the substituents may be more important than the dissociation effect. However, the involvement of charge-transfer phenomenon in drug-receptor interaction is reaffirmed.

$$\log [1/(ED_{30})_{cald}] = -1.771\,(\pm 0.56)\,\Sigma E_s - 0.401(\pm 0.12)\,(\Sigma E_s)^2 + 1.898$$
$$(\pm 1.09)\,\Sigma R + 5.129\,(\pm 1.67)\,E_{HOMO}\,(P) + 6.771\,(\pm$$
$$1.96)\,E_{exc} + 8.026$$
$$n = 27,\ r = 0.941,\ s = 0.33,\ F_{5,21} = 32.20 \tag{4}$$

Equation (4), however, was not found to adequately describe the activity of two meta-substituted analogues present in the series. Hence, when both the meta-substituted compounds were excluded, an appreciably improved correlation was obtained (r = 0.965, s = 0.26), which accounted better for the activity of 2-, 2,4-, or 2,4,6- substituted derivatives.

Initially upon dosing, clonidine also induces a transient peripheral effect due to stimulation of peripheral α-receptors in vasculature [20–22]. The relationship between centrally and peripherally mediated actions was studied [17, 23–26], but since penetration into the central nervous system (CNS) is related to the distribution coefficient and since antihypertensive effect is due to central α-stimulation, the quantitative correlation between them could be established only when the distribution coefficient was also taken into account. For a series of clonidine and its 12 analogues, Timmermans and van Zwieten [25] obtained:

$$\log (1/ED_{30}) = 0.84 \log (1/C_{100}) + 0.63 \log D - 0.30$$
$$n = 13, r = 0.912, s = 0.50 \tag{5}$$

where C_{100} is a measure of peripheral effect and stands for the dose (μmol/kg) causing a doubling in arterial pressure in the pithed rat (i.v.). In order to establish the general applicability of such a correlation, Timmermans et al. [26] derived Equation (6), exhibiting the correlation between the central and peripheral cardiovascular activities of a set of 21 structurally dissimilar α-adrenoceptor antagonists (Tab. 1), varying greatly in overall lipophilic characters. Equation (6), however, being quadratic in log D optimizes the effect of lipophilicity on central action, which, in fact, is a usual situation in *in vivo* assays.

$$\log (1/ED_{25}) = 0.887 \ (\pm \ 0.21) \log (1/C_{60}) + 0.895 \ (\pm \ 0.33) \log D$$
$$- 0.387 \ (\pm \ 0.16) \ (\log D)^2 - 0.098$$
$$n = 21, r = 0.945, s = 0.38, F_{3,17} = 47.03 \tag{6}$$

Based on these QSAR studies, Timmermans and van Zwieten proposed a hypothetical working model of the interaction of imidazolidines with the receptor as shown in Figure 1 and made the following suggestions [19].

(1) The aromatic phenyl ring of the imidazolidine possibly interacts by means of the electron donation with an electron-deficient area of the receptor.

Table 1.
Hypotensive potency and α-adrenoceptor binding affinities of structurally dissimilar α-adrenoceptor agonists [26, 36].

No.	Compound[a]	log $(1/ED_{25}$[b]$)$	log $(1/C_{60}$[c]$)$	log $[1/IC_{50}(\alpha_1)$[d]$]$	log $[1/IC_{50}(\alpha_2)$[e]$]$
1	44-549	2.77	2.40	1.22	2.80
2	Bay-a 6781	2.32	2.11	−0.13	2.22
3	lofexidine	2.09	1.99	0.18	2.60
4	clonidine	2.04	1.78	−0.08	2.51
5	Bay-c 6014	1.96	1.51	−0.57	2.00
6	UK-14, 304-18	1.55	1.56	−0.38	2.44
7	B-HT 920	1.43	0.69	−2.70	1.60
8	naphazoline	0.95	1.83	0.39	2.32
9	St-871	0.84	1.22	−0.10	2.19
10	tiamenidine	0.69	1.20	−0.69	2.04
11	St-1913	0.68	1.17	0.27	2.17
12	KUM 32	0.63	0.23	−0.53	1.32
13	xylazine	0.62	−0.22	−1.79	0.85
14	tramazoline	0.55	1.80	−0.04	1.80
15	xylometazoline	0.26	1.12	0.24	1.64
16	St-739	−0.02	0.65	−0.15	1.19
17	B-HT 933	−0.14	−0.41	−2.97	0.73
18	tetryzoline	−0.16	0.90	−0.20	1.52
19	St-889	−1.02	−0.26	−1.04	0.65
20	St-404	−1.31	−0.79	−1.72	0.23
21	St-1967	0.88	1.24	0.00	1.38

[a]For structures of compounds, see [26].
[b]Dose (μmol/kg) required to invoke a 25% decrease in mean arterial pressure in anesthetized, normotensive rats.
[c]Dose (μmol/kg) causing an increase in mean arterial pressure by 60 mm Hg in pithed, normotensive rats.
[d]Molar concentration leading to 50% inhibition of the specific [^{3}H]prazosin (0.2 nM) binding to α_1-adrenoceptor.
[e]Molar concentration leading to 50% inhibition of the specific [^{3}H]clonidine (0.4 nM) binding to α_2-adrenoceptor.

(2) A positively charged nitrogen of the imidazolidine nucleus interacts with the negatively charged site of the receptor.

(3) A third type of interaction is based upon the formation of a hydrogen bond with the bridge nitrogen, although this type of interaction is probably less important quantitatively.

(4) The optimal fit of the compound with the α-receptor is determined by one

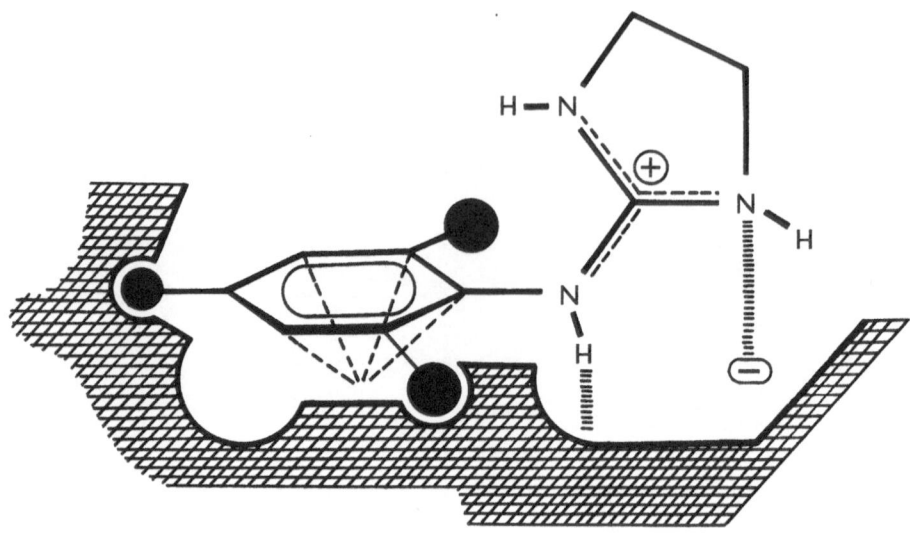

Fig. 1
Timmermans' hypothetical model of interactions of imidazolidines with central α-adrenoceptor [19].

side of the phenyl ring. On that side, an ortho substituent, chlorine or any other group whose steric bulk is close to that of chlorine, is preferably selected for this fit. The ortho substituent then possibly determines the orientation of the residual imidazolidine ring.

(5) Hypotensive activity is favoured when para position is left unsubstituted or it has a small substituent like fluorine or hydroxyl group.

These features of interactions suggested by Timmermans and van Zwieten for the interactions of imidazolidines with α-receptor are probably not much different from those proposed to be of importance for the peripheral situation [27–29].

The peripheral mechanism is explained by an α-sympathomimetic action. Quantitative correlations of peripheral α-mimetic action of some clonidine analogues as 3 with physicochemical parameters pointed out the critical role of the steric effects of ortho substituents [30, 31]. A correlation reported by Rouot et al. [30] was:

$$\log (1/D_2^*) = -1.93 \, (\pm 0.50) \, E_{s(2+6)} - 0.77 \, (\pm 0.20) \, [E_{s(2+6)}]^2 - 1.19$$
$$(\pm 0.52) \, E_{s(2)} - 0.70 \, (\pm 0.26) \, E_{s(3)} - 0.38 \, (\pm 0.36) \, F + 6.17$$
$$n = 22, \, r = 0.93, \, s = 0.29, \, F_{5,16} = 19.30 \tag{7}$$

where D_2^* refers to the molar concentration of the drug causing 50% of the maximal response and corrected for protonation (assuming the protonated species is active). This correlation expresses the major effect of steric factors and only a small effect of the field (inductive) factor F. These authors were, however, not able to find any correlation for the hypotensive activity of these compounds. This discrepancy led to the suggestion that central and peripheral adrenergic receptors are probably different.

Like β-adrenoceptors, α-adrenoceptors are also subdivided into α_1 and α_2 types. The terms α_1 and α_2 indicate only the preference of the receptors for agonists and antagonists and not localization with respect to the nerve ending and the synapse [32]. The acute blood pressure-lowering effect of α-adrenoceptors has been attributed to the participation of the α_2 type [26, 33–35]. This idea was further substantiated by Timmermans et al. by a QSAR study [36], in which they correlated their data [26] on hypotensive activity of a series of structurally dissimilar α-adrenoceptor agonists (Tab. 1) in anaesthetized, normotensive rats with *in vitro* binding affinities of compounds for α_1 and α_2 types, measured as the molar concentration (IC_{50}) inhibiting the specific [^{3}H]prazosin (0.2 nM) and [^{3}H]clonidine (0.4 nM) binding, respectively. The hypotensive activity C_{25} (as used in Eq. 6) was found to be poorly correlated with $IC_{50}(\alpha_1)$ (Eq. 8) but reasonably well correlated with IC_{50} (α_2) (Eq. 9).

$$\log (1/C_{25}) = 0.436 \, (\pm 0.45) \, \log [1/IC_{50}(\alpha_1)] + 1.063$$
$$n = 21, \, r = 0.422, \, s = 0.894, \, F_{1,19} = 4.1 \tag{8}$$
$$\log (1/C_{25}) = 1.265 \, (\pm 0.38) \, \log [1/IC_{50}(\alpha_2)] - 1.342$$
$$n = 21, \, r = 0.846, \, s = 0.578, \, F_{1,19} = 48.0 \tag{9}$$

For a small series of arylquinolizines (4), Huff et al. [37] recently demonstrated the existence of significant correlations between α-adrenoceptor affinities of the compounds and the lipophilicity of their aryl portion (Eqs. 10 and 11). Equation (10) was derived from [^{3}H]prazosin displacement data (α_1-adrenoceptor affinity) and Equation (11) for [^{3}H]clonidine displacement data (α_2-adrenoceptor affinity). This correlation study led Huff et al. to sug-

4; X = O/S/NH, R^1=R^2=O/H   **5**

gest that the structure of the aromatic ring plays an important role in determining the α-adrenoceptor affinity of arylquinolizines and exerts its influence primarily through the hydrophobic interaction.

$$\log (1/K_i) = 1.08 \ (\pm 0.28) \log P + 5.13 \ (\pm 0.36)$$
$$n = 8, \ r = 0.84, \ s = 0.62, \ F_{1,6} = 14.83 \tag{10}$$
$$\log (1/K_i) = 1.17 \ (\pm 0.24) \log P + 5.47 (\pm 0.31)$$
$$n = 8, \ r = 0.89, \ s = 0.53, \ F_{1,6} = 23.67 \tag{11}$$

However, the van der Waals type of interaction (dispersion interaction) has also been indicated in the binding of α-agonists to the receptors. Lee and Lien [38] found the [^{3}H]clonidine displacement activity of a mixed series of compounds on rat brain membrane to be correlated with molecular weight as

$$\log (1/K_i) = 9.869 \ (\pm 3.511) \ MW - 15.028 (\pm 3.511)$$
$$n = 18, \ r = 0.830, \ s = 0.684 \tag{12}$$

A considerable amount of work has gone into the study of clonidine and its analogues with fruitful results. Attempts have also been made to correlate the activity of clonidine and its analogues to their conformations. Following the conformational study of Pullman et al. [39, 40] and Wermuth et al. [41] on some sympathomimetic and sympatholytic amines, Hoefke [42] proposed that clonidine can assume a conformation mimicking that of noradrenaline (active form, **5**), with the phenyl and imidazolidine ring perpendicular.

In this conformation, the distance from the centre of the phenyl to the distant NH is 5.0–5.1 Å and that from the bridge nitrogen to the NH is

7; X=CH/N, n=0/1, Y=S/SO$_2$

6

8; X=S/O

1.28–1.36 Å. These distances compare very well with those in noradrenaline: 5.1–5.2 Å from the centre of the phenyl to N$^+$ and 1.2–1.4 Å from the plane of the phenyl to N$^+$. However, some quantum mechanical calculations [43, 44] showed that phenyl and imidazoline rings may not be perpendicular, and led to the proposition of an allene-like structure.

Compounds other than clonidine analogues were also studied for their central hypotensive action and subjected to QSAR analysis. For three different series of piperazines, **6–8**, the QSARs reported were as shown by Equations (13) [45], (14) [46], and (15) [47], respectively. In Equations 14 and 15, C has been used for % fall in BP/(100 – % fall in BP). The parameter D in Equation (14) refers to the distance between lipophilic regions in the molecule derived from molecular lipophilicity potential (MLP) [48]. In **7**, three important lipophilic regions were derived: region 1 is around the R-substituent of the phenyl ring 1 covering a substantial portion of the ring, region 2 surrounds the bridge group between the piperazine ring and the phenyl ring 2, and region 3 is in the neighbourhood of the basic nitrogen of piperazine. The D$_1$ refers to the optimum distance between regions 1 and 2. The use of D$_3$, the distance between regions 2 and 3, in place of D$_1$ had given equally significant correlation (Eq. 16) [46]. Thus in **7**, the distance of lipophilic region on either side of the piperazine ring is a controlling factor. Additionally, the resonance electronic effect of R^1-substituent at phenyl ring 2 also seems to play an import role in the hypotensive activity of the compounds. Such an elec-

67

$$\log (BP\ fall) = 4.789\ (0.391)\ \log P - 0.569\ (0.046)\ (\log P)^2 - 8.269$$
$$n = 23,\ r = 0.940,\ s = 0.09,\ F_{2,20} = 75.74 \tag{13}$$
$$\log C = 1.263\ (0.130)\ R_{R1} + 1.471\ (0.388)\ D_1 - 0.062\ (0.016)\ D_1^2 - 8.475$$
$$n = 14,\ r = 0.956,\ s = 0.12,\ F_{3,10} = 35.79 \tag{14}$$
$$\log C = 1.009\ (0.260)\ R_{R2} - 1.094\ (0.198)\ \sigma_{R2} - 0.491$$
$$n = 16,\ r = 0.875,\ s = 0.13,\ F_{2,13} = 21.26 \tag{15}$$
$$\log C = 1.174\ (0.133)\ R_{R1} + 1.132\ (0.326)\ D_3 - 0.084\ (0.023)\ D_3^2 - 3.528$$
$$n = 14,\ r = 0.954,\ s = 0.12,\ F_{3,10} = 34.17 \tag{16}$$

tronic effect in the series of **8** is shown to be exhibited by R^2-substituents at phenyl ring 1 (Eq. 15). The R^2-substituents also produce the electronic effect through the electron-donation described by the Taft electronic parameter σ. In the series of **8**, however, no lipophilic character was found to be important. On the contrary, for the series of **6**, only the lipophilicity of the compound could be found to govern the activity and no electronic properties could surface to have any effect (Eq. 13). In Equation (13), P stands for octanol-water partition coefficient describing the lipophilicity of the compound. These differences in the roles of physicochemical properties in the series of **6–8** may be attributed to the different conformational properties of each series.

The prazosin (**9**), which is frequently used in hypertension therapy, acts at α_1-adrenoceptors [49–51], but little QSAR studies have been made on prazosin-like drugs. However, drugs other than prazosin series were also studied for their α_1-adrenoceptor affinity against prazosin, and for a series of **10** studied by Winters et al. [52] a QSAR was reported [53]. The α_1-adrenoceptor bind-

9

10

ing constant (K_i) of these compounds was found to be related not only to lipophilic and electronic properties of the substituents but to their size also. The QSAR reported by Singh and Sharma [53] was as

$$\log (1/K_i) = 1.50 \, (\pm 0.18) \, V_w(R) - 1.35 \, (\pm 0.32) \, V_w(R^1) + 0.45 \, (\pm 0.39) \, \pi_4$$
$$- 0.98 \, (\pm 0.75) \, \sigma_x + 6.42$$
$$n = 38, \, r = 0.86, \, s = 0.41, \, F_{4,33} = 22.80 \tag{17}$$

where $V_w(R)$ and $V_w(R^1)$ refer to van der Waals volume of R- and R^1-substituents, respectively, π_4 is the lipophilic constant of 4-X substituent at the phenyl ring, and σ_x is the Taft electronic constant for X-substituent at any position of the ring. Thus, Equation (17) suggests that α_1-adrenoceptor binding of **10** will depend upon the size of R- and R^1-substituents and upon the lipophilic and electronic properties of X-substituents.

Some QSAR studies have also been made on peripherally acting α-adrenergic blocking agents. Following the discovery of the antihypertensive agent diazoxide (**11**) [54], its several analogues (**12**) were prepared for a study of structure-activity relationships [55, 56]. These compounds exist in two tautomeric forms, 2H (**12a**) and 4H (**12b**), with preference for the latter [57, 58].

A QSAR study was made of a few series of these compounds [59], in which both *in vitro* and *in vivo* activities were analyzed.

In vitro activity was based on the ability of the compound to block the noradrenaline-induced contractile response of the rat aortic ring and was determined experimentally in terms of ED_{50} [60]. This provides a measure of the effect of the compound on vascular reactivity which, according to the accepted mechanism of action of diazoxide, is directly related to its antihypertensive properties [60, 61]. For correlation purposes, a logarithmic parameter A was computed and then corrected for ionization and used as A* [59]. This A* was then correlated for two different series of **12**: one in which only X-substituents varied and Y was constant (CH_3) and the other in which mainly Y-substituents varied with only a little variation in X at the 6- and 7-positions, and the best correlations obtained for them were, respectively, as

$$A^* = 0.90\ (\pm 0.21) + 0.62\ (\pm 0.34)\ \pi_{x(6,7)} + 0.44\ (\pm 0.30)\ \sigma_{x(6,7)}$$
$$n = 29,\ r = 0.91,\ s = 0.29 \tag{18}$$
$$A^* = 0.42\ (\pm 0.33) + 1.28\ (\pm 0.31)\ \pi_{x(6,7)} + 0.72\ (\pm 0.47)\ \pi_Y$$
$$- 0.19\ (\pm 0.16)\ (\pi_Y)^2$$
$$n = 33,\ r = 0.91,\ s = 0.35 \tag{19}$$

We note that though the X-substituents were also located at the 5- and 8-positions, no physicochemical parameters for them were found to be relevant in Equation (18). Thus, the hydrophobic and electronic properties of only the 6- and 7- substituents were found to govern the activity. However, Equation (19) suggests that with little variation in 6- and 7-substituents, the electronic character of these substituents does not come into play and that, along with the hydrophobic character of 3-substituents (Y-substituents), their hydrophobic character alone is sufficient to account for the activity.

For a selected series of 3,6,7-substituted analogues of **12**, the *in vivo* data were also available, and the related activity parameter A' was found to be correlated with the hydrophobic properties of the substituents in the same manner as A* in Equation (19) (Eq. 20) [59]. A' is defined as log(1000/MED), where MED is the minimum effective dose producing a significant lowering of blood pressure.

$$A' = 1.23\ (\pm 0.40) + 0.43\ (\pm 0.22)\ \pi_{x(6,7)} + 1.42\ (\pm 1.14)\ \pi_Y - 0.81\ (\pm 0.78)\ (\pi_Y)^2$$
$$n = 14,\ r = 0.85,\ s = 0.25 \tag{20}$$

These QSAR studies thus show that in the case of peripheral α-antagonists the drug-receptor interactions mainly involve hydrophobic interactions.

3.2 Diuretics

In the treatment of hypertension, if not severe, diuretics have been found to be quite useful, and therefore attention has been focussed on the study of their structure-activity relationships. A QSAR study greatly helped in the design of potent, clinically useful diuretic, muzolimine (**13**) [62]. Some

13　　　　　**14**　　　　　**15**　　　　　**16**

azanaphthalene derivatives (**14**, **15**) were also studied for their diuretic activity, and a QSAR analysis was performed [63] by using urine volume (log V), amount of Na$^+$ and K$^+$ (log $U_{Na}V$ and log U_KV), and log (U_{Na}/U_K) at a dose of 30 mg/kg in rats as dependent variables. A Free-Wilson analysis on 37 derivatives of **14** was found to be quite significant for log V (r = 0.987, s = 0.06) and log (U_{Na}/U_K) (r = 0.979, s = 0.05), suggesting that the best substituents are X = phenyl, X′ = H and Y = Y′ = morphilino group (**16**) with Z = H in both cases. Similarly, a significant Free-Wilson analysis on 46 derivatives of **15** revealed the best substituents as

for log V: R = Me, X = phenyl, X′ = H, Y = Y′ = morphilino with Z = H/Me,
for log $U_{Na}V$: R = H, X = Et, X′ = H, Y = Y′ = morphilino with Z = H, and
for log U_KV: R = Me, X = Et, X′ = H, Y = Y′ = morphilino with Z = H/Me.

Compounds with these substituents were synthesized and many of them were found to be active.

For a set of different azanapthalene skeletons, a quantum mechanical calculation using the extended Hückel theory (EHT) was made [63], showing that diuretic activities can be correlated with quantum mechanical parameters as

$$\log V = 0.62\ N^*_{4a} - 5.01\ M_{4a,8a} + 4.98$$
$$n = 11,\ r = 0.891,\ s = 0.09 \tag{21}$$
$$\log U_{Na}V = 0.52\ N^*_{4a} - 6.13\ M_{4a,8a} + 6.16$$
$$n = 11,\ r = 0.836,\ s = 0.12 \tag{22}$$
$$\log U_KV = 0.53\ N^*_4 + 0.36\ N^*_{4a} - 0.22$$
$$n = 11,\ r = 0.835,\ s = 0.09 \tag{23}$$

71

where N^*_{4a} and N^*_4 are the sum of atomic populations of the highest and the next highest occupied molecular orbitals in the π system at positions 4a and 4, respectively, and $M_{4a,8a}$ refers to the atomic bond population between positions 4a and 8a.

Another quantum mechanical study on these azanaphthalenes was made by Singh and Gupta [64] using the Pariser-Parr-Pople method, in which they could satisfactorily correlate only log U_KV as shown by Equation (24).

$$\log U_K V = 0.345 - 2.888\ Q_{4a} - 0.528\ Q_{8a}$$
$$n = 10,\ r = 0.818,\ s = 0.12 \tag{24}$$

In this equation, Q_{4a} and Q_{8a} refer to the net charge at positions 4a and 8a, respectively. With these parameters, the other two diuretic measurements were found to be poorly correlated (logV, $r = 0.701$; log $U_{Na}V$, $r = 0.619$). Thus, the diuretic action can not be fully accounted for only by the electronic characteristics of the ring junction, but it does seem that the ring junction plays an important role in the action mechanism. The sulfhydryl reactivity of a series of acylphenoxyacetic acids (17), assumed to be responsible for ATPase inhibition, leading to diuresis, was found to be related to the electronic charge at the β-carbon of α,β-unsaturated ketonic moiety (Eqs. 25 and 26) [65]. The reactivity was measured in terms of time in minutes for half of the reaction ($t_{1/2}$) with mercaptoacetic acid (MAC) and cysteine. This correlation supports the idea that the drug-receptor interaction involves some kind of electronic interaction that is fairly strong. Among the other factors, lipophilicity has been found to be an important factor [66].

17

18

$$\log t_{1/2}\ (\text{MAC}) = 22.66 - 175.50\ Q_\beta$$
$$n = 13,\ r = 0.82,\ s = 0.28 \tag{25}$$
$$\log t_{1/2}\ (\text{Cys}) = 25.28 - 204.20\ Q_\beta$$
$$n = 13,\ r = 0.76,\ s = 0.29 \tag{26}$$

Inhibition of carbonic anhydrase (CA) also leads to diuresis, and sulfonamides (18) have been well studied for their enzyme inhibitory activity and
diuretic action. Regarding their structure-activity relationships, exhaustive
studies have been carried out by Kakeya et al. [67–70]. These authors showed
that the diuretic (excretion of urine) and natriuretic (excretion of Na^+) activities of sulfonamides, log (1/C), where C is the dose (mM/kg) required to
increase the excretion threefold, were well correlated with the *in vitro* enzyme
inhibition constant, log ($1/K_i$), with r = 0.955 and 0.953, respectively, for
monosubstituted derivatives [68]. The inclusion of some disubstituted compounds, however, slightly decreased this correlation. Both diuretic and natriuretic activities were found to be well correlated with electronic characteristics of the sulfamoyl group, such as the electron-withdrawing effect of substituents (σ factor), pK_a, nuclear magnetic resonance (NMR) chemical shift of
the sulfamoyl protons, and S = O valence-force constant [68]. A high mutual
correlation (r = 0.999) exists between the two activities; hence only one of
them, the natriuretic activity, was subjected to detailed QSAR study [70], and
the best correlations obtained were:

$$\log (1/C) = 0.283 + 1.497\,\Delta_{ppm} - 0.091\,\pi - 0.152\,\pi^2$$
$$n = 16,\ r = 0.939,\ s = 0.116 \tag{27}$$
$$\log (1/C) = 0.317 + 0.668\,\sigma - 0.106\,\pi - 0.175\,\pi^2$$
$$n = 16,\ r = 0.944,\ s = 0.113 \tag{28}$$
$$\log (1/C) = 0.335 - 0.674\,\Delta pK_a - 0.026\,\pi - 0.143\,\pi^2$$
$$n = 16,\ r = 0.965,\ s = 0.089 \tag{29}$$

In deriving these equations, however, only meta and para mono- or disubstituted analogues were included, and three ortho substituted analogues were
completely excluded because of their aberrant behaviour, which was attributed to the steric effects of ortho substituents. In isolation, the π factor was
not found to have any significant correlation – it simply improved the correlation with the electronic factors.

A positive coefficient of Δ^{ppm} (chemical shift) and σ and a negative coefficient of ΔpK_a in the equations suggest that the natriuresis (or diuresis) will
increase with a decrease in electronic density at the sulfamoyl group in sulfonamide derivatives.

The *in vitro* enzyme inhibition data were also found by Kakeya et al. [69]
to be significantly correlated with these electronic parameters, followed by

an improvement in the correlations with inclusion of π. The inhibition constants were measured at two different temperatures: 0.2 and 15°C. At both temperatures, highly significant correlations were obtained, for example with π and σ:

$$0.2°C: \quad \log(1/K_i) = 0.276\,\pi + 0.800\,\sigma + 0.413$$
$$n = 16, r = 0.965, s = 0.160 \tag{30}$$
$$15°C: \quad \log(1/K_i) = 0.223\,\pi + 0.839\,\sigma + 0.481$$
$$n = 16, r = 0.939, s = 0.212 \tag{31}$$

These correlations were obtained by Kakeya et al. with exclusion of ortho derivatives, but Lien et al. [71] used log P in place of π and obtained Equation (32) for all ortho, meta and para derivatives. Thus, the total lipophilicity of the molecule seems to absorb the steric effects of the ortho substituents. However, in a study on King and Burgen's data on the binding of sulfonamide to CA [72], Hansch et al. [73] observed, by deriving Equation (33), that not only the ortho substituents but also the bulky meta substituents can produce steric effects. These steric effects are accounted for by the two dummy parameters, I_1 and I_2, used in the equation with a value of 1 each for meta and ortho substituent, respectively, and zero for others. K here is a binding constant for the absorption of the compounds to human CA.

$$\log(1/K_i) = 0.259 \log P + 0.886\,\sigma + 5.314$$
$$n = 19, r = 0.923, s = 0.247 \tag{32}$$
$$\log K = 0.64\,(\pm 0.08)\log P + 1.55\,(\pm 0.38)\,\sigma - 2.07\,(\pm 0.22)\,I_1$$
$$- 3.28\,(\pm 0.23)\,I_2 + 6.94\,(\pm 0.18)$$
$$n = 29, r = 0.991, s = 0.204, F_{2,24} = 324 \tag{33}$$

$$0.2°C: \quad \log(1/K_i) = 3.069\,V_w - 0.096$$
$$n = 7, r = 0.958, s = 0.211 \tag{34}$$
$$15°C: \quad \log(1/K_i) = 2.741\,V_w + 0.038$$
$$n = 7, r = 0.902, s = 0.302 \tag{35}$$

Kumar et al. [74] analyzed the data of Kakeya et al. using only the van der Waals volume (V_w) and found that the activities of meta analogues at both temperatures were significantly correlated with V_w (Eqs. 34 and 35) but those of para analogues were not. This led Kumar et al. to suggest that meta substituent increases the binding affinity of the compound by involving itself in some secondary interaction with the receptor as shown in Figure 2. The primary interaction involves the sulfonamide group of the molecule and an active site of the enzyme that consists of Zn^{2+} with three ligands from the protein, all of which are histidyl residues [75–78]. The fourth ligand is either a water molecule or hydroxyl ion [79]. A good correlation between V_w and inhibition activity in the case of meta analogues suggests that the meta group comes in the vicinity of some amino acid residue near the primary binding site and interacts with it. Since the interaction depends on the molecular size, it may be of a van der Waals type.

Primary binding does involve the electronic character of the SO_2NH_2 group, which is influenced by the electronic nature of the substituents. Shinagawa and Shinagawa [80] made a Hückel molecular orbital (HMO) calculation on a series of sulfonamides studied by Krebs [81] and related CA inhibition activity with the formal charge Q^{NH} at the amide group position (Eq. 36). Several other QSAR studies [82–85] led to the same conclusion. However, Testa and Purcell [86] concluded in a QSAR study on King and Burgen's data [72] that the affinity constant of the sulfonamides for CA is massively structure-dependent, and depends only to a very limited extent on the partition properties of the ligand. The electronic characteristics of the substituents were not found by these authors to play any role, though their observations require further verification.

$$\log (1/C_{50}) = 11.2 \, Q_{NH} - 1.32$$
$$n = 22, \, r = 0.78 \tag{36}$$

3.3 Direct or peripheral vasodilators

Diazoxide (**11**) and its analogues, which have been discussed under peripheral α-antagonists, are treated as direct vasodilators, although their *in vitro* activity was measured as the ability of the compound to block the noradrenaline-induced contractile response of the rat aortic ring. In fact, the exact molecular mechanism by which clinically used diazoxide elicits its hypotensive activity is not yet fully known. However, Wohl et al. [60] have postulated

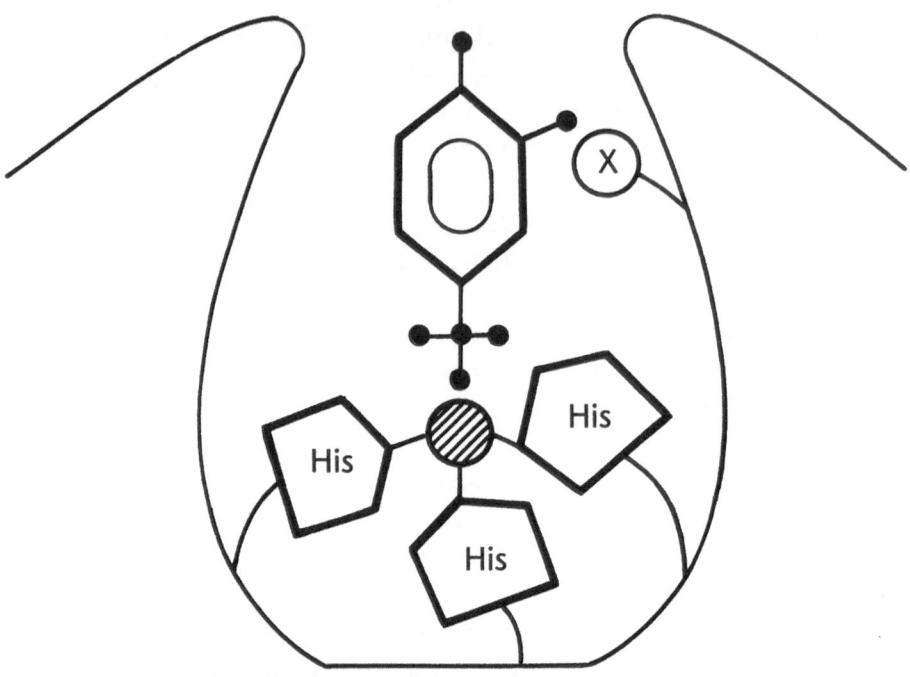

Fig. 2
Representation of binding of sulfonamids with carbonic anhydrase [74].

that diazoxide and its analogues probably act by occupying a receptor site at which Ca^{2+} is normally the operative stimulus in inducing arterial contraction. Accordingly, it was assumed that the molecule may have two strategically located electron-deficient regions that can substitute for Ca^{2+} at the receptor [87]. This picture was, however, not found to be compatible with the QSAR results of Topliss and Yudis (Eqs. 18–20), which suggest the importance of hydrophobic bonding at the regions of the drug molecule adjacent to the 6-, 7- and 3-positions. Therefore, Topliss and Yudis [59] conceived that the action of the drug may be indirect in that access of Ca^{2+} to its normal site may be prevented without direct action of the drug with this particular site. This prevention may be due to steric effects produced either directly by the drug or by induced receptor perturbation caused by the binding of the drug hydrophobically with the proximal sites.

19   **20**

$$\log (1/ED_{20}) = 0.28\,\pi - 0.24\,\pi^2 + 5.30$$
$$n = 12,\ r = 0.91,\ s \doteq 0.14 \tag{37}$$

The hypotensive activity of a series of **19** was also found to be correlated only with the hydrophobic constant (Eq. 37) [88]. But for a series of adenosine analogues (**20**) studied by Gangjee et al. [89], where R-substituents were varying sugar moieties, Bindal et al. [90] correlated vasodilator activity with Kier's first-order valence molecular connectivity index ($^1\chi^v$) and the van der Waals volume (V_w) as

$$\log (1/A) = 0.76\ ^1\chi^v + 22.03\ (1/^1\chi^v) + 2.98\ V_w - 11.08$$
$$n = 16,\ r = 0.77,\ s = 0.40 \tag{38}$$

Here A stands for the activity of the compound relative to adenosine. This correlation suggests the structural effect on the activity.

In an effort to develop antihypertensive agents with peripheral vasodilator activity, a fairly large series of 3-hydrazino-5-phenyl-1,2,4-triazines (**21**) were synthesized and evaluated for their activity in spontaneously hypertensive rat (SHR) by Heilman et al. [91]. But these authors failed in their attempts to correlate the antihypertensive activity of these compounds with any physicochemical parameters.

The vasodilating and antihypertensive activities have also been found to be associated with potassium channel activators, and many compounds of this class are under development for hypertension therapy [92], among which the cromakalim (**22**) is in the final stage of trials. Several studies on compounds structurally related to cromakalim [93–98] have shown that the presence of an electron-withdrawing group at the 6-position and of a *gem*-dialkyl group (preferably methyl) at the 2-position of benzopyran nucleus is essential for good biological activity. In a series of **23**, Almansa et al. [99]

21

22

23

found a rough parallelism existing between the portal vain relaxation activity (in rat) of the compounds and the electron-withdrawing ability of the 6-position substituents. Earlier studies [93–98] had also indicated that a five- or a six- membered cyclic amide ring at the 4-position would be equally beneficial and so would be a trans-hydroxyl group at the 3-position or a double bond between positions 3 and 4. A new beneficial modification of benzopyran ring by replacing pyran by a carbonyl group was envisaged by Almansa et al. [99].

For a set of structurally diverse potassium channel activators, the vasorelaxation activity (IC_{50}: the concentration causing 50% inhibition of spontaneous activity in rat portal vein) was shown to be significantly correlated with the receptor binding constant K_i (Eq. 39) [100]. A similar correlation has been recently obtained between the two by Atwal et al. [101] for a series of pinacidil (24) analogues (Eq. 40). Pinacidil is being tried as an antihypertensive agent.

$$\log (1/IC_{50}) = 0.88 (\pm 0.08) \log (1/K_i) + 1.04$$
$$n = 13, r = 0.96 \tag{39}$$
$$\log (1/IC_{50}) = 1.092 \log (1/K_i) + 0.035$$
$$n = 11, r = 0.84 \tag{40}$$

24

$$HS(CH_2)_n\overset{\overset{X}{|}}{C}H-R-COOH$$

25

3.4   ACE and renin inhibitors

The ACE inhibitors hold a great promise in the treatment of hypertension. Mercaptoacyl amino acids and analogues (**25**) have been widely studied for their ACE inhibition activity by the Ondetti group. For a series of 27 derivatives studied by these authors [102], Prabhakar and Gupta [103] correlated the inhibition activity with the hydrophobicity as

$$\log (1/IC_{50}) = 1.765 + 1.733 \log P - 0.244 (\log P)^2 + 0.831\ I_1 + 1.555\ I_2$$
$$n = 27, r = 0.915, s = 0.62, F_{4,22} = 28.31 \qquad (41)$$

where the indicator variable I_1 has been used with a value of 1 for the R moiety capable of forming a hydrogen bond with the receptor and I_2 with a value 1 for X = CH_3 in the S-configuration (above the plane). These authors performed QSAR studies on other types of ACE inhibitors also [103] but the results on them were not so encouraging. Several other qualitative and quantitative SARs are available on *in vitro* data of ACE inhibitors [104–108], but no SAR studies are available on *in vivo* data of these agents. *In vitro* binding studies have suggested that three requirements are essential for successful inhibition of ACE: (1) a functional group capable of binding to zinc at the active site of the enzyme, (2) a carbonyl oxygen to form the hydrogen bond with the receptor and (3) an ionizable C-terminal carboxylate moiety that can interact with a positively charged residue.

Like ACE inhibitors, renin inhibitors can also be exploited for hypertension therapy. However, little QSAR studies are available on their *in vivo* data. Only a few QSAR studies have been reported on *in vitro* enzyme inhibition data of some renin inhibitors. Gupta et al. [109] made a QSAR study of two series of peptide analogues of angiotensinogen (**26** and **27**) and for both series

26

Boc = (CH$_3$)$_3$C–O–CO
AA$_1$, AA$_2$ = amino acid residues
X = S, O, SO$_2$ or CH$_2$

27

R = varying alkyl/aryl groups
R$_1$ = Boc-like moiety
R$_2$ = varying alkyl groups

they found significant correlations between the potency of compounds against human renin and the connectivity index $^1\chi^v$ or the molecular weight as shown by Equations (42) and (43) for the series of **26** and by Equations (44) and (45) for the series of **27**.

$$\log (1/IC_{50}) = 0.394 \ (\pm 0.086) \ ^1\chi^v - 0.793 \ (\pm 0.346) \ D_1 - 0.564$$
$$(\pm 0.389) \ D_2 + 0.348$$
$$n = 31, \ r = 0.90, \ s = 0.34, \ F_{3,27} = 36.67 \tag{42}$$

$$\log (1/IC_{50}) = 1.410 \ (\pm 0.375) \ MW - 0.941 \ (\pm 0.320) \ D_1 - 0.575$$
$$(\pm 0.333) \ D_2 - 1.844$$
$$n = 31, \ r = 0.92, \ s = 0.31, \ F_{3,27} = 46.05 \tag{43}$$

$$\log (1/IC_{50}) = 0.233 \ (\pm 0.161) \ ^1\chi^v + 1.652 \ (\pm 0.514) \ D + 1.886$$
$$n = 20, \ r = 0.98, \ s = 0.28, \ F_{2,17} = 154.77 \tag{44}$$

$$\log (1/IC_{50}) = 0.752 \ (\pm 0.413) \ MW + 1.673 \ (\pm 0.415) \ D + 1.155$$
$$n = 20, \ r = 0.98, \ s = 0.26, \ F_{2,17} = 187.44 \tag{45}$$

In Equations (42) and (43), D_1 and D_2 are two dummy variables which have been used with a value of unity each for R = an aryl group and X = SO$_2$, respectively. The negative coefficients of these variables suggest that such moieties are not favourable for activity; otherwise, activity increases with an increase in the bulk of the molecule.

In Equations (44) and (45), the dummy parameter D was used with a value of unity for R$_2$ = c-hexylmethyl group. The positive coefficient of this parameter shows an additional positive effect of a cyclohexylmethyl group on the potency of the compound along with the bulk of the molecule. In neither series was the activity found to be correlated with hydrophobicity.

In a series of pepstatin analogues with the general formula A-X-Y-Sta-Ala-Sta-R, where A and R are protecting groups like Boc and OH, respectively, X and Y are amino acid residues and Sta stands for statine [(3S, 4S)-4-amino-3-hydroxy-6-methylheptanoic acid], Nisato et al. [110] performed a Free-Wilson analysis and reported, with a value of r = 0.979, that most favourable to the activity were the Y amino acid residues in the order: valine > cyclopentyl-glycine > norvaline > histidine. These authors also identified the crucial physicochemical parameters of Y that were important for the activity. They were the NMR chemical shift of the α-carbon, inductive effect and van der Waals radius-related steric parameter.

3.5 Miscellaneous

In the case of miscellaneous groups of antihypertensive agents, the inhibitors of various enzymes as mentioned in section 2.5, namely, cAMP phosphodiesterase, monoamine oxidase, tyrosine kinase and dopamine-β-hydroxylase have been studied mostly for their *in vitro* enzyme inhibition activity and little for their any *in vivo* activity. Hence, QSARs on their *in vivo* data are scarcely available. QSARs on their *in vitro* data are, however, more or less available [9], but since in no case sufficient reports are available to establish that *in vitro* enzyme binding data have significant bearing on antihypertensive effects, any discussion on QSARs of only *in vitro* data would be totally irrelevant.

The platelet aggregation inhibition activity of a series of dihydropyridazinones (28) was found to be coupled with antihypertensive action [111]. However, while platelet aggregation activity was shown to be satisfactorily correlated with the V_w of the R^3NH group (Eq. 46), antihypertensive activity was found to have slightly poorer correlation (Eq. 47) [112]. The indicator

28

variables I_1 and I_2 were used with a value of unity each for R_1- and R_2-substituents being CH_3, respectively. Both equations show an optimum effect of the size of the R^3NH, but if there is a CH_3 group at the R^1-position, it will lead to a decrease in activity, while the same at the R^2-position will enhance activity. I_1 does not appear in Equation (47) because all the compounds for which antihypertensive activities were available had R^1 = H. RA in both equations refers to relative activity based on acetylsalicylic acid.

$$\log (RA)_{aggr} = 4.245\ V_w - 3.262\ (V_w)^2 - 1.102\ I_1 + 0.900\ I_2 + 1.225$$
$$n = 32,\ r = 0.857,\ s = 0.47 \tag{46}$$
$$\log (RA)_{antihyp} = 3.771\ V_w - 3.818\ (V_w)^2 + 0.578\ I_2 - 0.539$$
$$n = 20,\ r = 0.724,\ s = 0.42 \tag{47}$$

4 Concluding remarks

Since the inception of the QSAR studies, the design and development of drugs have been greatly facilitated and it became easier to understand even the most complicated mechanisms in the actions of several drugs. QSAR studies have led to excellent results in the design of antihypertensives. A number of successful predictions have been made on clonidine-like drugs, and a potent diuretic, muzolimine, owes its development greatly to only QSAR technologies.

In the case of centrally acting clonidine-like drugs, the present review has suggested that their activity will be primarily governed by the lipophilic and steric properties of the molecules and at the receptor level the molecules may form the charge-transfer complexes. Somewhat similar suggestions have emerged for other kinds of centrally acting antihypertensives also, e.g. piperazines. But for the latter, the conformational properties of the molecules could also appear to play effective roles in their actions.

For peripherally acting diazoxide-like α-antagonists, however, the prime role was found to be of only lipophilicity (Eqs. 18–20), but in the case of diuretics it appeared to be of little importance. Instead, the electronic characters of molecules or substituents emerged to be the major factors governing the activity of diuretics (Eqs. 21–29). However, for *in vitro* enzyme inhibition activity of carbonic anhydrase inhibitors, which could also act as diuretics, both lipophilicity and electronic properties could be found important (Eqs. 30–33) and even the molecular size of the substituents appeared to control the inhibition potency (Eqs. 34 and 35).

For direct vasodilators also, both lipophilic and electronic properties appear to be important. Similarly, for ACE inhibitors, too, their enzyme inhibition potency is indicated, in general, to depend upon both lipophilic and electronic characters of the molecules, but for renin inhibitors the activity seems to depend more upon the structural properties of the molecules than upon the physicochemical properties. Among the miscellaneous groups of antihypertensive agents, the platelet aggregation inhibitors are found to base their activity on the molecular size of the compounds.

As to the final conclusion, one would find that the fundamental property of the molecules that is overwhelmingly involved in the majority of antihypertensive agents is lipophilicity. The greatest contribution of QSAR study is that it has provided a systematic and fairly complete understanding in quantitative terms of the role of lipophilicity in drug action. Lipophilicity is not only related to the absorption or distribution phenomena but also to the interactions with the receptors. The critical role of lipophilicity in *in vitro* activity has provided valuable information about receptor sites. Receptors may have both hydrophobic (lipophilic) and electronic sites, but the extent of hydrophobic or electronic interaction of drug molecules with them will depend upon the orientation and accessibility of these sites to the hydrophobic and electronic fragments of the drug molecules. The steric fit of these fragments into the active sites of the receptor also influences the interactions.

Acknowledgement

The assistance rendered in the preparation of the manuscript by one of my students, M. Suresh Babu, is gratefully acknowledged.

References

1   A.C. Guyton, T.G. Coleman, A.W. Cowley, R.D. Manning, Jr., R.A. Norman, Jr. and J.D. Ferguson: Circ. Res. 35, 159 (1974).
2   A.C. Guyton, D.B. Young, J.W. DeClue, J.D. Ferguson, R.E. McCaa, A.Gevise, N.C. Trippado and J.E. Hall, in: G. Berglund, L.Hansson and L. Werkö (eds.): Pathophysiology and Management of Arterial Hypertension, Astra Pharmaceuticals A.B., Sweden 1975, p. 78.

3   B. Folkow, M. Hallbäck, Y. Lundgren, R. Sivertsson and L. Weiss: Circ. Res. *32* (Suppl. I), I-2 (1973).

4   M.J. Peach: Physiol. Rev. *57*, 313 (1977).

5   M.A. Ondetti and D.W. Kushman : J. Med. Chem. *24*, 355 (1981).

6   E.A. Murphy: Circ. Res. *32/33* (Suppl. I), I-129 (1973).

7   M. Thyes, H.D. Lehman, J. Gries, H. Konig, R. Kretzschmar, J. Kunze, R. Lebkücher and D. Lenke: J. Med. Chem. *26*, 800 (1983).

8   S.P. Gupta, P. Singh and M.C. Bindal: Chem. Rev. *83*, 633 (1983).

9   S.P. Gupta: Chem. Rev. *87*, 1183 (1987).

10   S.P. Gupta: Chem. Rev. *89*, 1765 (1989).

11   S.P. Gupta: Chem. Rev. *91*, 1109 (1991).

12   S.P. Gupta: Chem. Rev. *94*, 1507 (1994).

13   S.P. Gupta: Prog. Drug Res. *45*, 67 (1995).

14   S.P. Gupta: Current Pharm. Des. *4*, 455 (1998).

15   S.P. Gupta: Chem. Rev., communicated.

16   S.P. Gupta, H. Gao, R. Garg, M.S. Babu and C. Hansch: Chem. Rev., communicated.

17   P.B.M.W.M. Timmermans and P.A.van Zwieten: Eur. J. Pharmacol. *47*, 391 (1977).

18   P.B.M.W.M. Timmermans, A. Brands and P.A. van Zwieten: Naunyn Schmiedebergs Arch. Pharmacol. *300*, 217 (1977).

19   P.B.M.W.M. Timmermans and P.A. van Zwieten: J. Med. Chem. *20*, 1636 (1977).

20   P.A. van Zwieten and P.B.M.W.M. Timmermans: Trends Pharmacol. Sci. *1*, 39 (1979).

21   P.A. van Zwieten: Br. J. Clin. Pharmacol. *10*, 135 (1980).

22   P.B.M.W.M. Timmermans: Proc. Pharmacol. *3*, 25 (1980).

23   W. Hoefke, W. Kobinger and A. Walland: Arzneim.-Forsch. *25*, 786 (1975).

24   A. Walland and W. Hoefke: Naunyn Schmiedebergs Arch. Pharmacol. *282*, R104 (1974).

25   P.B.M.W.M.Timmermans and P.A.van Zwieten: Eur. J. Pharmacol. *45*, 229 (1977).

26   P.B.M.W.M. Timmermans, A. De Jonge, J.C.A. van Meel, F.P. Slothorst-Grisdijk, E. Lam and P.A. van Zwieten: J. Med. Chem. *24*, 502 (1981).

27   B. Belleau, in: K.J. Burnings (ed.): Proceedings of the First International Pharmacological Meeting, Stockholm 1961, Vol. 7, Pergamon Press, Oxford 1963, p. 75.

28   B. Bellaeu: Ann. NY Acad. Sci. *139*, 580 (1967).

29   R.B. Barlow: Introduction to Chemical Pharmacology, 2nd ed., John Wiley, New York 1963.

30   B. Rouot, G. Leclerc, C.-G. Wermuth, F. Miesch and J. Schwartz: J. Med. Chem. *19*, 1049 (1976).

31   B. Rouot, G. Leclerc, C.-G. Wermuth, F. Miesch and J. Schwartz: J. Pharmacol. *8*, 95 (1977).

32   P.A. van Zwieten and P.B.M.W.M. Timmermans: Adv. Drug Res. *13*, 209 (1984).

33   W. Kobinger and L. Pichler: Naunyn Schmiedebergs Arch. Pharmacol. *315*, 21 (1980).

34   A. De Jonge, F.P. Slothorst-Grisdijk and P.B.M.W.M. Timmermans: Eur. J. Pharmacol. *71*, 411 (1981).

35   A. De Jonge, P.B.M.W.M. Timmermans and P.A. van Zwieten: J. Pharmacol. Exp. Ther. *222*, 705 (1982).

36   P.B.M.W.M. Timmermans, A. De Jonge, M.J.M.C. Thoolen, B. Wilffert, H. Batink and P.A. van Zwieten: J. Med. Chem. *27*, 495 (1984).

37   J.R. Huff, J.J. Baldwin, S. DeSolms, J.P. Guare, Jr., C.A. Hunt, W.C. Randall, W.S. Sanders, S.J. Smith, J.P. Vacca and M.M. Zrada: J. Med. Chem. *31*, 641 (1988).

38   J.D. Lee and E.J. Lien: Acta Pharm. Jugosl. *36*, 211 (1986).

39   B. Pullman, J.L. Coubeils, P. Courriére and J.P. Gervois: J. Med. Chem. *15*, 17 (1972).

40   J.L. Coubelis, P. Courriére and B. Pullman: J. Med. Chem. *15*, 453 (1972).

41   C.-G. Wermuth, J. Schwartz, G. Leclerc, J.P. Garnier and B. Rouot: Clin. Ther. *1*, 115 (1973).

42   W. Hoefke: ACS Symp. Ser. No. *27*, 27 (1976).

43   C.M. Meerman-van Benthem, K. van der Meer, J.J.C. Mulder, P.B.M.W.M. Timmermans and P.A. van Zwieten: Mol. Pharmacol. *11*, 667 (1975).

44   P.B.M.W.M. Timmermans, P.A. van Zwieten, C.M. Meerman-van Benthem, K. van der Meer and J.J.C. Mulder: Arzneim.-Forsch. *27*, 2266 (1977).

45   A. Murti, K. Bhandari, S. Ram, Y.S. Prabhakar, A.K. Saxena, P.C. Jain, A.K. Gulati, R.C. Srimal, B.N. Dhawan, S. Nityanand and N. Anand: Indian J. Chem. *28B*, 934 (1989).

46   A.K. Saxena, J. Rao, R.C. Srimal, E. Audry and A. Karpy: Indian J. Chem. *32B*, 1249, (1993).

47   N. Sinha, S. Jain, M.P. Dubey, A.K. Saxena and N. Anand: Indian J. Chem. *35B*, 213 (1996).

48   E. Audry, J.P. Dubost, Ph. Dallet, M.H. Langlois and J.C. Colleter: Eur. J. Med. Chem. *24*, 155 (1989).

49   R.M. Graham, H.F. Oates, L.M. Stoker and G.S. Stoker: J. Pharmacol. Exp. Ther. *201*, 747 (1977).

50   J.C. McGrath: Biochem. Pharmacol. *31*, 467 (1982)

51   F. Gross: Br. J. Clin. Pharmacol. *13* (Suppl. 1), 5 (1982).

52   G. Winters, A. Sala, D. Barone and E. Baldoli: J. Med. Chem. *28*, 934 (1985).

53   P. Singh and R.C. Sharma: Quant. Struct.-Act. Relat. *9*, 29 (1990).

54   A.A. Rubin, F.E. Roth, M.M. Winbury, J.G. Topliss, M.H. Sherlock, N. Sperber and J. Block: Science *133*, 2067 (1961).

55   J.G. Topliss, M.H. Sherlock, H. Reimann, L.M. Konzelman, E.P. Shapiro, B.W. Petterson, H. Schneider and N. Sperber: J. Med. Chem. *6*, 122 (1963).

56   J.G. Topliss, L.M. Konzelman, E.P. Shapiro, N. Sperber and F.E. Roth: J. Med. Chem. 7, 269 (1964).

57   F.C. Novello, S.C. Bell, E.L.A. Abrams, C. Ziegler and J.M. Sprague: J. Org. chem. *25*, 970 (1960).

58   A. J. Wohl: Mol. Pharmacol. *6*, 189 (1970).

59   J.G. Topliss and M.D. Yudis: J. Med. Chem. *15*, 394 (1972).

60   A.J. Wohl, L.M. Hausler and F.E. Roth: J. Pharmacol. Exp. Ther. *158*, 531 (1967).

61   A.A. Robin, F.E. Roth, R.M. Taylor and H. Rosenkilde: J. Pharmacol. Exp. Ther. *136*, 344 (1962).

62   H. Horstmann, E. Moller, E. Wehinger and K. Meng: ACS Symp. Ser. No. *83*, 125 (1978).

63   E. Mizuta, K. Nishikawa, K. Omura and Y.Oka: Chem. Pharm. Bull. *24*, 2078 (1976).

64   P. Singh and S.P. Gupta: Indian J. Med. Res. *69*, 804 (1979).

65   M.C. Bindal, Y.M. Chopra, P.Singh and S.P. Gupta: Indian J. Pharm. Sci. *43*, 47 (1981).

66   G. Satzinger: Arzneim.-Forsch. *27*, 1742 (1977).

67   N. Kakeya, M. Aoki, A. Kamada and N. Yata: Chem. Pharm. Bull. *17*, 1010 (1969).

68   N. Kakeya, N. Yata, A. Kamada and M. Aoki: Chem. Pharm. Bull. *17*, 2000 (1969).

69   N. Kakeya, N. Yata, A. Kamada and M. Aoki: Chem. Pharm. Bull. *17*, 2558 (1969).

70   N. Kakeya, N. Yata, A. Kamada and M. Aoki: Chem. Pharm. Bull. *18*, 191 (1970).

71   E.J. Lien, M. Hussain and G.L. Tong: J. Pharm. Sci. *59*, 865 (1970).

72   R.W. King and A.S. Burgen: Proc. Roy. Soc. London B *193*, 107 (1976).

73   C. Hansch, J. McClarin and R. Langridge: Mol. Pharmacol. *27*, 493 (1985).

74   K. Kumar, M.C. Bindal, P. Singh and S.P. Gupta: Int. J. Quantum Chem. *20*, 123 (1981).

75   K.K. Kannan, in: R. Srinivasan (ed.): Biomolecular Structure, Conformation, Function and Evaluation, Vol. 1, Pergamon Press, Oxford, New York 1980, p. 165.

76   S. Lindskog, L.E. Henderson, K.K. Kannan, A. Liljas, P.O. Nyman and B. Strandberg, in: P.D. Boyer (ed.): The Enzymes, 3rd ed., Vol. 5, Academic Press, New York 1971, p. 587.

77   K.K. Kannan, I. Waara, B. Notstrand, S. Lovgren, A. Borell, K. Fridborg and M. Petef, in: G.C.K. Roberts (ed.): Drug Action at the Molecular Level, University Park Press, Baltimore 1977, p. 73.

78   J.E. Coleman: Annu. Rev. Pharmacol. Toxicol. *15*, 221 (1975).

79   A. Vedani and F.E. Meyer, Jr.: J. Pharm. Sci. *73*, 352 (1984).

80   Y. Shinagawa and Y. Shinagawa: Int. J. Quantum Chem., Quantum Biol. Symp. No. *1*, 169 (1974).

81   H.A. Krebs: Biochem. J. *43*, 525 (1984).

82   S.N. Subbarao and P.Bray: J. Med. Chem. *22*, 111 (1979).

83   P.G. De Benedetti, M.C. Menziani and C. Frassineti: Quant. Struct.-Act. Relat. *4*, 23 (1985).

84   P.G. De Benedetti, M. C. Menziani, M. Cocchi and C. Frassineti: Quant. Struct.-Act. Relat. *6*, 51 (1987).

85   M.C. Menziani, P.G. De Bendetti, F. Gago and W.G. Richards: J. Med. Chem. *32*, 951 (1989).

86   B. Testa and W.P. Purcell: Eur. J. Med. Chem. *13*, 509 (1978).

87   A.J. Wohl: Mol. Pharmacol. *6*, 195 (1970).

88   G. Leclerc, C.-G. Wermuth, F. Miesch and J. Schwartz: Eur. J. Med. Chem. 11, 107 (1976).

89   A. Gangjee, H.P.C. Hogencamp and J.M. Kitzen: J. Pharm. Sci. *67*, 121 (1978).

90   M.C. Bindal, P. Singh, R.P. Bhatnagar and S.P. Gupta: Arzeim.-Forsch. *30*, 924 (1980).

91   W.P. Heilman, R.D. Heilman, J.A. Scozzie, R.J. Wayner, J.M. Gullo and Z.S. Ariyan: J. Med. Chem. *22*, 671 (1979).

92   G. Edwards and A.H. Weston: Trends Pharm. Sci. *11*, 417 (1990).

93   D.G. Smith: J. Chem. Soc., Perkin Trans. *1*, 3187 (1990).

94   G. Burrel, F. Cassidy, J.M. Evans, D. Lightowler and G. Stemp: J. Med. Chem. *33*, 3023 (1990).

95   M.R. Attwood: Current Drugs: Potassium Channel Modulators KCK-B 39 (1991).

96   P.J. Sanfilippo, J.J. McNally, J.B. Press, L.J. Fitzpatrick, M. Urbanski, L.J. Katz, E. Giardino, R. Falotico and J. Salata: J. Med. Chem. *35*, 4425 (1992).

97   V.A. Ashwood, F. Cassidy, J.M. Evans, S. Gagliardi and G. Stemp: J. Med. Chem. *34*, 3261 (1991).

98   D.R. Buckle, D.S. Eggleston, C.S.V. Houge-Frydrych, I. Pinto, S.A. Readshaw, D.G. Smith and R.A.B. Webster: J. Chem. Soc., Perkin Trans. *1*, 2763 (1991).

99   C. Almansa, L.A. Gomez, F.L. Cavalcanti, R. Rodriguez, E. Carceller, J. Bartrol, J. Garcia-Rafanell and J. Forn: J. Med. Chem. *36*, 2121 (1993).

100   P.W. Manley, U. Quast, H. Andres and K. Bray: J. Med. Chem. *36*, 2004 (1993).

101   K.S. Atwal, G.J. Grover, N.J. Lodge, D.E. Normandin, S.C. Traeger, P.G. Sleph, R.B. Cohen, C.C. Bryson and K.E.J. Dickinson: J. Med. Chem. *41*, 271 (1998).

102   M.E. Condon, E.W. Petrillo, Jr., D.E. Ryono, J.A. Reid, R. Neubeck, M. Puar, J.E. Heikes. E.F. Sabo, K.E. Losee, D.W. Kushman and M.A. Ondetti: J. Med. Chem. *25*, 250 (1982).

103   Y.S. Prabhakar and S.P. Gupta: Indian J. Biochem. Biophys. *22*, 318 (1985).

104   W.W. Petrillo, N.C. Trippodo and J.M. DeForrest: Annu. Rep. Med. Chem. *25*, 51 (1990).

105   D.G. Hangauer, in: T.J. Perun and C.L. Propst (eds.): Computer-Aided Drug Design: Methods and Applications, Marcel Dekker, New York 1989, p. 253.

106   M.R. Saunders, M.S. Tute and G.A. Web: J. Comput.-Aided Mol. Des. *1*, 133 (1987).

107   D. Mayer, C.B. Naylor, I. Motoc and G.R. Marshall: J. Comput.-Aided Mol. Des. *1*, 3 (1987).

108   C.L. Waller and G.R. Marshall: J. Med. Chem. *36*, 2390 (1993).

109   S.P. Gupta, J.K. Gupta, A.N. Nagappa, V. Jagannathan and D. Gangwal: Drug Des. Deliv. *5*, 73 (1989).

110   D. Nisato, J. Wagnon, G. Callet, D. Mettefeu, J.-L. Assens, C. Plouzane, B. Tonnerre, V. Pliska and J.-L. Fauchère: J. Med. Chem. *30*, 2287 (1987).

111   M. Thyes, H.D. Lehman, J. Gries, H. Konig, R. Kretzschmar, J. Kunze, R. Lebkucher and D. Lenke: J. Med. Chem. *26*, 800 (1983).

112   S.P. Gupta, D.G. Shewade, C. Garg, A. Handa and Y.S. Prabhakar: Indian J. Biochem. Biophys. *22*, 122 (1985).

Progress in Drug Research, Vol. 53 (E. Jucker, Ed.)
©1999 Birkhäuser Verlag, Basel (Switzerland)

Combinatorial chemistry: Polymer supported synthesis of peptide and non-peptide libraries

Bijoy Kundu, Sanjay K. Khare and Shiva K. Rastogi

Division of Medicinal Chemistry, Central Drug Research Institute, Lucknow 226001, India

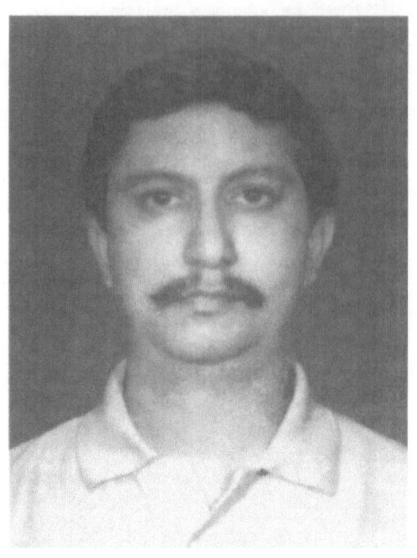

Bijoy Kundu

was born in India in 1955, studied chemistry at the University of Gorakhpur and in 1983 obtained his doctorate from Kanpur University, India. He spent four years in the United States as a postdoctoral fellow, first at the College of Staten island (CUNY) from 1982–83, and then at the University of Illinois, Urbana-Champaign from 1989–1991. In 1997, he received a WHO research grant and went on to work in the area of combinatorial chemistry at the University of Tubingen, Germany. He has been working as a scientist at Central Drug Research Institute, Lucknow, India since 1985. His research deals with the design and synthesis of oligopeptides and small organic molecules of biological interest.

Sanjay K. Khare

was born in Gorakhpur, India, in 1969. He received his masters degree in chemistry from the University of Gorakhpur in 1991, and a Ph.D. from the University of Faizabad under supervision of Dr. B. Kundu.

Shiva K. Rastogi

was born in 1975 in Lucknow, India. He received his masters degree in chemistry from Lucknow University and is currently in the first year of his Ph.D. programme under supervision of Dr. B. Kundu.

Summary

In recent years, combinatorial chemistry has emerged as a powerful tool for accelerating drug discovery. While industry is rapidly embracing the technology, researchers continue to develop novel library methods including resins, linkers, tagging and deconvolution techniques. Newer strategies involving computer-customized combinatorial libraries offer enormous potential for the design of more "focused" and "smart" chemical libraries with maximal diversity. In addition, miniaturized systems for synthesizing chemical libraries are also being developed, which has made it possible to carry out reactions at submicroliter volumes.

Contents

Bijoy Kundu, Sanjay K. Khare and Shiva K. Rastogi

Keywords

Combinatorial libraries, solid phase resin, linkers, peptides, small organic molecules, coding, deconvolution

Glossary of abbreviations

GC, gas chromatography; ESMS, electrospray mass spectrometry; ELISA, enzyme linked immunoadsorbent assay; HPLC, high pressure liquid chromatography; TG, tentagel resin; PyBrOP, bromo-tris-pyrrolidino-phsosphonium hexafluorophosphate; DCR, divide couple and recombine; TFA, trifluoroacetic acid; NK, neurokinin

1   Introduction

High-speed combinatorial synthesis of peptides and small organic molecules using solid phase chemistry is emerging as a powerful tool in the drug discovery process. Compared to traditional drug discovery approach which requires many days of work to synthesise and analyse a single new compound, combinatorial chemistry can produce and screen one million compounds over a period of weeks for the discovery of novel drug entities against various disease targets. The continuous development of high throughput bioassay screening formats coupled with human genomics as a potential source of new biological targets [1] has created an acute need for a large number of structurally diverse molecules. The practical application of combinatorial chemistry to drug discovery is expected to fulfil this need, and hopefully in turn reverse the problem by creating a demand for more efficient screening strategies.

Thus, at a time when the pharmaceutical market has slowed and average research and development expenditures have accelerated, combinatorial chemistry coupled with high throughput screening (HTS) provides a cheaper and faster way to discover drugs. This is evident by world-wide acceptance of this new technology by various pharmaceutical companies. Every company now has some aspect of this in-house to the extent that combinatorial chemistry is becoming primarily a commercial, as opposed to an academic, endeavour.

2   Historical perspective

Historically combinatorial chemistry began with the libraries of linear, oligomeric peptides whose synthesis was based on the reliable amide bond forming solid phase chemistry pioneered by Merrifield in the 1960s. In 1980s Geysen et al. were the first to synthesise a limited array of peptides on polyethylene or polypropylene pins [2], and later Houghten et al. [3] developed a technique for creating peptide libraries in tiny mesh tea bags by solid phase parallel synthesis. Subsequently, in the 1990s three groups independently reported methods to divide, couple and recombine [4], portioning-mixing [5] and split synthesis [6] for preparing libraries of peptides based on combinatorial concept. The introduction of combinatorial libraries made up of millions of individual peptide sequences led to a revolution in drug discovery and basic research involving peptides. In fact, many laboratories have found it easy to generate impressive libraries comprising 10^5 or more compounds by capitalising on the principles of combinatorial mixture synthesis. The most widely used technique for mixture synthesis is the split/combine method which assures that each component of the mixture is present in approximately equimolar concentration. But despite some acknowledged success, the outcome of screening these libraries has often been less successful than hoped for.

Thus, initial enthusiasm for high order mixtures has now largely waned and most laboratories are preparing a mixture of not more than 10–40 compounds per mixture or libraries of single compounds by parallel synthesis. While both methods have advantages and disadvantages, when employed in concert they provide the medicinal chemist with powerful tools in lead discovery and optimisation. The structures of the bound ligands are determined either through an iterative or recursive deconvolution strategy or through the use of encoded libraries.

Though the initial success with combinatorial peptide libraries had been very encouraging as it led to the identification of several interesting "hits", their inherent limitation as effective therapeutic agents shifted interest from amide bond formation to small organic molecules that are more attractive as pharmaceutical leads. To achieve this new solid phase organic reactions are being explored vigorously with several new publications on new resins, linkers, chemical libraries, purification and analytical techniques and encoded libraries etc. This review deals with the various resins used for solid support, new linkage strategies, synthesis of chemical libraries, some issues pertaining to solid phase organic reactions, analytical techniques and miniaturised system for synthesis.

3   Solid supports and linkers

The ability to synthesise compounds on an inert polymeric resin bead, to force a reaction to completion by the addition of excess reagents and monomers, and to then remove all the unwanted material by a suitable filtration and wash, forms the core of most library synthesis. However, for the successes of organic synthesis on solid support, the correct choice of supports as well as bound anchors is of utmost importance. Pioneering work by Merrifield and others in peptide synthesis has made 1% cross-linked polystyrene the standard support for solid phase organic reaction. However, synthesis of small organic molecules necessitated the search for solid supports which are compatible with a large number of different chemical reactions so as to get a large variety of structurally diverse compounds. This is in contrast to standard solid phase peptide synthesis where one is dealing with a set number of reaction types. The earliest form of polystyrene resin being completely hydrophobic in nature severely limits synthetic access to the exposed end of a growing chain hence alternative conditions have been explored to obviate these effects.

Different solid supports were then developed which exhibited less variation when exposed to various polar and/or aqueous solvents. The various solid supports developed recently have been summarised in Table 1. For routine solid phase organic synthesis polystyrene and tentagel (TG) resins have been one of the most widely used solid supports. Both resins are robust and have been found to be compatible with a wide range of reaction conditions. TG resins are particularly recommended for use with the one bead/one com-

Table 1.
Various solid supports used in organic synthesis

Name of solid support	Composition	Loading capacity	Ref.
Kieselguhr-polyacrylamide composite	Polyacrylamide gel trapped in the porous structure of Kieselguhr	0.1–0.2 mmol amine/g	7
Polystyrene-polyacrylamide composite	10–50% cross-linked polystyrene containing covalently or noncovalently attached polyacrylamide	0.1–0.2 mmol amine/g	8
Tentagel (Rapp Polymere)	Ethylene oxide polymerised onto a primary alcohol located on the cross-linked polystyrene	0.2–0.3 mmol amine/g	9, 10
PEG-PS (perspective)	Amino terminal of PEG chain linked by amide bond to 1% cross-linked polystyrene	0.2–0.3 mmol amine/g	11
Polyethylene glycol-polyacrylamide composite (PEGA)	comprises N,N'-dimethyl-acrylamide, bis-2-acrylamido-prop-1-yl-PEG and sarcosine ethyl ester	0.4-0.8 mmol amine/g	12
Controlled pore glass (CPG)	Highly porous form of nearly pure silica having pore diameter in the range of 40–2500 Å	0.06-0.17 mmol amine/g	13
Kieselguhr (Novasyn)	Silica based support containing alumina	0.05–0.13 mmol amine/g	14
Polyethylene based support composite	Polystyrene-polyethylene	1 mmol/g	15
Cellulose supports	Paper sheets and cotton	0.5–0.6 mmol/cm^2	16
Branched support	Lysine branched Tentagel with high loading capacity	0.76 mmol amine/g	17
Branched support	"High-load" PEG-PS	0.3–0.5 mmol/g	18
Branched support	Argo-gel-two PEG chains branching from single carbon attachment point	0.5 mmol amine/g	19
Carboxylated polystyrene support	Derivatised cross-linked polystyrene	2–3 mmol COOH/g	20
Poly[N-[2-(4-hydroxy-phenyl)ethyl]acryl-amide] support	Ultra high loading	5.0 mmol hydroxyl/g	21

pound approach. The beads have a narrow size distribution and readily swell in water, facilitating biological assay in aqueous system. In addition, these supports also assist in the monitoring of solid phase organic reaction using gel-phase carbon and proton NMR.

Anchors that covalently link the substrate to the resin beads are one of the most decisive factors with regard to the design of combinatorial library. The anchor must be stable to all of the reagents used during synthesis and should be cleavable under mild conditions without damaging the final products. Additionally, anchors should be also able to reveal greater range of functionality after the cleavage step. This is in contrast to solid phase peptide synthesis where release of carboxylic acid or carboxamide functionality after the cleavage step is well served by a range linking groups. Several suitable and most widely used anchors have been summarized in Table 2.

4   Combinatorial synthesis of compounds on solid phase

Progress in the fields of biotechnology, molecular biology, robot techniques and automation have led to the development of new screening assays which are capable of testing a series of substances for receptor binding and biological activities in the cell test system in a remarkably short time. Therefore the usual methods of synthesis are insufficient to meet the demand for new compounds. Combinatorial chemistry on solid phase provides an alternative which uses a new type of fully automated multiple reactors for the synthesis of libraries within a short time. Various techniques used for the synthesis of chemical libraries have been summarized below.

4.1   Split and mix method

One of the most widely used methods for generating chemical libraries is the divide, couple and recombine technique pioneered by Furka [5]. The method has been described below with the solid phase synthesis of a 27 compound trimer library as an example: the resin is first divided into three equal portions and is then allowed to react individually with first components. After

Table 2.
Anchors commonly used for immobilization of chemical compounds on solid support

Structure of the anchor	Description, cleavage conditions, utility	Ref.
	• R=H, Wang linker; 95% TFA • R=OMe, Sarsin linker; 1% TFA • Immobolization of carboxylic acids	22, 23
	• R=H, tritylchloride anchor; weak acid • R=Cl, 2-chlorotritylchloride anchor; weak acids (AcOH, TFE) • Immobolization of nucleophilic compounds	24
	• PAM anchor • HF, TFMSA • Immobilization of carboxylic acids	25
	• X=OH, Rink acid anchor, X=NH-Fmoc, Rink amide anchor • TFA-DCM • Immobilization of carboxylic acids, cleavage yields amides	26
	• Benzhydrylamine (BHA) anchor • TFMSA • Immobilization of carboxylic acids, cleavage yields amides	27
	• Sieber amide anchor • TFA in DCM • Immobilization of carboxylic acids, cleavage yields amides	28
	• DBU • Piperidine • Immobilization of carboxylic acids	29

Table 2 (continued)

Structure of the anchor	Description, cleavage conditions, utility	Ref.
	• Cleavage with NaOH • Coupling of alcohols or amines by irreversible coupling	30
	• Silicon based linkers • Cleavage with Bu4NF • Immobilization of carboxylic acids	31
	• Photolysis (h$\sqrt{}$ = 350 nm) RT, 72 h • Stable in 50% TFA and labile in hydrazine hydrate • Immobilization of carboxylic acids	32
	• X = halogen, OH, NH_2 • Photolysis (h$\sqrt{}$ = 350 nm) under inert atmosphere • Immobilization of carboxylic acids	33
	• Hydroxyethyl linker • Stable to both TFA and piperidine • Immobilisation of carboxylic acids	34
	• Photolysis (h$\sqrt{}$ = 350 nm) • Labile in piperidine/DMF • Immobilization of carboxylic acids	35
	• Kenner's safety catch linker • Nucleophile mediated cleavage • Immbolisation of carboxylic acids	36
	• Trichloroacetamide activated Wang resin • LiOBn in THF, RT, 2 h • Formation of resin bound carboxylic, esters and thioesters	38

Table 2 (continued)

Structure of the anchor	Description, cleavage conditions, utility	Ref.
	• "Clean-break" indole based linker • TFA-DCM, 4 h, RT • Immobilization of N containing compounds, yields secondary amides, ureas and sulfonamides	39
	• Imidazolide carbamates • TFA-^{i}Pr$_3$SiH-DCM • Generation of alkyl-acyl- and arylguanidines as an attachment point in SPOS	40
	• Weinreb amides, stable under acidic and basic conditions • Cleavage yields aldehydes and ketones	41
	• Safety catch peptide resin linkage based on glycolic acid anchor • 10 mM NaOH • Immobilization of carboxylic acids	42
	• Multireleasable linkers based on combination of two molecules of iminodiacetic acid • Yields peptied molecules in two equimolar portions in two distinct steps	43
	• Activated diazo linkers • TFA-water, RT, 20 min • Chemoselective immobilization of functionlisation carboxylic acids	44
	• Phosgenated p-nitrophenyl (Polystyrene) ketoxime or resin • Thermolytic cleavage • Immobilization of amines	45

Table 2 (continued)

Structure of the anchor	Description, cleavage conditions, utility	Ref.
	• Diversifiable thiophenoxy carbonyl linker • Amine, Et₃N, THF, acetonitrile 60°C, 24–72 h • Immobilization of primary amines and secondary amines , yields urea libraries	46
	• 9-phenylfluoren-9-yl based linkers • TFA-DCM/MeOH (9:1) • Immobilization of nucleophiles	47
	• 9-phenylfluoren-9-yl acetic acid linker • TFA, overnight • Immobilization of nitrogen and oxygen nucleophiles	48
	• Phthalimide based linker • Hydrazine induced cleavage • Immobilization of primary alcohols via Mitsonobu reaction	49
	• Sulfonamide functional group as an anchor • TFA in DCM, 15 min • Sufficiently stable to a variety of reactions used in SPOS, yields functionalised sulfonamide	50
	• Carbamate linker • Based catalysed cyclisation/cleavage strategy • Immobilization of amines	51
	• Dihydropyran functionalised resin • 95% TFA-water, 20 min • Immobilization of alcohols	52

completion of the reactions and washings to remove excess reagents, the individual resins are thoroughly mixed and divided equally into three portions. Subsequently, with reaction with the next set of building blocks, one obtains nine different compounds after two steps. The whole process is then repeated to finally get three mixtures each consisting of nine compounds. Thus, depending on the number of individual blocks and synthetic steps, thousands of different compounds can be synthesized in each reaction vessel, which can then be screened either as polymer-bound products or as polymer free libraries. Identification and structural elucidation of the most active compounds from combinatorial libraries relies on deconvoluting the active mixtures through further synthesis and screening.

4.2 Premix method

Mixture positions have been incorporated by coupling mixtures of side chain protected Fmoc/Boc-amino acids by several groups for the generation of peptide libraries. Houghten et al. [53] have used protected amino acid mixtures in a predetermined molar ratio which compensated for the different coupling rates of amino acids. Hudson and co-workers [54] balanced the reaction rates of Fmoc-amino acids by competitive reaction of each residue in the presence of an equimolar amount of Nle. An alternative approach for one pot synthesis was described by Kramer et al. [55] and later modified by Quesnel et al. [56]. In each synthetic cycle, a mixture containing 19 different amino acids (0.8 equivalent) was allowed to react with a peptidyl resin. With extended coupling times, slower acylating derivatives could be incorporated in good yields. Kramer acetylated unreacted amino groups with acetic anhydride, whereas Quesnel capped with biotin to remove truncated peptides from the libraries by affinity chromatography. Complex nona and hexapepitde mixtures generated by premix method have been successfully screened for the identification of antigenic peptides and MHC-class II binding peptides.

4.3 Spatially addressable parallel chemical synthesis

For rapid optimization of previously identified lead compounds, parallel synthesis of a large number of individual compounds is a very attractive proposition. Since the amino acid sequences of peptides are predetermined, structural identification of the active compound is not required. The screening of these libraries of single compounds can also be performed in parallel format both while attached to the solid support or after cleavage from the support for solution phase assay. The various techniques based on parallel strategy for preparing libraries of single compounds have been described below.

4.3.1 Multipin synthesis

The concept was originally developed for the parallel synthesis of several hundred single peptides in a reusable form. The peptides are synthesized on polyacrylate-grafted polyethylene pins arranged in a standard 96 well microtiter plate format. The peptides remain attached to the pin after the synthesis and only side chain protecting groups are removed. The screening is performed by ELISA while peptide remain bound to the pins. After completion of each assay a thorough disruption procedure is used to remove bound antibodies, allowing reuse of the peptide pins (50 times or more). Though the technology was originally developed for epitope mapping, subsequently it was also applied for T cell proliferation studies [57], substance P receptor binding studies [58], endothelin receptor antagonist [59] and for inhibitors of human heart chymase [60]. In recent years the technology has been modified which allows both increase in the loading capacity of the pins as well as synthesis of small organic molecules [61, 62].

4.3.2 Light directed synthesis of chips

Fodor et al. [63] introduced this method for generating peptides. The technique combines the miniaturisation of solid phase peptide synthesis with the process of photolithography. It allows parallel synthesis of thousands of peptides at the defined sites on aminoalkylated glass sheet using photolabile nitroveratryloxy group for the protection of amino group. A mask was used to control the irradiation of predefined regions of the surface to reveal free amino group for further acylation. Screening was performed on the chip by fluorescence microscopy [64] and structure of the active compound(s) read by their position on the surface. The technique has been used in an epitope mapping studies at Affymax [65].

4.3.3 Spot synthesis

Frank et al. [66] developed a simple and an inexpensive procedure for the synthesis of polymer bound peptides. Synthesis of peptides was carried out on the functionalized cellulose paper. Solution of protected amino acids and coupling reagents are applied as droplets of liquid onto the membrane that spreads over a restricted circular area resembling a "spot". The entire sheet can then be immersed in an appropriate solvent bath for washing and deprotection. The miniaturized technique could accommodate up to 100 peptides/cm^2. The peptide bound paper can be used either directly for ELISA assay or after punching out the spot, cleaving it individually and then screening in solution. The technique has been used for epitope mapping [67] and for the synthesis of random libraries [68]. An automatic synthesiser based on SPOT technique has been developed and is available commercially.

4.3.4 Double combinatorial approach

Recently, two different groups have independently demonstrated chemical synthesis of libraries using double combinatorial technique. Though both the approaches provide basis for the synthesis of a very large number of molecules their concept is based on entirely different schemes. Pavia et al. [69] demonstrated their approach by synthesizing a large number of highly functionalized biphenyl libraries by initially introducing various functional groups (e.g. alkyl, aryl, alcohols, amines etc.) onto the first scaffold building block. The second scaffold building block is then incorporated followed by additional rounds of introduction of functional groups on solid support. The libraries prepared in parallel format is then cleaved from the resin to afford desired product for screening. Nielsen et al. [70] on the contrary have used a different approach which is based on the chemical ligation of one library with another library to yield library with an exponential increase in library members. This has been explempified by the synthesis of a small [6+3] member model library. Though the double combinatorial chemistry technique offers a powerful tool for synthesizing large libraries, its efficacy has yet to be proven in terms of lead generation and optimisation.

5 Identification of active compounds from combinatorial libraries

The search for active compounds from combinatorial libraries, whether based on split synthesis or random incorporation format, requires a sensitive target-based assay, deconvolution, decoding or other special methods to get back to original discrete compounds. The first step in screening combinatorial libraries is similar to those in any biological screen. For initial screening the mixtures are assayed for activity at a higher concentration of 1.25 to 2.5 mg/ml using serial dilutions in order to determine their IC_{50} values. Once a subset of compounds is found, the challenging task of identifying the structures of these compounds remains by way of deconvolution. Therefore, discovering activity in combinatorial mixtures comprises screening and deconvolution.

5.1 Methods for assaying combinatorial libraries

5.1.1 Microplate activity assay

Screening of combinatorial mixtures in 96- or 384-well microplate is one of the most popular and widely used technique as the various biochemical, cellular or ligand binding assays routinely used are compatible with this format. Testing combinatorial mixtures of higher magnitude may result in solubility problems while maintaining total mixture concentration to a certain maximal level. High concentration during initial screening of compound libraries is needed to achieve adequately high concentrations of each compound in the mixture. Beside this there are other pitfalls in using this method such as screening artifacts and non-specific activity. In spite of these variables, screening of combinatorial libraries for lead generation and optimization remains a proven method. Many examples of successful use for this strategy have been reviewed [71].

5.1.2 Gel diffusion assay

This screening technique is highly compatible with combinatorial libraries made by split synthesis format. It involves configuring an assay so that the components are in an agarose gel. Active components released from a particular bead exhibit a zone of activity or inhibition in the gel. Thus, a very large number of beads can be screened in one Petridish by spreading them either randomly or in ordered arrays. The techniques have been successfully used with cell based screens for G-protein coupled receptors [72], cytotoxicity [73] and enzyme assays using a fluorescence read out [74].

5.1.3 Affinity selection

The affinity selection method is based on the fact that protein targets are used to purify those library mixtures that have a sufficiently high affinity for the target away from the rest of the libraries. As a result, only one predominant motif, rather than multiple distinct motifs is identified. Thus affinity column procedure may be particularly useful for large combinatorial mixtures or for libraries made by random incorporation. However, like other assays affinity selection too has some shortcomings. First, a compound obtained from affinity selection of libraries must be obtained in sufficient quantity to allow structural elucidation. And secondly, one needs to have targets of high purity available along with methodologies for separating the bound compounds from the rest of the library. Recently, on-line, one-step selection and structural identification of candidate ligands from a small mixture has been developed using electrospray ionisation mass spectrometry [75]. These developments make affinity selection one of the most interesting methods as it involves both screening and structural elucidation in one-step. However, further studies are needed to allow its application to larger mixtures.

5.1.4 One bead/one compound concept

The one bead/one compound concept or the selectide process uses the solid phase split/mix method to generate random libraries such that only one compound is displayed on a single bead. The random library of millions of beads is then screened in parallel for a specific acceptor molecule. The beads that bind with the acceptor molecule are then identified using enzyme linked colorimetric assay. The colour beads are then isolated and structures of compound determined by microsequencing, mass spectrometry, NMR or coding. Lam et al. [6] first reported the synthesis and screening of the one bead/one compound library of pentapeptide and identified ligands for anti-β-endorphin monoclonal antibody and streptavidin. To develop a solution phase screen and maintain the one bead/one compound concept, Lebl et al. modified the library and applied a dual releasable linker technology so that the peptide can be released from beads and screened [78, 79]. Recently numerous investigators have applied this concept to nonpeptidyl oligomers and to small organic molecule libraries for a variety of different targets. Over the last 3 to 4 years, several important developments have been made to screen bead libraries more efficiently. They include use of fluorescent labled protein domains and antibodies, receptors labelled with dyes, dual colour method and whole cell on bead binding assay.

5.2   Deconvolution

The structure/lead identification of a library member by deconvolution can be carried out with both mixture libraries or from those generated by split synthesis. Four general deconvolution methods used frequently have been summarized below.

5.2.1 Iterative approach

Iterative approach for deconvolution remains one of the most widely used methods for lead identification. In this approach mixtures of compounds are resynthesized and tested. The result of the biological assay determines the next step. This method has resulted in the successful identification of antigenic determinants [80], opioid peptides [81], antimicrobial peptides [82] and enzyme inhibitors.

5.2.2 Positional scanning

In order to shorten the time required for structural identification from a large peptide mixture, positional scanning method was introduced by Houghten et al. In this method peptide libraries are composed of individual peptide mixture in which a single position is defined with a single amino acid while the remaining positions are composed of mixtures of amino acids. For a hexa-peptide library constructed from 20 amino acids the following mixtures can be synthesized: $Ac-O_1XXXXX-NH_2$, $Ac-O_1O_2XXXX-NH_2$ to $Ac-O_1O_2O_3O_4O_5X-NH_2$ and $Ac-O_1O_2O_3O_4O_5O_6-NH_2$ (120 peptide mixture in total). After screening, the most active amino acid residue at each position is defined [83]. The approach has been used to study monoclonal antibody interaction, opioid ligands, mellitin inhibitors. Recently a two-dimensional positional scan library has been reported from which a novel inhibitor of acetylcholine esterase has been identified and confirmed through resynthesis of the individual compounds [84].

5.2.3 Orthogonal partition

An alternative library format, an orthogonal library was described by Tartar et al. [85]. In this method a group of 25 different amino acids is divided in a 5×5 matrix format of five groups in one direction labelled as A_1–A_5 and orthogonally in another direction labelled as B_1–B_5. Each library resulted from the incorporation of one group of amino acids. A_n for library A and B_n for library B, at each of the three variable positions. Thus two orthogonally different but related libraries, A_n, A_n, A_n and B_n, B_n, B_n (125 sublibraries) are synthesized. The utility of this format has been demonstrated in a V2 vasso-pressin receptor binding assay.

5.2.4 Recursive deconvolution

This approach was introduced by Erb et al. to shorten the time required for the identification of active peptide sequences from a library. They described this method using a pentapeptide library synthesized by split/mix method. In this modified iteration method, at each step a portion of resin from each reaction vial is held back and labelled; the remaining resin from each vial is combined and redistributed [86]. After the synthesis of library, the sublibraries of which the N-terminal amino acid has defined are screened and the amino acid of the sublibrary that demonstrated the highest activity is then coupled to the partial libraries set aside in the previous split synthesis. This recursive deconvolution is repeated until the most active peptides are identified.

5.3   Coding

An alternative to deconvolution technique which requires resynthesis of several sublibraries, is the encoded bead method that has been widely used for structure identification of compounds. The indirect and simple method for determining the structure of a compound synthesized on a single bead can be used with both the testing methods that involve bead bound ligands as well as polymer free ligands in solution. The technique employs a readable chemical tag that is simultaneously attached to the individual bead for each step in the synthesis of the actual molecule on the bead. Codes can be also used to identify a particular reaction history thereby enabling tracking of any unforeseen chemical products. Four encoding or tagging methodologies are generally used and have been described below.

5.3.1 Peptides encoding library

Lam and co-workers first described the concept of encoding libraries using peptide molecules to facilitate structural determination of nonsequenceable compounds [87]. In this technique each step of building the nonsequeaceable structure is followed by the independent incorporation of one or two amino acid as coding strand onto a separate point on the solid phase particle. This alternate synthesis of coding strand and compound can be carried out on the N^α and N^ϵ amino groups of Lysine residue using an orthogonal protecting group approach. Selectide have devised a multiple linker that includes Lysine as a branch point on the resin so as to attach both sequences. The peptide code can then be sequenced using Edman degradation, mass spectrometry or HPLC and the structure of the organic molecule can be recalled.

5.3.2 Oligonucleotides encoding library

The concept of using DNA as an encoding strand was first prepared by Berner and Lerner [88] and later pioneered by Needels et al. [89]. The method has been mainly used for tagging peptide libraries. In this process, alternating parallel combinatorial synthesis is used to encode individual members of a large library of compounds with unique nucleotide sequence. Thus to each bead is covalently attached many copies of a single peptide sequence and, additionally, copies of a unique single stranded oligonucleotide that effectively records the process by which the encoded peptide sequence is assembled. The beads are then screened for binding to acceptor molecule (target) using a fluorescence-activated sorting technique. The beads to which acceptor molecules are bound tightly are isolated and the oligonucleotide tag attached to individual sorted beads are amplified by PCR. Sequence of amplified DNAs are then determined to recall the identity of peptide sequences. However, the method suffers from the drawback with regard to the limitations of protection strategies for the DNA strand and its compatibility with the reagents and conditions used for the synthesis of non-oligomeric libraries.

5.3.3 Molecular tags as an encoding strategy

Molecular tag encoding system has been one of the most widely used methods and has been successfully applied to the synthesis of both peptides and large nonoligomeric libraries. Unlike peptide and nucleotide encoding, the tags are not built into a parallel chain, but instead are added onto the free amino terminal of growing peptides. Approximately 0.5 to 1% of the amino groups of each amino acid synthon at each stage of synthesis are blocked by molecular tags. The tagging molecules used are halophenoxy derivatives of aliphatic alcohols [90], diazomethane derivatives[91] and secondary amines [92]. The identities of active compounds are then determined by analysing the tags cleaved either by UV irradiation followed by GC or by acid hydrolysis followed by ESMS or by oxidation followed by EC-GC.

5.3.4 Radio frequency encoding

Introduction, removal, and decoding of chemical tags as discussed above comprise a large portion of the effort to generate and screen the library. Beside the coding structure, an on bead screening may also interfere with the interaction between the target and the test compound. This necessitated the search for an alternative encoding strategy which resulted in the identification of radio frequency encoding as a novel method for tagging. In this non-chemical method commercially available RF transponders are used to tag each compound in the library. These transponders are preencoded with a unique ID, and are glass encased, and thus are stable to most solvents and reagents. In practice, glass encased microchips, each having a unique binary encoded ID, are added to individual bags containing appropriate resin. The tea bags are then subjected to the chemical steps required for the build up of the desired library using split-mix procedure. At each stage of the synthesis, the microchips are RF-scanned and the unique ID number is recorded. After the synthesis is complete, each bag is introduced to individual wells of a microtiter plate and the products are deblocked from the polymer. The histogram of the ID for each well is then used to assign the structure of every product in the library [93]. The transponders are useable and can be scanned directly through standard laboratory glassware, even while immersed in a solvent. A library of 64 compounds [94] using Wang's resin and a 125 membered tripeptide library [95] using Rink resin have been successfully synthesized using glass encased microchips with unique encoded ID.

6 Analytical methods for the characterisation of combinatorial libraries

Issues pertaining to the quality of combinatorial libraries such as following a solid phase reaction, characterisation of libraries etc. have always been a subject of immense interest and discussion. Many different analytical techniques have been developed and successfully used for the quality control of chemical libraries. Some of the most widely used methods have been described below.

6.1 Functional group titration

This method has often been used to monitor reactions on solid phase. For example for amines: Kaiser test [96], picric acid test [97], bromophenol blue test [98] and trinitrobenzenesulfonic acid [99] test are some of the best known methods. Similarly Ellman's test [100] for free thiols and nitrophenylisothiocyanate-O-trityl for sterically hindered or nonbasic amines have been also reported.

6.2 UV measurements

The quantitative measurement of Fmoc release from derivatized amino group is one of the most commonly used method for measuring loadings [101]. In addition UV-active byproducts resulting from protecting group cleavage such as dimethoxytrityl ether cleavage with acid [102], nitrophenylethyloxy group cleavage with [103] base and Fmoc group cleavage with piperidine [104] have been reported to monitor solid phase reactions.

6.3 IR methods

FTIR methods are routinely used to monitor the course of a reaction on solid phase. FTIR measurements can provide both qualitative as well as quantitative data on the reaction. It has also been used to estimate yield [105]. Measurements of loaded and unloaded resin under identical conditions give rise to absorption bands which otherwise are seen as weak shoulders. Calibrating measurements can be also performed for monitoring the completion of reaction [106].

6.4 HPLC

Reverse phase analytical HPLC has been widely used to assess the purity of the products formed at every step of solid phase synthesis. At every step 7–8 mg of resin is removed from the reaction vessel and the product cleaved from the resin using TFA or other methods recommended. The cleavage mixture is then lyophilized using t-BuOH-Water or acetonitrile-water mixture and residue subjected to RP-HPLC to assess its purity. This technique is particularly useful when reaction conditions are being optimized during solid phase organic synthesis. Further before synthesizing libraries, a number of model compounds are synthesized and in practice the purity of model compounds are routinely estimated by analytical HPLC. At times it is also recommended to even prepare a small library of 6–9 compounds by split-mix method and then establish the presence of all components of the resulting mini library by RPHPLC before proceeding for the synthesis of a large library. Recently rapid RPHPLC analytical and preparative HPLC methods have been developed for application to parallel synthesis of libraries. Gradient method, short columns, and high flow rates allow analysis of over 300 compounds per day on a single system, or purification of up to 200 compounds per day on a single preparative system. Hardware and software modifications allow continuous use for maximum efficiency and throughput [107]. MDS Panlabs in collaboration with Biotage, Inc have developed the Parallex high throughput preparative HPLC system for providing compounds of high purity. In addition, they have also developed new protocols and methodologies to support preparation, characterisation and plating of the purified libraries as well as data tracking of samples moving through the purification process [108].

6.5 NMR

NMR techniques have been used to characterise support bound compounds. Natural abundance gel phase ^{13}C NMR spectroscopy has been used for assessing intermediate structures in solid phase synthesis [109] but unfortunately it requires long acquisition times and may not find wide application. However, use of ^{13}C labelled starting materials in conjunction with ^{13}C gel phase NMR, to follow multistep reaction has been quite successful [110–112]. Gel phase ^{31}P is very useful in following the reaction involving phosphorous containing moieties [113]. Magic angle spinning (MAS) solid state NMR [114], MAS ^{13}C-1H correlation [115] and MAS HMQC and TOCSY experiments [116–117] have been carried out for compounds attached to TG or other resins. Fluorinated linkers for monitoring solid-phase synthesis using gel-phase ^{19}F NMR spectroscopy has been recently described [118]. Application of NMR methods to combinatorial chemistry has been reviewed by Shapiro and Wareing [119].

6.6 Mass spectrometry

Electrospray and MALDI/TOFMS have been used with adequate sensitivity for single bead detection of molecular weight and structural information [120]. Single bead MS using TFA cleavage and MALDI/TOF analysis is now a well established and widely used technique [121–124]. Mass spectromerty has been used to characterise reaction products in conjunction with other analytical techniques: HPLC-MS, GC-MS and MS-MS [125–127]. A new ultra-high throughput method for characterizing combinatorial libraries incorporating a multiple probe autosampler coupled with flow injection mass spectrometry analysis has been described [128]. Similarly sequential mass spectrometry of combinatorial libraries by using automated matrix assisted laser desorption mass spectrometry has been also reported [129].

7 Application of combinatorial library using solid phase chemistry

Much of the early work in combinatorial chemsitry and molecular diversity approaches laid emphasis on the preparation of large mixtures of peptides. Synthetic peptide combinatorial libraries comprising peptide mixtures or randomized peptides or combination of defined positions have been extensively used in all areas of biomedical research in the search for new leads. These mixtures have been screened either in solution or while immobilized on solid phase supports. A range of structurally diverse combinatorial peptide libraries have been prepared and successfully used to identify potent peptide lead sequences of therapeutic interest. However, in recent years much of the focus of combinatorial libraries is on the synthesis of small organic molecules other than peptides. To achieve this, novel combinatorial organic synthesis (COS) is appearing at an increasing rate along with relatively high order of diversity in contrast to peptides. The remainder of the section deals with the application of combinatorial approach for synthesizing libraries of peptides and small organic molecules.

7.1 Library of peptides

Polymer bound and soluble libraries of linear peptides ranging from tetrapeptide to pentadecapeptide have been prepared and screened to identify a range of bioactive products including antigenic determinants [80, 130], antimicrobials [131], enzyme inhibitors [132] and ligands for opioid receptors [81, 133]. A number of reviews have appeared covering the areas of libraries based on peptides [134, 135]. To illustrate the various library types, as well as the utility of the library approach in general, a number of different peptide libraries and their use in identifying new leads against different targets have been summarized in Table 3. Combinatorial peptide libraries containing all L amino acids, all D-amino acids or a mixture of L, D and unnatural amino acids have been reported by several laboratories.

7.2 Library of cyclic peptides

Libraries of cyclic peptides have been reported by various groups. The method of cyclisation includes: disulfide bond [151], side chain lactam [152] and head to tail amide bond formation [153]. Several cyclic penta-, hexa- and heptapeptide libraries using split-mix and premix method have been prepared and characterized [154, 155]. One bead/one compound disulfide cyclic peptide libraries have yielded ligands which bind to gp IIb/IIIa integrin [156]. Potent and selective α-glucosidase inhibitors have been identified from the iterative synthesis and screening of 26 cyclic libraries of varying size [157]. Cellulose immobilized cyclic hepta- and octapeptide libraries have been screened for ligands that bind to TGFβ [152].

7.3 Library of peptidomimetics

Beside libraries of peptides, a number of groups have synthesized libraries of peptidomimetics for the purpose of lead generation against various targets. Terett et al. identified an endothelin receptor antagonist 1 from the peptidomimetic library of 30 000 compounds [158]. Similarly a library of 900 compounds of peptidylphosphonic library based on 2 yielded compounds with less than 100nM activity [159]. An on-resin tag coded peptidomimetic

Table 3.
Lead peptides identified from libraries

Peptide library	Target	Peptide(s) identified	Ref.
Hexapeptide	19B10 mab	Ac-DVPDYA-NH2, IC_{50} 30 nM	5
Hexapeptide	125–10F3 mab	Ac-PYPNLP-NH$_2$, IC_{50} 4 nM	132
Hexapeptide	μ-receptor	Ac-RFMWMK-NH$_2$ IC_{50} 5 nM	81
Hexapeptide	3E7	YGGFMT-NH$_2$, IC_{50} 3 nM	80
Hexapeptide	S. aureus	Ac-RRWWCR-NH$_2$, IC_{50} 3.4 μM	5
Hexapeptide	C. albicans	Ac-RRWWRR-NH$_2$, IC_{50} 28 μg	136
Hexapeptide	Mellittin hemolytic	Ac-IVILLW-NH$_2$, IC_{50} 5 μg/mL	137
Hexapeptide	HIV integrase	HCKFYY-NH$_{52}$, IC_{50} 2 μM	138
Hexapeptides with with D amino acids	μ-receptor	Ac-rfwink-NH$_2$	139
Tetrapeptide	MMP-2 & MMP-9	H-εAhx-βAla-H	140
Tetrapeptide	Zinc endopeptidase	Z-$_{(L,D)}$PheΨ(PO2CH2)$_{L,D}$ARF	141
Tetrapeptide with L,D amino acids	S. aureus	(αFmoc-εLys) WfR-NH$_2$, IC_{50} 4–8 μg/mL	142
Statine tetrapeptide	HIV protease	AcWV-Statine-I-NH$_2$, IC_{50} 200 nM	143
Nonapeptide	Src SH3	RALPPLPRY-NH$_2$, IC_{50} 7.8 μM	144
Nonapeptide	Thrombin	fPRPFGYRV-βAla, IC_{50} 40 μM	145
Dodecapeptide	Trypsin	AcYYGAKIYRPDKM, IC_{20} 10 μM	134
Pentadecapeptide	HLA class II	QLWVILLAKAVTAPDT	146
Tetrapeptide derivatives	Thrombin	Dihydroxybenzoyl-KIFR, IC_{20} 2 μM	147
Pentapeptide	Dopamine D2	ELFKA	148
Cyclic octapeptide	Streptavidin ligand	Cyclo (AHPQFPAE)K-NH$_2$, IC_{50} 128 nM	149
Inverted tripeptide	Dansylated tweezer	Z-Glu(Obut)-Ser(0But)-Val, Kassoc = 4×10^5	150

library of 1.1 million oligomers designed to identify amide based structure **3** that binds to the Src domain has been reported with micromolar active leads [160]. A phosphodiester based library **4** was used to identify LTB$_4$ and PLA$_2$ binding inhibitors from a library of 20 000 compounds [161]. A library of β-turn mimetics based on **5** has been synthesized using α-amino acids, aminoalkyl thiols and α-halo acids [162] (Fig. 1).

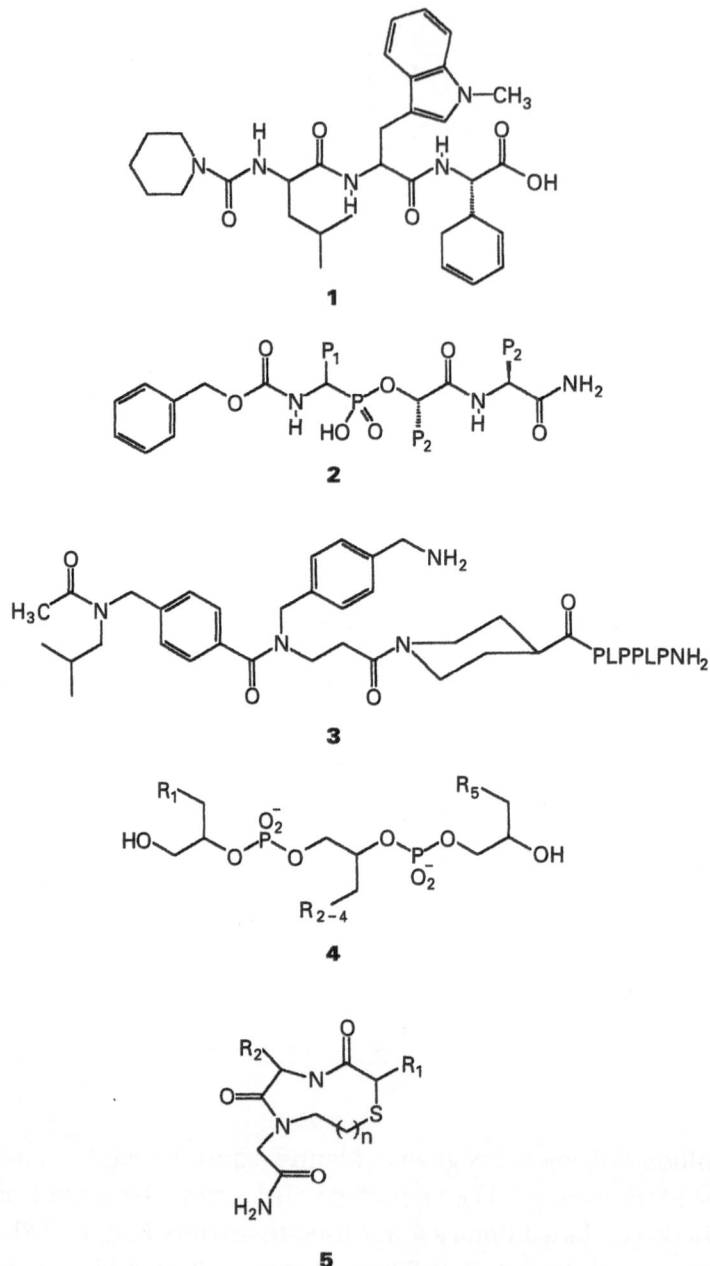

Fig. 1
Structure of peptidomimetics identified from libraries

7.4   Library of peptoids

Peptoids are unnatural oligomers made up of non-amino acids with backbone resembling that of the peptide backbone except that peptoids are devoid of amide protons (Fig. 2a). The tertiary nature of amide bonds makes these molecules less susceptible to proteolysis than the native peptides and may also increase their oral bioavailability. Zuckerman et al. at Chiron for the first time reported libraries of N-substituted glycines using conventional solid phase peptide synthesis method [163]. An alternative approach [164] utilises an automated cycle of Rink amide resin, haloacetylation followed by displacement with a wide range of primary amines followed by further acylation of new secondary amine (Scheme 1). Synthesis and screening of 204 membered peptoid trimer library have led to the discovery of nanomolar ligands (Fig. 2b) for seven trans membrane G-protein receptors. These include CHIR 2279 (α-adrenergic receptor, Ki 5nM) and CHIR-4531 (μ-opiate receptor, Ki 6 nM) [165, 166].

Recently a biased mini tetrapeptoid library has been constructed and screened for ZAP-70 antagonism. The studies resulted in the identification of a novel selective monodentate ZAP-70 antagonist (Fig. 2c) as a lead in the search for new immunosuppressant [167].

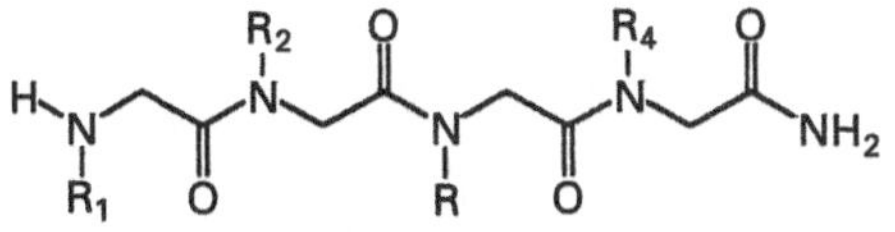

Fig. 2a
Structure of peptoids

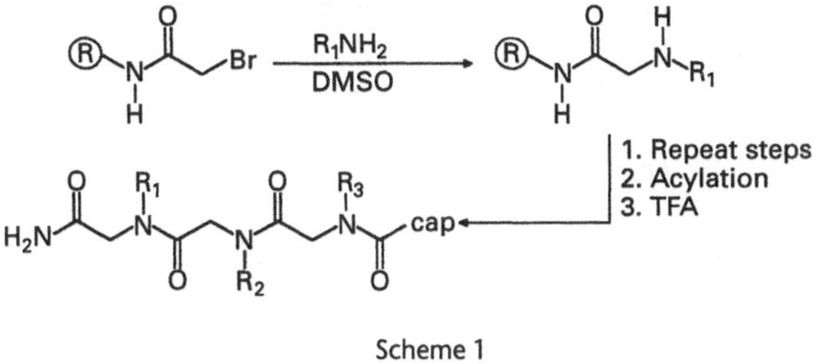

Scheme 1

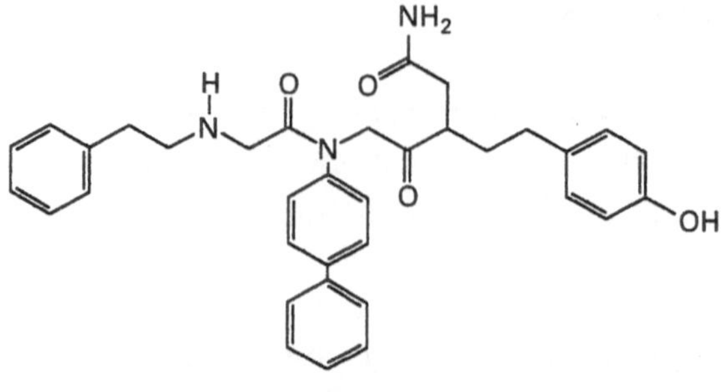

CHIR 2279

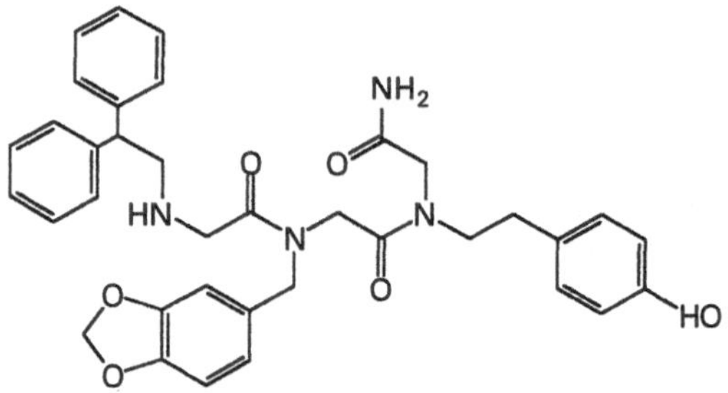

CHIR 4531

Fig. 2b
Structure of ligands for seven transmembrane G proteins

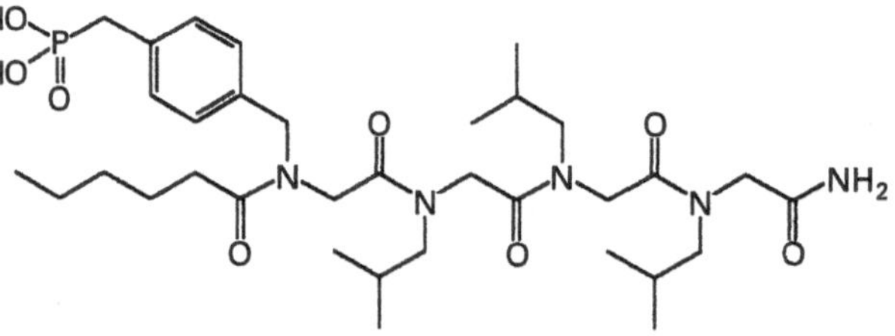

Fig. 2c
Structure of a novel selective monodentate ZAP-70 antagonist

7.5 Library of oligocarbamates

Oligocarabamates offers another new source of unnatural oligomers for the search of lead structures. It comprises chiral ethylene units connected by relatively rigid carbamate units (Fig. 3).

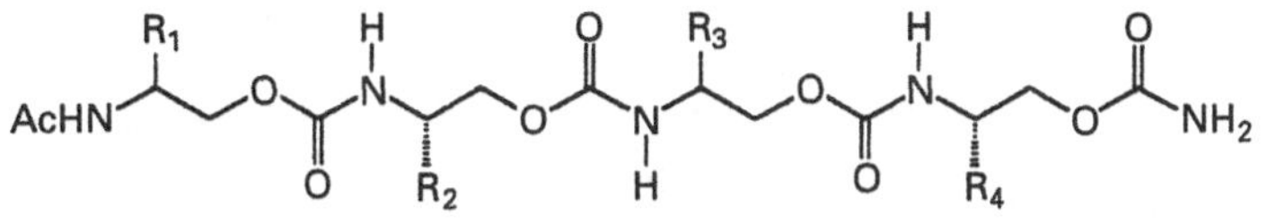

Fig. 3
Structure of oligocarbamates

When compared with peptides, oligocarabamates are more hydrophobic and more stable against enzymatic degradation. At Affymax, a total of 256 oligocarbamates that express every deletion combination of the sequence AcY^{c}F^{c}A^{c}S^{c}K^{c}I^{c}F^{c}L^c (where X^c is the carbamate equivalent of the amino acid X) were synthesized [63]. The library was screened against an antibody prepared using a conjugate of the sequence AcY^{c}K^{c}F^{c}L^{c}G^c and several products were observed to bind.

7.6 Library of oligoureas

Obstacles associated with the therapeutic use of peptides have led to the efforts to develop new oligomeric backbone with improved pharmacological properties related to peptides. In this direction oligoureas provide an opportunity to generate unnatural polymers with new class of folded polymers and properties. These oligomers have backbone with H-bonding groups, chiral centres, a significant degree of conformational restriction and sites for the introduction of additional side chain groups that may modulate the physical and biological properties of the oligoureas. Burgess et al. [168] for the first time reported solid phase synthesis of oligoureas using monophthalimide protected isocyanates as monomers. Recently Schultz et al. [169] developed an efficient and improved method for solid phase synthesis of oligoureas from optically active azido-4-nitrophenyl carbamate monomers (Scheme 2).

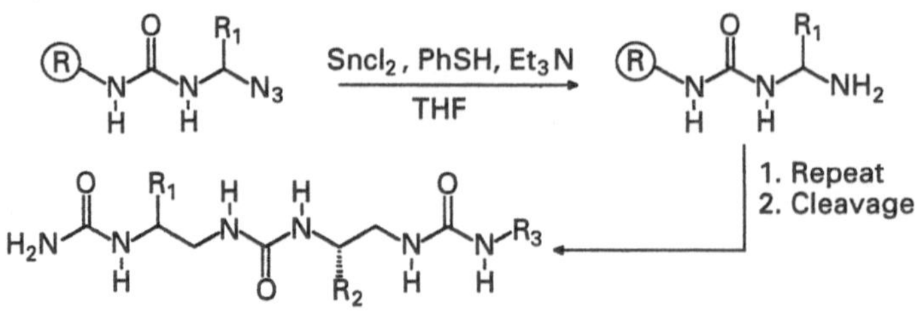

Scheme 2

7.7 Library of small organic molecules

7.7.1 Library of molecules with drug-like structure

The preponderance of heterocyclic frameworks in historical samplings of known drug structures (privileged structures) provides strong rationale for the inclusion of these scaffolds in lead discovery programs. Library synthesis involving both combinatorial and parallel synthesis strategies, is now evolving from linear polymeric scaffolds towards nonoligomeric small organic compounds including heterocycles. Libraries of diverse compounds have been prepared and tested in high throughput biological assays. In recent years this has resulted in a tremendous impact on both the rate discovery of biologically active lead structures, as well as lead structure optimisation.

One of the earliest libraries, based on known drugs such as benzodiazepines, was reported by Ellman et al. The most interesting aspect of benzodiazepines is their acceptance in the clinic as oral medication for a wide range of activities despite their somewhat peptide-like character. The classical benzodiazepine libraries were constructed using bead bound strategies [170]. In the first step benzenoid ring was affixed to a resin via a phenolic group through an arm terminating in a benzyl alcohol moiety. This was followed by six chemical steps resulting in a series of benzodiazepines comprising 1680 members in 85–100% yield (Scheme 3). When screened for binding to CCK-A receptor, a novel analogue was identified as a potent CCK ligand library memeber [171]. Subsequently the size of the library was increased to 11 200 members [172] through the generation of biphenylketone moiety by adopting Stille coupling chemistry. On the other hand, Dewitt et al. treated 2-

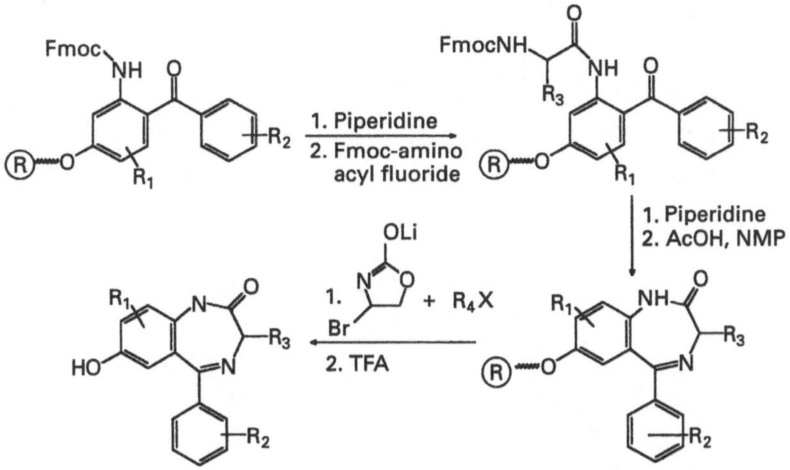

Scheme 3

aminobenzophenone imine to commercially available α amino acids on Wang resin followed by intramolecular cleavage to yield the desired benzodiazepine. Starting with five different amino acids and eight different benzophenone imines, 40 benzodiazepine were produced in 9–63% yield [173] and SAR data were generated in a bioassay based on the inhibition of fluoronitrazepam.

Boojamra et al. developed a method for the synthesis of 1,4 benzodiazepine-2,5-diones [174]. First an amino ester was reductively aminated with an aldehyde derivatized support. The secondary amine was then acylated with anthranilic acid and the resulting amide was treated with lithium salt of acetanilide followed by *in situ* alkylation to yield the cyclic product. Treatment of the resin with TFA afforded the desired benzodiazepine (Scheme 4) which offers a fast, convenient and mild method for the synthesis of benzodiazepine library on solid phase.

Recently synthesis of a diverse library comprising 120 compounds with three points of diversity has been reported using a cleavage-conjugate addition protocol as the key step [175].

Another interesting class of privileged structure for generating libraries is that of the hydantoins, primarily known to be active as anticonvulsant. Dewitt and Czarnik prepared a 40-member library of hydantoins by the condensation of a variety of isocyanates to Wang resin bound amino acids [176]. The cyclative cleavage leading to the hydantoin product was carried out by heating the resin bound urea in 6M HCl (Scheme 5).

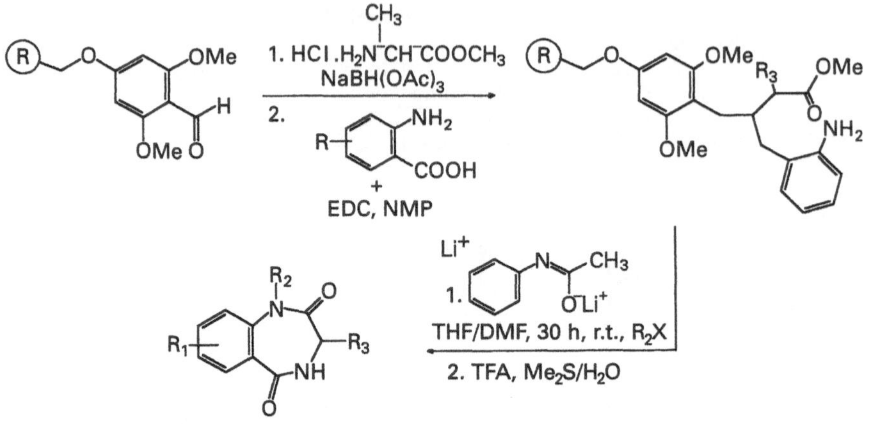

Scheme 4

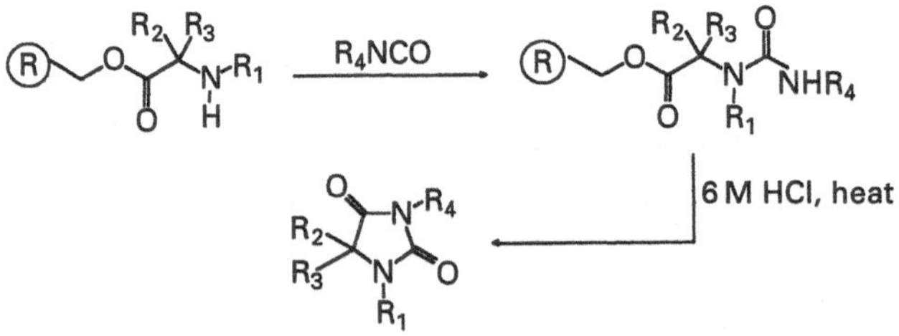

Scheme 5

Later a hydantoin library of 800 compounds using 20 different amino acids and over 80 primary amines has been reported (Scheme 6) by Dressmann et al. [177]. Beside this several alternative methods have also been reported in the literature for the combinatorial synthesis of hydantoins [178, 179].

Piperazine moieties are found in many bioactive compounds and therefore have been extensively studied for generating diversity. Diketopiperazine libraries, being relatively easier to prepare from amino acids, have been synthesized by various groups. Gordon and Steele reported synthesis of 1000 diketopiperazines using DCR method [180]. Their strategy is based on reductive amination of support bound amino acid with an aldehyde. The resulting secondary amine was then coupled with Boc-amino acids employing

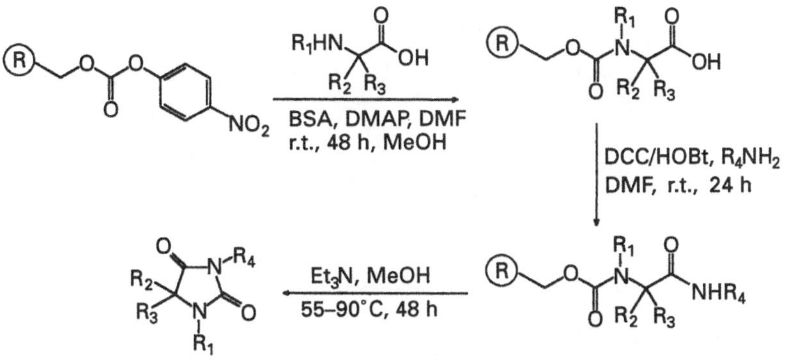

Scheme 6

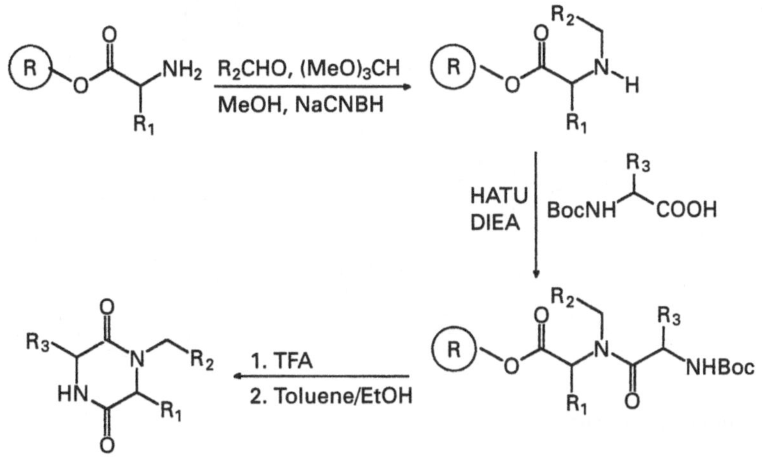

Scheme 7

PyBrOP as an activating agent. Following TFA treatment cyclisation was accomplished by heating at reflux in toluene (Scheme 7). Several diketo-piperazines have been identified from libraries with significant biological activity including affinity for NK2 receptor.

In addition several groups [181–184] have also developed newer routes to diketopiperazine libraries by extending diversity at other position as well (Fig. 4).

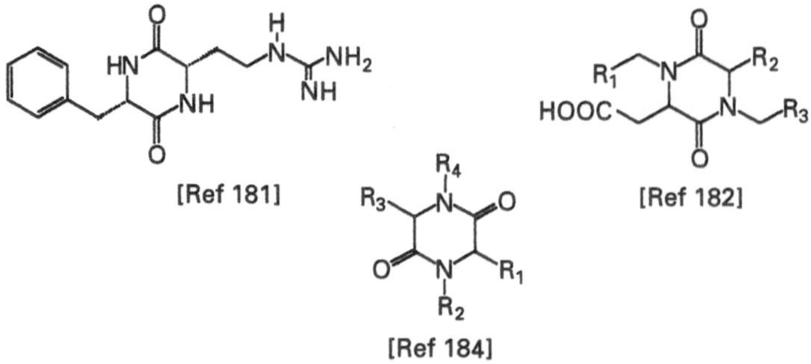

[Ref 181]

[Ref 182]

[Ref 184]

Fig. 4
Structure of diketopiperazines libraries

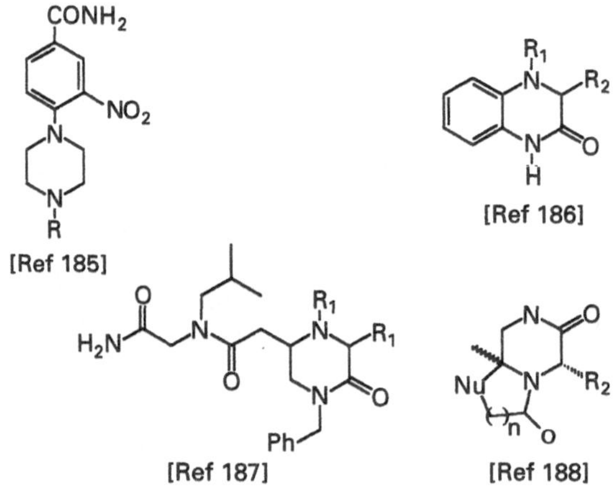

[Ref 185]

[Ref 186]

[Ref 187]

[Ref 188]

Fig. 5
Structurally diverse piperazines

Also, several groups [185–188] have developed synthetic routes for the libraries of benzyl, benzo, phenyl and 1-acyl-3-oxo piperazines on solid phase (Fig. 5).

Another pharmacophore of interest is the dihydropyridine template which has been found to be present in numerous molecules spanning a wide range of bioactivity. Its synthesis involves a promising multicomponent condensation and could be an excellent choice for library preparation [189, 190]. At Affymax, a 100-member library of dihydropyridine using 10 structurally diverse β keto esters and 10 aromatic aldehydes has been synthesized (Scheme

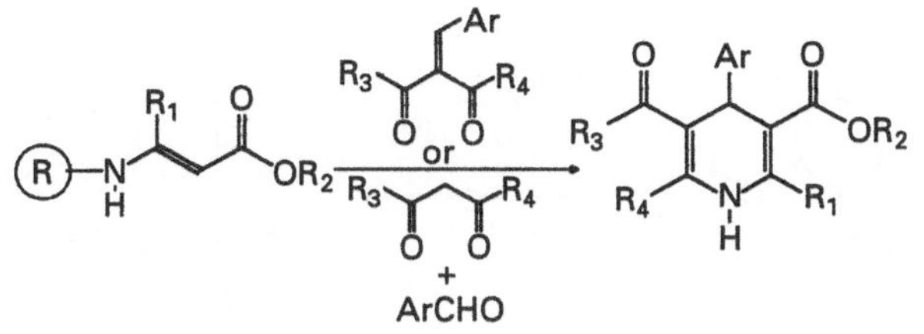

Scheme 8

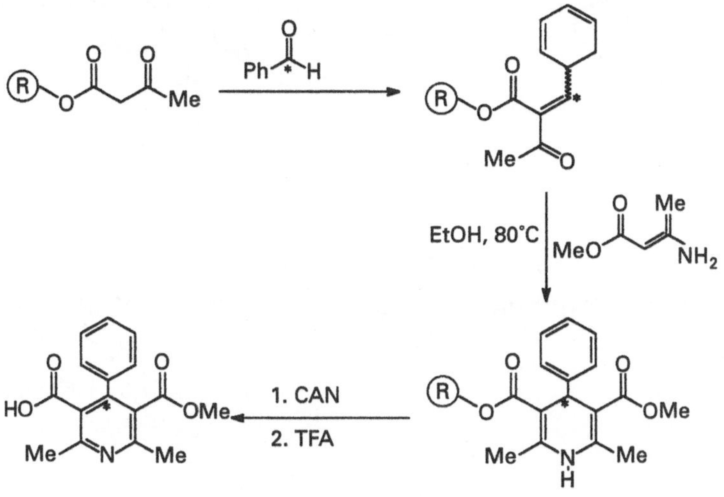

Scheme 9

8). Screening of these libraries for calcium blockade activity led to the identification of Nifedipine [191] (a known antihypertensive drug) and its closely related ethyl ester analogue as some of the most active members. An alternate strategy for synthesis involves attachment on solid support via the ester side chain instead of nitrogen atom. Thus the N-atom of the DHP ring system formed on the solid support is available for oxidation to pyridines and other synthetic modifications (Scheme 9).

Further using the above strategy, another class of combinatorial diversity has been synthesized [189, 190] by replacing the enamino ketone component

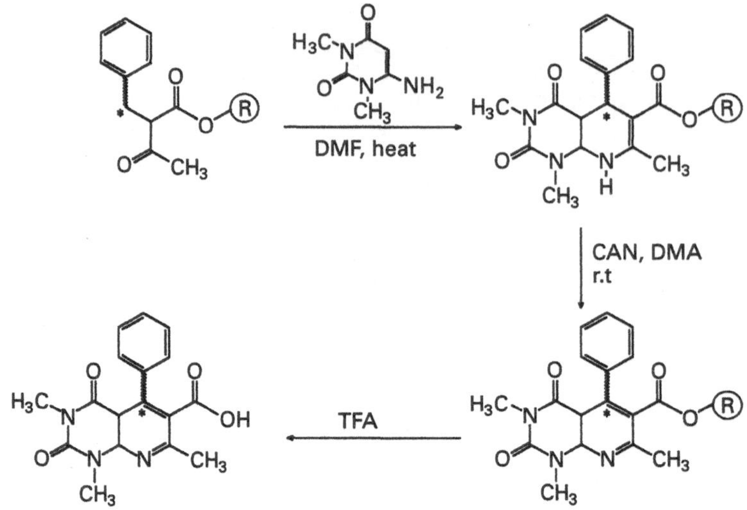

Scheme 10

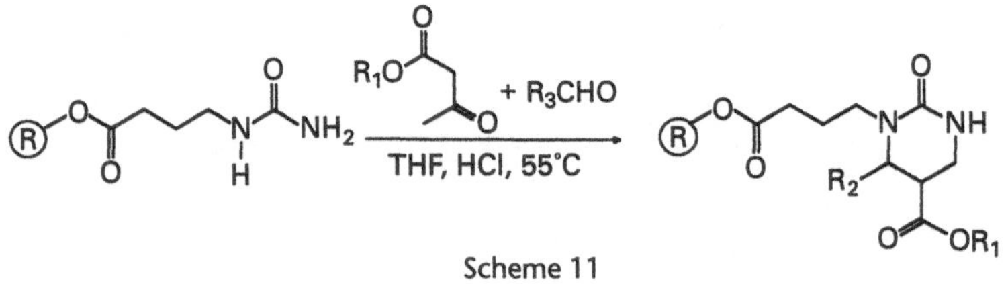

Scheme 11

with 6 amino uracil in the immobilized β-keto ester which led to the formation of pyrido[2,3-d] pyrimidine in excellent yield purity (Scheme 10).

Another privileged class of heterocycles, the Bignelli dihydropyrimidines [192] has been synthesized on solid support from β-keto esters, aldehydes and ureas in one pot reaction (Scheme 11).

Further, Kolodzieg and Hamper [193] reported synthesis of a series of 1,3-disubstituted-5,6-dihydropyrimidine-2,4-diones starting from commercially available amines and isocyanates (Scheme 12).

γ-lactones, commonly encountered in many natural products are of importance in insect pheromones and antifungal substances. Hetet et al. [194] reported synthesis of functionalized γ and δ-lactones from the polymer bound epoxides as precursors (Scheme 13).

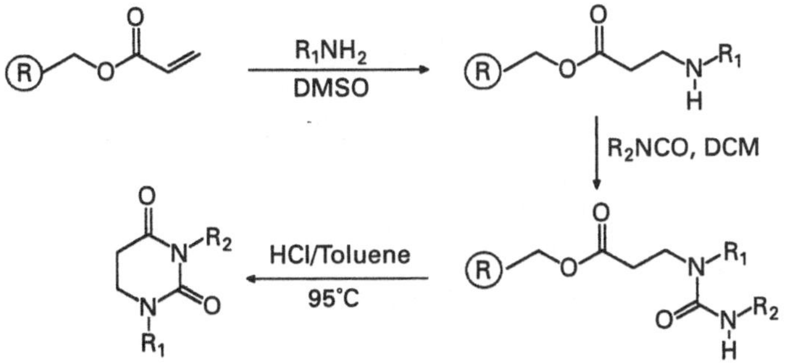

Scheme 12

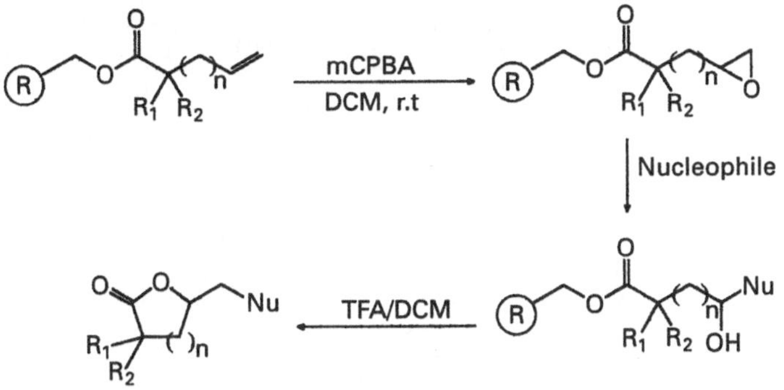

Scheme 13

Therapeutic use for γ-lactam such as cholestrol absorption modulators, analgesics and bronchodilators have led to the development of highly efficient route for their synthesis. Mjalli et al. [195] reported a combinatorial method for the synthesis of lactam via the condensation of ω-keto acids, isocyanides and amines (Scheme 14).

Scott et al. [196] reported a diketomorpholine library of 980 compounds from seven acids, 20 amines and seven aldehydes, using divide, couple and recombine method. The cyclisation of resin bound bromides to diketomorpholine was induced by treatment with TFA. Recently Szardenings et al. [197] described a simple procedure for diketomorpholine on tentagel resins using multicomponent Ugi reaction. Cyclisation was carried out under mild basic condition yielding desired diketomorpholine (Scheme 15).

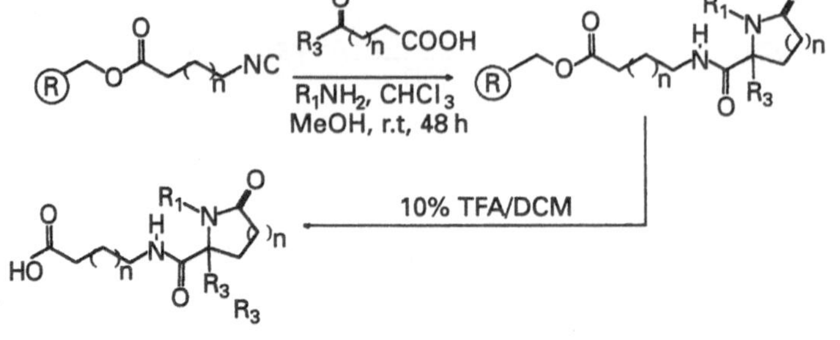

Scheme 14

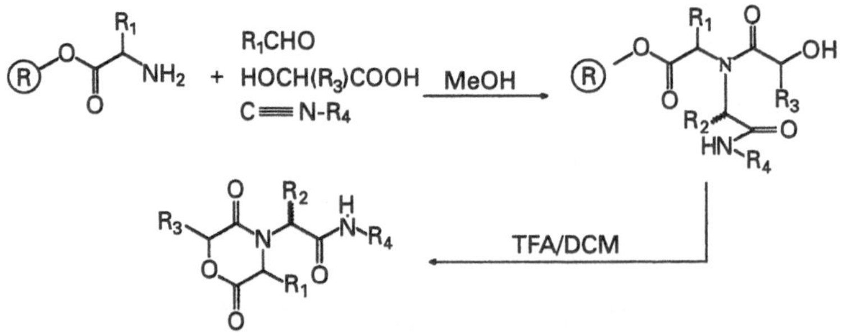

Scheme 15

A number of groups [198–200] have reported solid phase synthesis of β-carbolines which are known to exhibit significant bioactivity. In general, a library of 1,2,3,4-tetrahydro-β-carboline derivatives can be prepared through a support bound diamine which is coupled with tryptophan derivatives either by acylation or reductive amination.

The final product can then be obtained by condensation with an aldehyde/ketone followed by Pictet-Spengler cyclisation (Scheme 16).

Combinatorial library of tetrahydroisoquinoline comprising 4300 compounds [201] has been constructed using DCR method from 11 amino acids, 38 aldehydes and 51 amines in three steps. Meutermans and Alewood [202] reported a convenient route for the synthesis of dihydro- and tetrahydroisoquinolines in good yield and high purity via Bischler-Napieralski approach in one pot (Scheme 17). The scope and limitation of the method has been established by constructing a mini library.

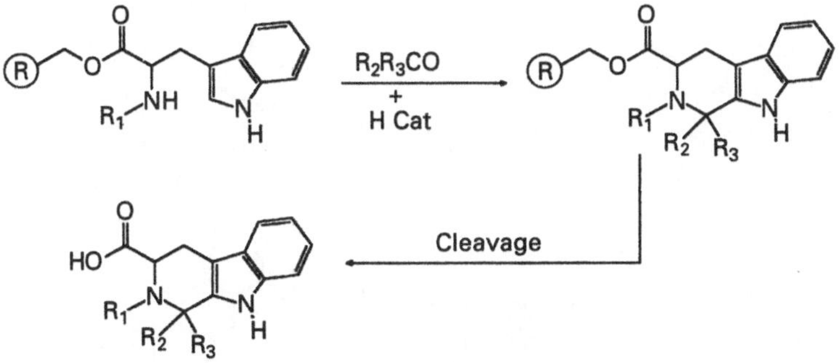

Scheme 16

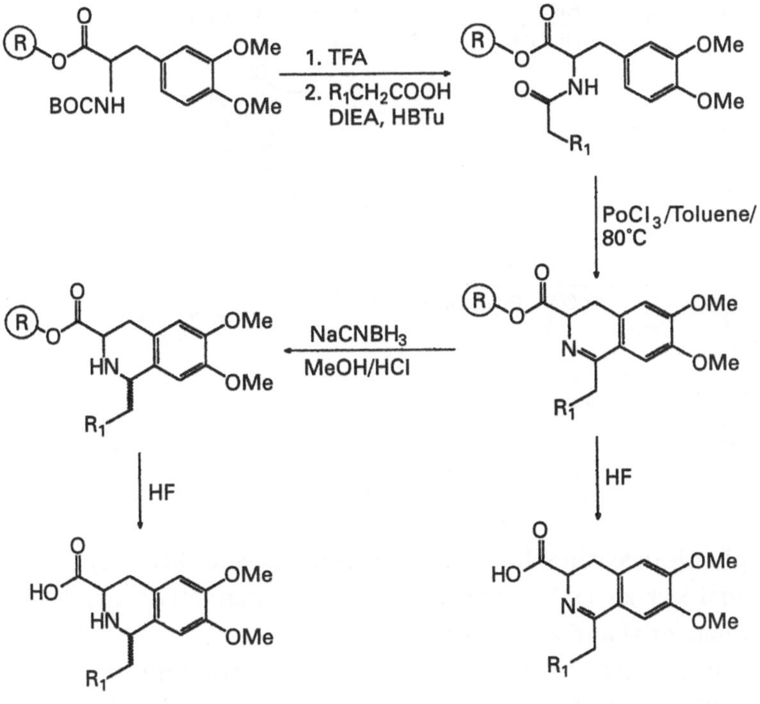

Tetrahydroisoquinoline

Dihydroisoquinoline

Scheme 17

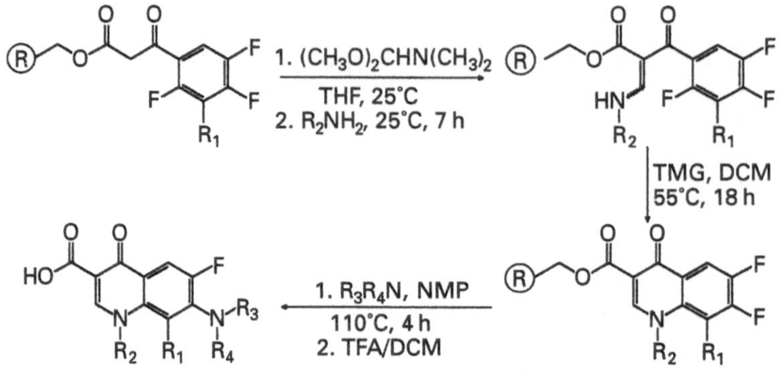

Scheme 18

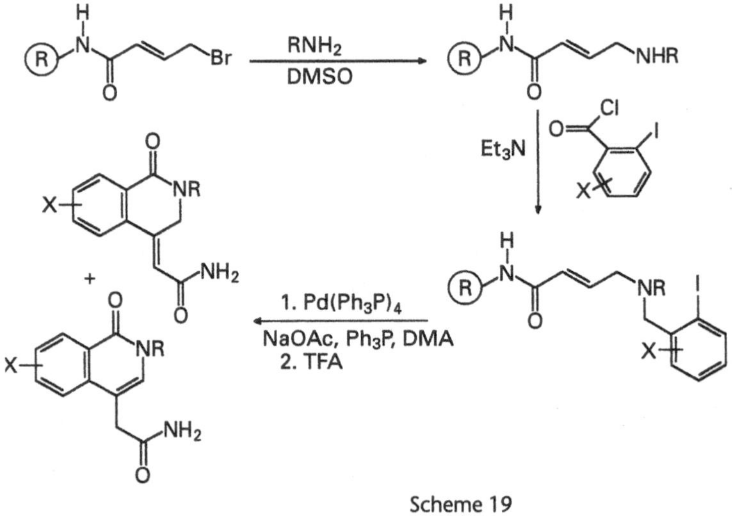

Scheme 19

Eight quinolones using diversomer technology have been reported [203] by MacDonald et al. (Scheme 18). Quinolones derivatives are known to exhibit antibacterial and antibiotic properties.

Isoquinoline derivatives are an important class of compounds with diverse biological activities such as bronchodilators, skeletal muscle relaxants and antiseptics. Goff and Zuckerman [204] generated isoquinolines using intramolecular Heck reaction on solid phase as shown in Scheme 19. Isomerisation has been observed due to a subsequent readdition of PdH. Elimi-

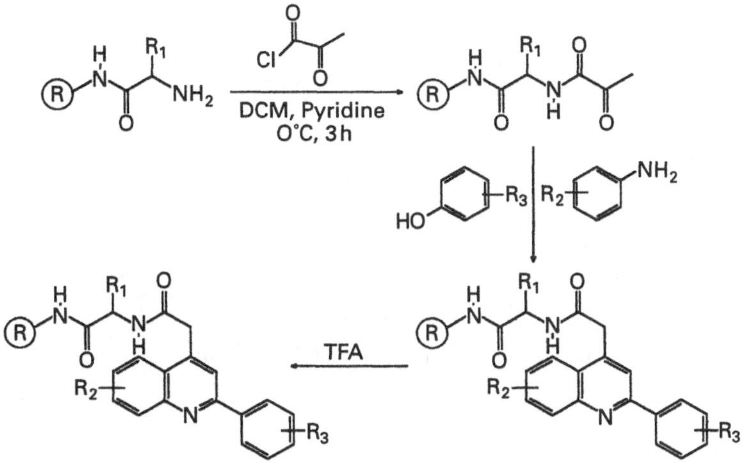

Scheme 20

nation in the opposite direction gives rise to another isomer which is thermodynamically more stable.

2-phenylquinoline-4-carboxylic acid and its derivatives have shown a variety of biological effects such as antimalarials, antimicrobials, antitumor, antioxidant and cardiovasular agents. Recently Gopalsamy and Pallai [205] reported synthesis of eight 2-aryl-quinoline-4-carboxamides using multicomponent condensation approach (Scheme 20) based on Doebner reaction [206]. The versatile method can be readily adopted for combinatorial synthesis by mix and split method or parallel synthesis.

A library of 4140 dihydroquinolinones from amino acids aldehydes and acid chlorides has been constructed [207] through the rearrangement of β-lactam intermediate on the solid phase (Scheme 21).

An efficient method for the synthesis of quinazolinediones [208] which is amenable to combinatorial synthesis and offers broad scope for structural and chemical diversity has been reported (Scheme 22).

A small library of variably substituted pyrazoles and isoxazoles has been reported [209] using a four-step reaction sequence as described in Scheme 23.

A highly substituted imidazole library [210] using aldehyde, amine and 1,2-dione has been reported as shown in Scheme 24.

Recently a mini library of 2,4,5-triarylimidazoles, where the three substitutents has been independently varied on solid support has been constructed.

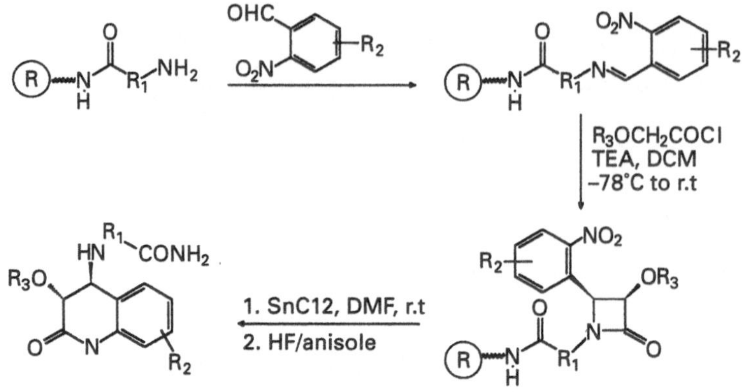

Scheme 21

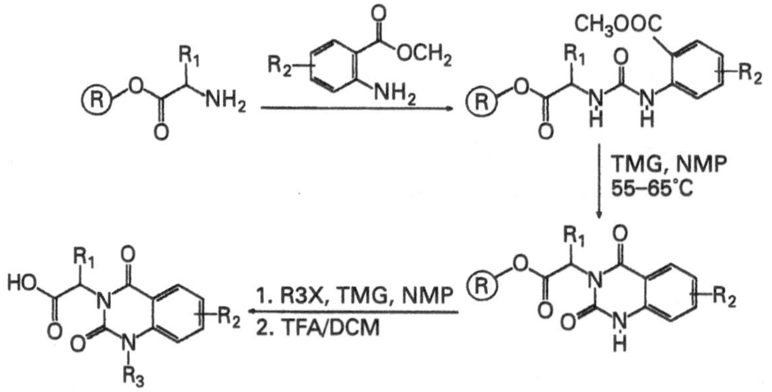

Scheme 22

The method also includes a strategy for the purification of the imidazoles on resin before cleavage [211].

A 1760 member combinatorial synthesis of structurally diverse β-lactams [212] have been carried out via [2+2] cycloaddition reaction of ketens with resin bound amino acids (Scheme 25).

Mohan and Yun [213] reported solid phase synthesis of indole analogues via an intramolecular Heck reaction of polymer bound aryl halides as depicted in Scheme 26.

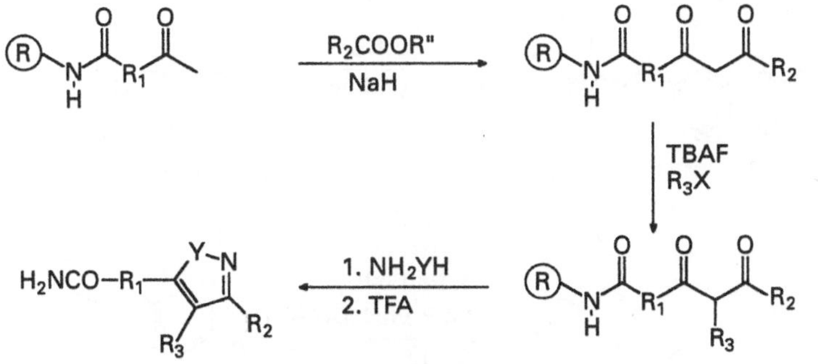

Scheme 23

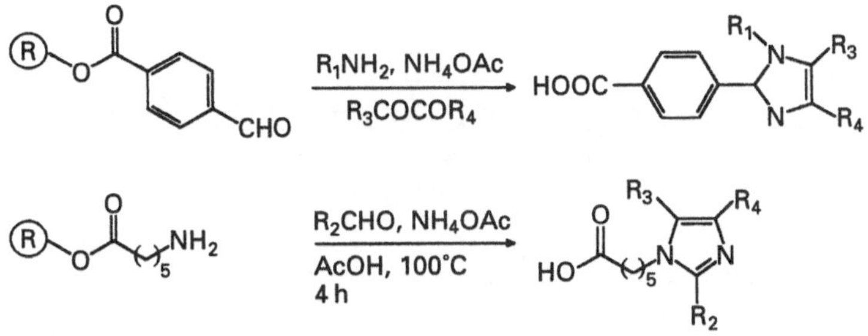

Scheme 24

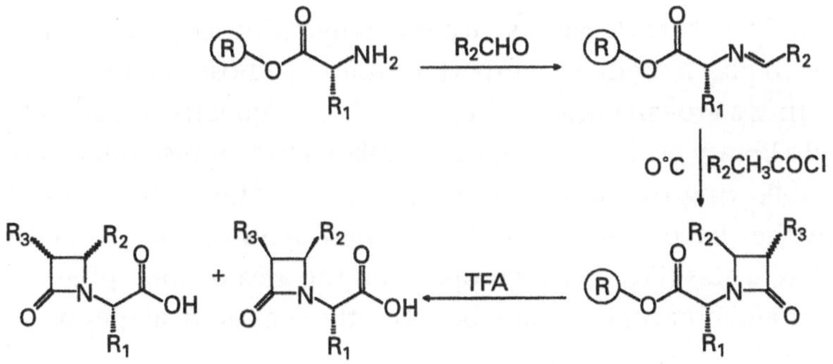

Scheme 25

133

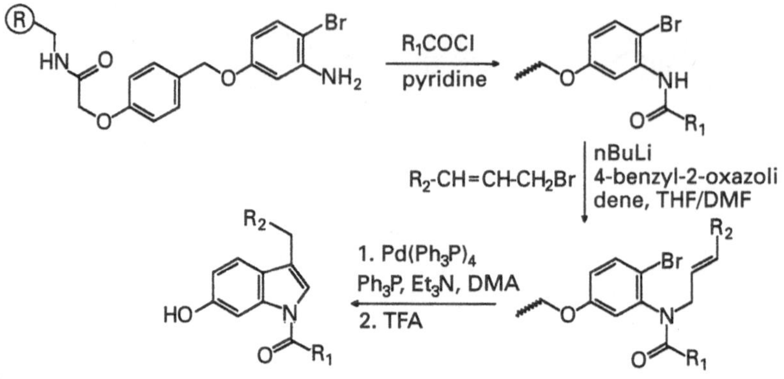

Scheme 26

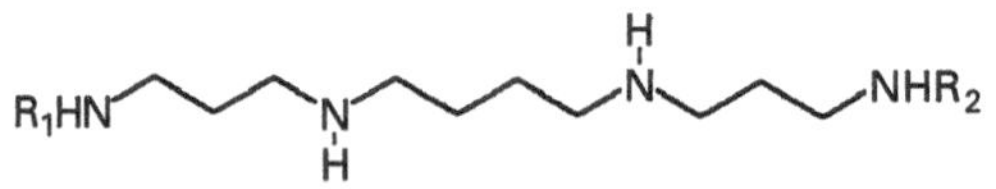

Fig. 6
Structure of symmetrical spermine conjugates

Recently Zhang et al. reported synthesis of diverse trisubstituted indoles in good yield via Pd mediated hetroannulation of internal alkynes on solid phase [214].

Naturally occurring and synthetic polyamine conjugates have been observed to play a myriad of important roles in a host of biological systems. There is thus a growing interest in polyamine conjugates. Bradely et al. [215] reported a library of 10 000 compounds related to N,N-bis(glutathionyl) spermidine following the immobilization of spermidine onto a solid support. Recently they have demonstrated solid phase synthesis of symmetrical sper-imine conjugates (Fig. 6) which opens up the area of solid phase spermine chemistry and library generation based on the symmetrical spermine scaffold [216].

Tetramic acid nucleus is found in many biologically active compounds such as antimicrobials and inhibitor of glycolic acid oxidase [217]. Mathews

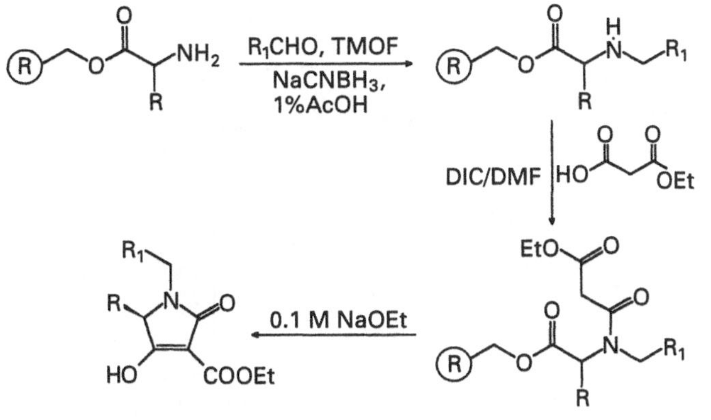

Scheme 27

et al. [218] reported a three-step solid phase synthesis of diverse libraries of 1,3,5-trisubstituted tetramic acid derivatives as depicted in Scheme 27.

7.7.2 Library based on lead structures

Combinatorial synthesis of small organic molecules have also been carried out from lead optimisation point of view. Based on the structure of captopril, a 500 member mercaptoacyl proline library (Scheme 28) was synthesized [219]. The screening resulted in the identification of a novel, highly potent ACE inhibitor analogue of captopril which was found to be about three times more potent than captopril.

Similarly a mini library comprising 24 hydroxystilbene derivatives has been synthesized by coupling hydroxybenzaldehyde and benzylphosphonate anions (Scheme 29). Screening of these compounds in a cell based estrogenic assay led to the identification of several analogues with IC_{50} in the range of 5–15 µM [220].

A library of 60 compounds and 600 phenolic compounds based on the structure of Lavendustin, a known inhibitor of tyrosinekinases has been reported by two groups independently [221, 222].

A modest library based on COX-1 inhibiting thiazolidinones [223] as lead structure has been synthesized and deconvoluted in the search for more

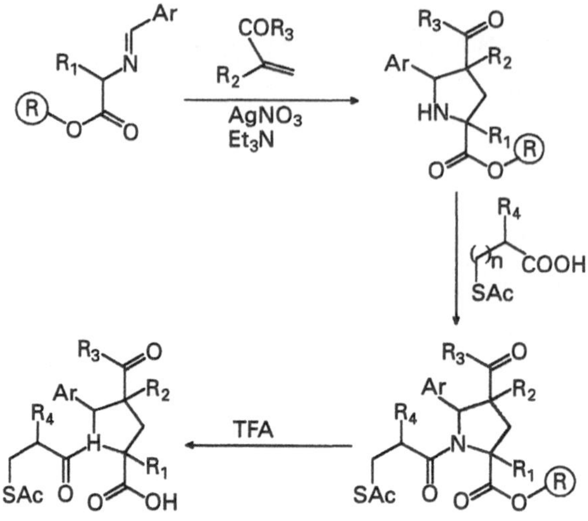

Scheme 28

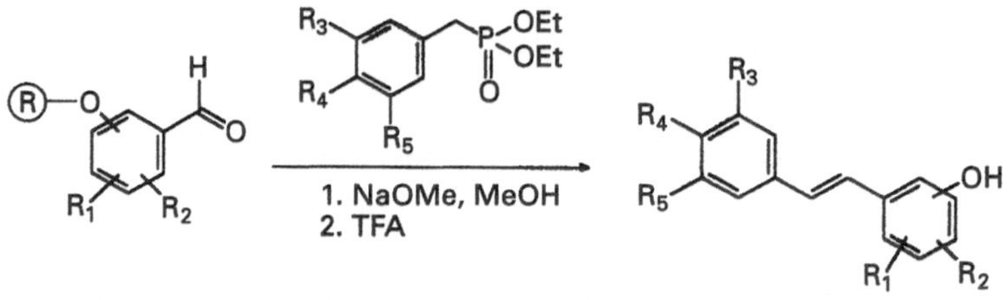

Scheme 29

potent analogues. The studies led to the identification of active compounds upon which the libraries were based.

The purine ring is a common structural element of a large number of agonists, antagonists and effectors that play key roles in many cellular processes. An example is Olomoucine which exhibits moderate inhibitory activity but good selectivity for the CDK/cyclin protein kinases. Schultz et al. [224] used combinatorial chemistry to increase the affinity and specificity of Olomoucine through the introduction of diversity at the 2,6 and 9 position of purine ring. Hence a method for the combinatorial synthesis of 2,9 substi-

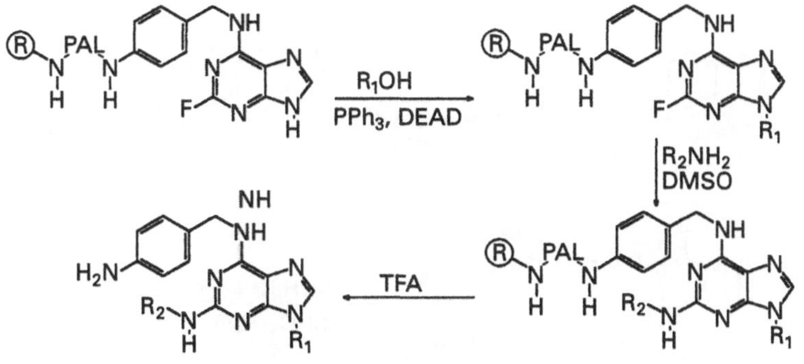

Scheme 30

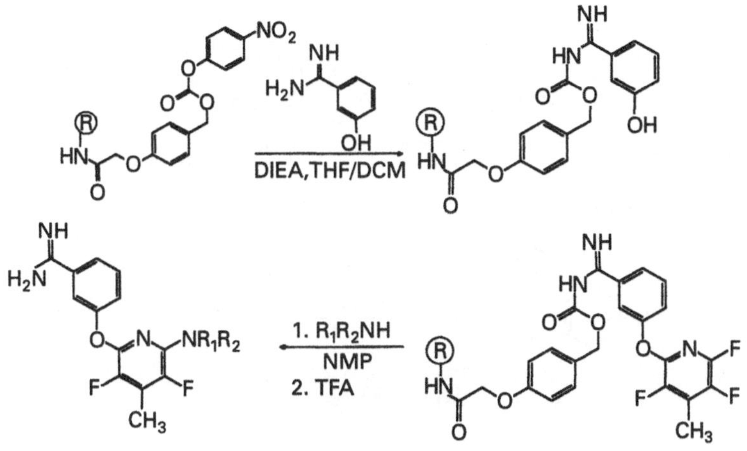

Scheme 31

tuted purines using a Mitsunobu reaction to alkylate the N-9 position and an amination reaction to install amine at c-2 position has been developed as shown in Scheme 30.

Based on the structure of biamidine ZK80563 [225], Mohan et al. [226] embarked upon a program to find a replacement for one of the benzamidine ring and accordingly generated a library of 400 N-substituted amidino-phenoxy pyridine analogues (Scheme 31). All compounds were assayed for their inhibiting activity against Fxa which led to the identification of two compounds with k_i values of 560 and 495 nM.

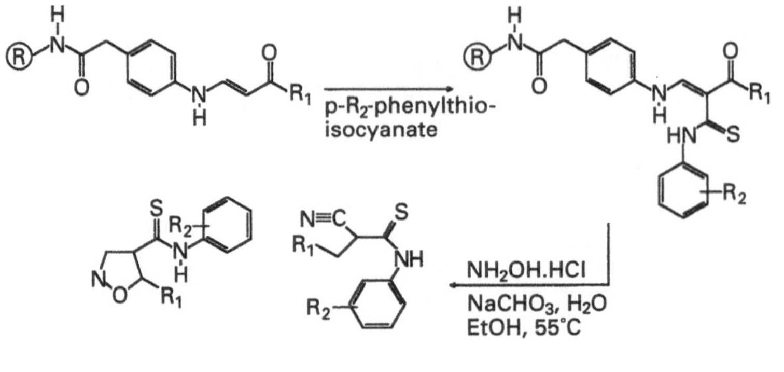

Scheme 32

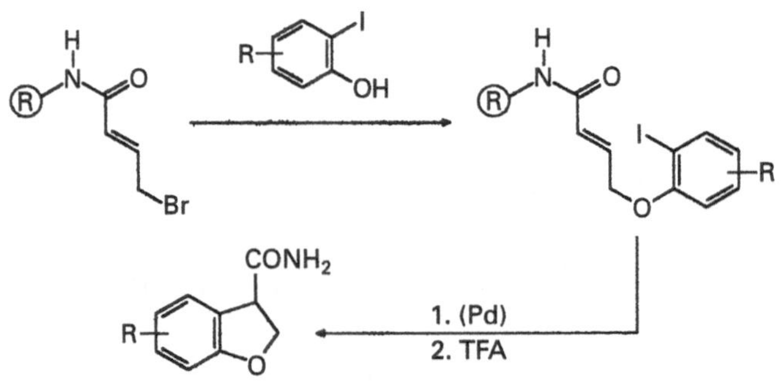

Scheme 33

Recently a library of thioamide derivatives of Leflunomide and its bioactive metabolite, a known immunosuppressant, have been synthesized on solid phase (Scheme 32). *In vitro* evaluation of these compounds demonstrated that the amide thioamide isologous substitution was detrimental of the biological activity [227].

Syntheses of benzofurans were carried out using the methodology developed earlier for solid phase indole formation. Alkylation of the substituted 2-iodophenol followed by palladium mediated intramolecular cyclisation afforded the desired benzofuran (Scheme 33) derivatives in excellent yields and purity [228]. Recently Marzanik and Felder [229] reported an elegant method for the combinatorial assembly of four different templates on the solid phase namely pyrimidines, dihydropyrimidines, pyridines and pyra-

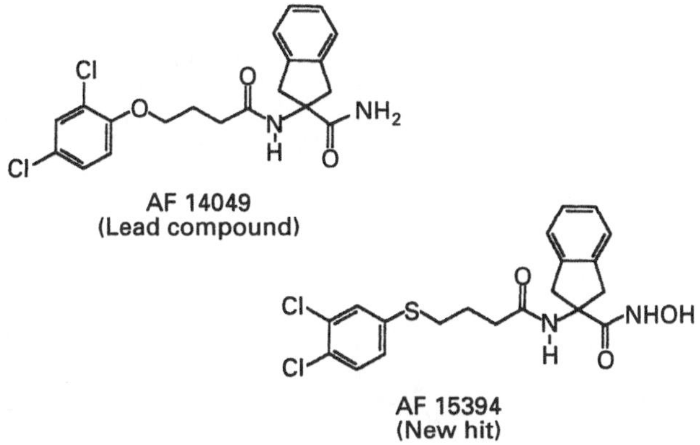

AF 14049
(Lead compound)

AF 15394
(New hit)

Fig. 7
Structure of PMI inhibitors with weal antifungal activity

zoles by using α,β unsaturated ketones as the key intermediate. Thus the method may find wide application for the efficient preparation of combinatorial small molecule libraries.

Substituted 2-amino and thiobenzimidazoles have proven to be important as drug leads in several drug discovery programmes and have relevance as antiarrhythmic and antiviral agents. A minilibrary of substituted 1-phenyl-2-methyl amino-benzimidazole and 2-methyl thiobenzimidazole [230] has been reported on solid phase in good yield.

Bhandari et al. [231] optimized the activity of PMI inhibitor AF 14049 by synthesizing combinatorial libraries of approximately 30 000 compounds which resulted in the identification of AF 15394 as a moderately selective PMI inhibitor with weak antifungal activity (Fig. 7).

7.7.3 Library of novel structures

Initial combinatorial libraries were based on drug like scaffolds or template. However, in recent years much emphasis has been given to searching for novel pharmacophores by synthesizing combinatorial libraries of novel structure rather than of known pharmacophores. These libraries may find application in the generation of new leads against various targets and will be

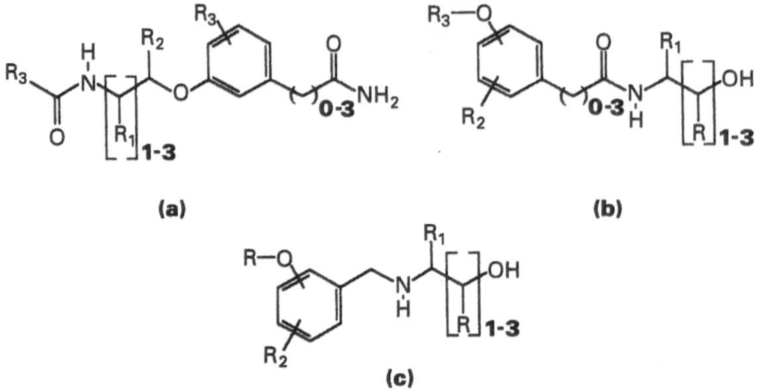

Fig. 8
Structure of libraries of novel prototypes

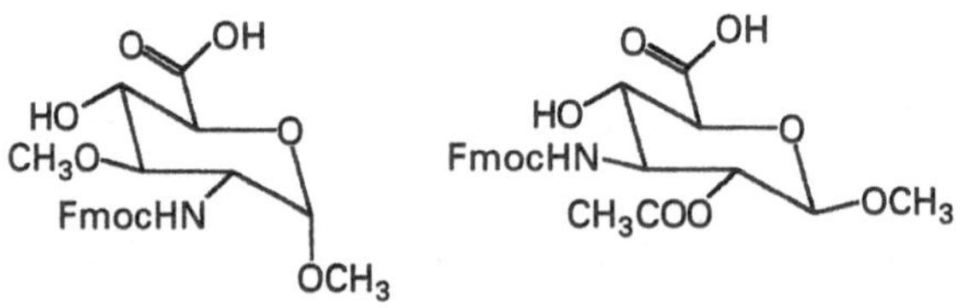

Fig. 9
Structure of monosaccharide scaffolds with three sites of diversification

reviewed next. Lebl et al. [232] designed and synthesized structurally heterogeneous libraries built of structurally unrelated bifunctional building blocks (Fig. 8). Polymer supported N-acylation, etherification, esterification, reduction amination and nucleophilic displacement have been carried out to synthesise several novel libraries. In three randomization steps, a complexity of 125 000 compounds has been generated.

Recently Sofia et al. reported [233] an elegant synthesis for carbohydrate-based universal pharmacophore mapping libraries as a new strategy for identifying novel receptor ligands. Two monosaccharide scaffolds with three sites of diversification (amino, carboxyl and hydroxyl functionality) were synthesized (Fig. 9). This was then followed by synthesis of 1648 member sublibraries using isocyanates, amino acids and carboxylic acids as building blocks.

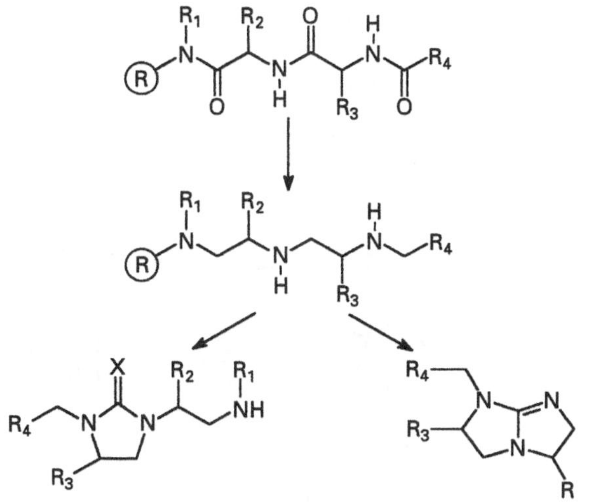

Fig. 10
Structure of libraries of heterocycles prepared from dipeptide precursors

7.7.4 Libraries from libraries

The concept was first demonstrated through the successful N-permethylation of hexapeptide combinatorial library [234]. Houghten has shown that it is possible chemically to transform the peptide libraries whilst they are still attached to the solid phase to give mixtures of novel nonpeptidic compounds. For example, a 10-fold excess of sodium hydride in dimethylsulfoxide followed by a 30-fold excess of methyl iodide was successful in converting peptides to their fully methylated derivatives. Recently this concept has been used for the preparation of hydantoins and cyclic ureas from dipeptide precursor [235–237]. Mixture based combinatorial libraries of both polyamines and bicyclic guanidines each having three positions of diversity and made up of more than 100 000 compounds have been synthesized (Fig. 10).

Out of the various libraries reported above some of them have been evaluated in a variety of *in vitro* assays and several lead compounds have been identified. Some of the lead compounds identified have been summarized in Table 4.

Table 4.
Leads identified from various libraries of small organic molecules

Name of library	Lead identified	Target/ligand	Ref.
Benzodiazepines		CCK ligand IC_{50} 80 nM	171
Benzodiazepines		Fluoronitrazepam inhibitor IC_{50} 21 nM	173
Thiazolidinones		COX-1 inhibitor IC_{50} 3.7 mM	223
Aminopurine Glycinamide		CDK2 ligand IC_{50} 0.6 µM	238
Dihydrobenzopyran		Carbonic anhydrase II activity K_D 15 nM	239
β-mercaptoacyl pyrolines		ACE inhibitor Ki 160 pM	219
Diketopiperazines		NK2 ligand IC_{50} 313 nM	180

Table 4. (continued)

Leads identified from various libraries of small organic molecules

Name of library	Lead identified	Target/ligand	Ref.
Dihydropyridines		Calcium channel blocker IC_{50} 18 nM	190
1,3 diols		Antioxidant ferricthiocyanate assay	240
Stilbenes		Estrogen ligand	220
Cinnamic acid		Phosphatae inhibitor IC_{50} 4 µM	241
Tetrahydroacridines		Acetylcholinestrase Ki 10 nM	242
Novel prototype		Thrombin inhibitor Ki 0.2 nM	243

8 Solid phase organic reactions

An increasing number of organic reactions are being demonstrated on the solid support. These reactions can be categorized into carbon-heteroatm bond forming reactions, carbon-carbon bond forming reactions, cycloadditions and multicomponent reactions etc. Much of the work pertaining to solid phase organic reactions developed over the years has been extensively reviewed by several authors [244–246] and are regularly updated on the internet (*www. 5z.com*). It will be out of the scope of this review to discuss all the solid phase organic reactions reported to date, however, for the convenience of the readers some interesting examples of solid phase reactions have been depicted in Table 5.

9 Software for combinatorial chemistry

Over the years computer software has come to play a very important role in combinatorial chemistry. These software packages help to construct desired libraries from the lists of selected monomers. In addition different databases are commercially available in which one can either find hundreds of thousands of compounds and their source or find information about the reactions by which the chemical transformations can be realised. Software is also available for the purpose of bookkeeping wherein one can store information pertaining to synthesis, analysis and activity profile in different test systems of hundreds of thousands of compounds prepared by combinatorial methods. Finally genetic algorithms have also been applied with success in the design and automated synthesis of combinatorial libraries [260]. The various commercially available and widely used software has been summarized in Table 6.

Beside this software computational methods have been developed that can emphasise diversity or similarity [261] in libraries. Using these methods one can design more "focussed" and "smart" libraries instead of synthesizing compounds *en masse* and screening them all. However, the efficacy of computational methods for custom combinatorial libraries has yet to be established.

Table 5.
Examples of solid phase organic reactions

Solid phase organic reactions	Reaction type	Ref.
	Friedal craft reaction	247
	Heck reaction	248
	Knoevenagel reaction	249
	Nucleophilic substitution reaction	250
	Suzuki reaction	251
	Aldol condensation	252

Table 5. (continued)
Examples of solid phase organic reactions

Solid phase organic reactions	Reaction type	Ref.
	Claisen Schmidt condensation	253
	Enamine formation	254
	Knoevenagel condensation	255
	Cycloaddition	212
	Diels-Alder reaction	256
	Dieckman cyclisation	257
	Reductive amination reaction	258

Table 6.
Various software packages available for combinatorial libraries

Databases	Library building softwares programme	Structure focussing
MDL ISIS, Chime	MDL Project Library and central library	R. Pearlman Diverse selectors
Tripos Unity	Tripos Legion	Tripos Selector
Oxford Molecular group	R. Pearlman combine DBMaker	Molecular simulations Cerices^2-Diversity
Cambridge software chem finder	Wave function spartan	
	OMG ChemDiverse	

10 Miniaturized systems for the synthesis of libraries

Beside rapid developments in the area of combinatorial chemistry, automation has also been the subject of immense interest. Several fully automatic as well as semiautomatic organic synthesisers have been developed and are now commercially available for the rapid synthesis of libraries based on either parallel format or combinatorial approach. These synthesisers are equipped with temperature-controlled reaction blocks having 24 to 96 reaction wells in an inert atmosphere. However, in recent years the focus has been more on the miniaturisation of the technique so as to keep the equipment size and reagent quantities to a minimum. Miniaturized combinatorial synthesisers have been developed that offer preparation and screening of over 30 000 discrete compounds. Another interesting and elegant synthesis involves a microfluidic chip-based system that can be used to carry out chemical reactions at sub-microliter volumes in 144-well arrays [262].

11 Conclusion

It is thus evident that combinatorial chemistry has become an integral part of drug discovery process. Several libraries of drug-like molecules as well as of novel structures have been published. In addition many advances continue to be made in the synthesis of small molecule libraries on solid support.

Bijoy Kundu, Sanjay K. Khare and Shiva K. Rastogi

Combinatorial optimization based on computational methods is also being developed in order to restrict the large size of libraries to smart, small-sized libraries having both diversity as well as adequate representation of useful subgroups. The field continues to grow exponentially and with serious commitment from drug companies world-wide, in coming years one can look forward to the emergence of numerous new leads and drug candidates from combinatorial chemistry.

References

1   S.J. Rhodes and R.C. Smith: Drug Dis. Today *3*, 361 (1998).

2   H.M. Geysen, R.H. Meloen and S.J. Barteling: Proc. Natl. Acad. Sci. USA *81*, 3498 (1984).

3   R.A. Houghten: Proc. Natl. Acad. Sci. USA *82*, 5131 (1985).

4   R.A. Houghten, C. Pinilla, S.E. Blondelle, J.R. Appel, C.T. Dooley and J.H. Cusrvo: Nature *354* 84 (1991).

5   Furka, F. Sebestyen, M. Asgedom and G. Dibo: Int. J. Peptide Protein Res. *37*, 487 (1991).

6   K.S. Lam, S.E. Salmon, E.M. Hersh, V.J. Hruby, W.M. Kazmiersky and R.J. Knapp: Nature *354*, 82 (1991)

7   C.Minganti, K.N. Ganesh, B.S. Sproat and M.J. Gait: Anal. Biochem. *147*, 63 (1985)

8   N.K. Bhaskar, B.W. King, P. Meyers and J.P. Wetlake, in: R. Epton (ed.): Innovation and Perspective in Solid Phase Synthesis, 3rd International Symposium. Mayflower Worldwide, Birmingham, U.K. 1994, 451.

9   E. Bayer and W. Rapp: Chem. Pept. Proteins *2*, 3 (1986)

10   E. Bayer: US patent 4908 405, (1990).

11   S. Zalipsky, F. Albericio and G. Barany, in: V.J. Hruby, C.N. Deber and K.D. Kopple (eds.): Peptides: Structure and Function (Proc. of IXth Am. Pept. Symp) Pierce Chemical Co., Rockford, USA 1985, 257–260.

12   M. Renil and M. Meldal: Tet. Lett. *33*, 4647 (1995).

13   B.P. Zhao, G.B. Panigrahi, P.D. Sadowski and J.J. Kreprinsky: Tet. Lett. *37*, 3093 (1996).

14   E. Atherton, E. Brown, R.C. Sheppard and A. Rosevear: J. Chem. Soc. Chem. Commun. *1151* (1981).

15   L. Winther, C.S. Nielsen, W.B. Pedersen and R.H. Berg: Peptides 1994, 23rd European Peptide Symposium, Braga, Portugal, Sept. 4–10 (1994).

16   R. Frank and R. Doring: Tetrahedron *44*, 6031 (1988).

17   S.Butz, S. Rawer, W. Rapp and U. Birsener: Peptide Res. *7*, 20 (1994).

18   B.F. McGainness, S.A. Kates, G.W. Griffin, L.W. Herman, N.A. Sale, J. Vagner, F. Alberico and G. Barany, in: P.T.P. Kaumaya and R.S. Hodges (eds.): Peptides (Proc. 14th Am. Kept. Symp.) Mayflower Worldwide, Birmingham, U.K. 1996, 125–126.

19   ArgoGel is a product of Argonaut Technologies Inc.

20   H.V. Heyers, G.J. Dilley, T.L. Durgin, T.S. Powers, N.A. Winssinger, H. Zhu and M.R. Pavia: Mol. Diversity *1*, 13 (1995).

21   R.E. Epton, D.A. Wellings and A. Williams: React. Polym. *6*, 143 (1987).

22   R.B. Wang: J. Amer. Chem. Sci. *95*, 1328 (1972).

23   M. Mergler, R. Tanner, J. Gosteli and P. Grogg: Tet. Lett. *29*, 4005 (1988).

24   K. Barlos, D. Gatos, S. Kapolos, G. Paphotin, W. Schafer and Y. Wen Ging: Tet. Lett. *30*, 3947 (1989)

25   A.R. Mitcehll, B.W. Wrickson, M.N. Raybtsev, R.S. Hodges and R.B. Merrifield: J. Amer. Chem. Sci. *98*, 7357 (1976).

26   H. Rink: Tet. Lett. *28*, 3787 (1987).

27   J. Tam, R.D. DiMarchi and R.B. Merrifield: Tet. Lett. *22*, 2851 (1981).

28   P. Sieber: Tet. Lett. *28*, 2107 (1987).

29   F. Albericio, E. Giralt and R. Eritja: Tet. Lett. *32*, 1515 (1991).

30   J.W. Apsimon and D.M. Dixit: Synth. Commun. *12*, 113 (1982).

31   R. Ramage, C.A. Barron, S. Bielecki and D.W. Thomas: Tet. Lett. *28*, 4105 (1987).

32   F.S. Tjoeng and G.A. Heavner: J. Org. Chem. *48*, 355 (1983).

33   R.P. Hammer, F. Albericio, E. Giralt and G. Barany: Int. J. Pept. Protein Res. *28*, 31 (1990).

34   A product of Affymax Research Institute.

35   D. Bellof: Chimia *39*, 10 (1985).

36   B.J. Backes and J.A. Ellamn: J. Am. Chem. Soc. *116*, 11171 (1994).

37   B. Sauerbrei, V. Jungmann and H. Waldmann: Angew. Chem. Intl. Engl. *37*, 1143 (1998).

38   C.W. Phoon, S.F. Oliver and C. Abell: Tet. Lett. *39*, 7959 (1998).

39   K.G. Estep, C.E. Neipp, L.M.S. Stramiello, M.D. Adam, M.P. Allen, S. Robinson and E.J. Roskamp: J. Org. Chem. *63*, 5300 (1998).

40   J.A. Josey, C.A. Tarlton and C.E. Payne: Tet. Lett. *39*, 5899 (1998).

41   J.A. Fehrentz, M. Paris, A. Heitz, J. Velek, C.F. Liu, F. Winternitz and J. Martinez: Tet. Lett. *36*, 7871 (1995).

42   S. Hiffman and K. Frank: Tet. Lett. *35*, 7763 (1994).

43   P. Kocis, V. Krchnak and M. Lebl: Tet. Lett. *34*, 7251(1993).

44   G. Bhalay and R.A. Dunstan: Tet. Lett. *39*, 7803 (1998).

45   M.A. Seialdone, S.W. Shuey, P. Sauper, Y. Hamuro and D.M. Burns: J. Org. Chem. *63*, 4803 (1998).

46   B.A. Dressman, U. Singh and S.W. Kaldor: Tet. Lett. *39*, 3631 (1998).

47   K.H. Bleichor and J.R. Wareing: Tet. Lett. *39*, 4587 (1998)

48   K.H. Bleichor, J.R. Wareing: Tet. Lett. *39*, 4591 (1998).

49   A.M. Aronov and M.H. Gelb: Tet. Lett. *39*, 4947 (1998).

50   K.A. Beaver, A.C. Siegmund and K.L. Spear: Tet. Lett. *37*, 1145 (1996).

51   B.A. Dressman, L.A. Spangle and S.W. Kaldor: Tet. Lett. *37*, 937 (1996).

52   L.A. Thompson and J.A. Ellman: Tet. Lett. *35*, 9333 (1994).

53   J.Eichler and R.A. Houghten: Biochemistry *32*, 11035 (1993).

54   J.A. Buettner, D. Hudson, C.R. Johnson, M.J. Ross and K. Shoemaker, in: R. Epton (ed.): Innovations and Perspectives in Solid Phase Synthesis: Peptides, Proteins and Nucleic Acids. Mayflower Worldwide Ltd., Birmingham, U.K. 1994, 169–174.

55   A. Kramer, R. Valkmer-Engert, R. Malin, U. Reineke and J. Schneider-Mergener: Peptide Res. *6*, 314 (1993).

56   A. Quesnel, A. Delmas and Y. Trudelle: Anal. Biochem. *231*, 182 (1995).

57   N.J. Mayi, A.M. Bray and H.M. Geysen: J. Immunol. Methods *134*, 23 (1990).

58   J.-X. Wang, A.M. Bray, A.J. Dipasquals, N.J. Maeji and H.M. Geysen: Bioorg. Med. Chem. Lett. *3*, 447 (1993).

59   D.C. Spellmeyer, S. Brown, G.B. Stauber, H.M. Geysen and R. Valerio: Bioorg. Med. Chem. Lett. *3*, 519 (1993).

60   M. Bastos, N.J. Maeji and R.H. Abeles: Proc. Natl. Acad. Sci. USA *92*, 6738 (1995).

61   A.M. Bray, D.S. Chiefari, R.M. Valerio and N.J. Maeji: Tet. Lett. *36*, 5081 (1995).

62   D.H. Drewry, S.W. Gerritz and J.A. Linn: Tet. Lett. *38*, 3377 (1997).

63   S.P.A. Fodor, J.L. Read, M.C. Purung, L. Stryer, A.T. Lu and D. Salas: Science *251*, 767 (1991).

64   S.P.A. Fodor, R.P. Rava, X.C. Huang, A.C. Pease, C.P. Holmes and C.L. Adams: Nature *364*, 555 (1993).

65   C.P. Holmes, C.L. Adams, L.M. Kochersperger, R.B. Mortensen and L.A. Aldwin: Biopolym. Pept. Sci. Sect. *37*, 199 (1995).

66   R. Frank: Tetrahedron *48*, 9217 (1992).

67   W. Tegge, R. Frank, F. Hofmann and W.R.G. Dostmann: Biochemistry *34*, 10569 (1995).

68   R. Frank: J. Biotechnol. *41*, 259 (1995).

69   M.R. Pavia, M.P. Cohen, G.J. Dilley, G.R. Dubuc, T.L. Durgin, F.W. Forman, M.E. Hediger, G. Milat, T.S. Powers, I. Sucholeiki et al.: Bioorg. Med. Chem. *4*, 659 (1996).

70   J. Neilsen, F.R. Jensen: Tet. Lett. *38*, 2011 (1997).

71   R.A. Houghten: Gene *137*, 7 (1993).

72   C.K. Jayawickreme, G.F. Graminski, J.M. Quillan and M.R. Lerner: Proc. Natl. Acad. Sci. USA *91*, 1614 (1994).

73   S.E. Salmon, R.H. Liu-Stevens, Y. Zhao, M. Lebl, V. Krchnak, K. Werlman, N. Sepetav and K.S. Lam: Mol. Div. *2*, 57 (1996).

74   Z. Yuan: High Density Assay Formats for Screening Large Combinatorial Chemical Libraries. Society for Biomolecular Screening 2nd Annual Conference, Basel, Switzerland, Oct. 14–17 (1996).

75   X. Chang, R. Chen, J.E. Bruce, B.L. Schwartz, G.A. Anderson, S.A. Hofstadler, D.C. Gale, R.D. Smith, J. Gao, G.B. Sigal et al.: J. Amer. Chem. Soc. *117*, 8859 (1995).

76   K.S. Lam, V.J. Hruby, M. Lebl, R.J. Knapp, W.M. Kazimierski, E.M. Hersh and S.E. Salmon: Bioorg. Med. Chem. Lett. *3*, 419 (1993).

77   K.S. Lam, M. Lebl, V. Krchnak, S. Wade, F. Abdul-Latif, R. Ferguson, C. Cuzzocera and K. Wertman: Gene *137*, 13 (1993).

78   M. Lebl, M. Patek, P. Kocis, V. Krchnak, V.J. Hruby, S.E. Salmon and K.S. Lam: Int. J. Peptide Protein Res. *41*, 301 (1993).

79   P. Koces, V. Krchnak and M. Lebl: Tet. Lett. *34*, 7251 (1993).

80   C. Pinilla, J.R. Appel and R.A. Houghten: Gene *128*, 71 (1993).

81   C.T. Dooley, N.N. Chung, P.W. Schiller and R.A. Houghten: Proc. Natl. Acad. Sci. USA *90*, 10811 (1993).

82   S.E. Blondelle and R.A. Houghten: Ann. Rep. Med. Chem. *27*, 159 (1992).

83   C.Pinilla, J.R. Appel, P. Blanc and R.A. Hoghten: Biotechniques *13*, 901 (1992).

84   M.C. Pirrung and J. Chen: J. Am. Chem. Soc. *117*, 1240 (1995).

85   B. Deprez, X. Williard, L. Bourel, H. Coste, F. Hyafil and A. Tartar: J. Am. Chem. Soc. *117*, 5405 (1995).

86   E. Erb, K.D. Janda and S. Brenner: Proc. Natl. Acad. Sci. USA *91*, 11422 (1994).

87   V. Nikolaiev, A. Stierandova, V. Krchnak, B. Seligmann, K.S. Lam, S.E. Salmon and M. Lebl: Peptide Res. *6*, 161 (1993).

88   S. Berner and R.A. Lerner: Proc. Natl. Acad. Sci. USA *89*, 5381 (1995).

89   M.C. Needels, D.G. Jones, E.H. Tate, G.L. Heinkel, L.M. Kochersperger, W.J. Dower, R.W. Barrett and M.A. Gallap: Proc. Natl. Acad. Sci. USA *90*, 10700 (1993).

90   M.H.J. Ohlmeyer, R.N. Swanson, L.W. Dillard, J.C. Reader, G. Asouline, R. Kabayashi, M. Wigler and W.C. Still: Proc. Natl. Acad. Sci. USA *90*, 10922 (1993).

91   H.P. Nestler, P.A. Batlett and W.C. Still: J. Org. Chem. *59*, 4723 (1994).

92   Z. Ni, D. Maclean, C.P. Holmes, M.M. Murphy, B. Ruhland, J.W. Jacobs, E.M. Gordon and M.A. Gallop: J. Med. Chem. *39*, 1601 (1996).

93   K.C. Nicolaou, X.Y. Ziao, Z. Parandosh, A. Senyei and M.P. Nova: Angew. Chem. Int. Ed. Engl. *34*, 2289 (1995).

94   R.W. Armstrong, P.A. Tempest, J.F. Cargil: Chimia *50*, 258 (1996).

95   E.J. Moran, S. Sarshar, J.F. Cargil, M.M. Shahbaz, A. Lio, A.M.M. Mjalli and R.W. Armstrong: J. Am. Chem. Soc. *117*, 10787 (1995).

96   V.K. Sarin, S.B.H. Kent, J.P. Tam and R.B. Merrifield: Anal. Biochem. *117*, 147 (1981).

97   B. Gisin: Analytical Chimie *58*, 248 (1972).

98   V. Krchnak, J. Vagner, P. Safar and M. Lebl: Czech. Chem. Comm. *53*, 2542 (1988).

99   W.S. Hancock and J.E. Battersby: Anal. Biochem. *71*, 260 (1976).

100   G.L. Ellman: Arch. Biochem. Biophys. *82*, 70 (1959).

101   Z. Ni, D. Maclean, C.P. Holmes, M.M. Murphy, B. Ruhland, J.W. Jacobs, E.M.Gordon and M.A. Gallop: J. Med. Chem. *39*, 1601 (1996).

102   M.H. Caruthers, A.D. Barone, S.L. Beaucage, D.R. Dodds, E.F. Fisher, L.J. McBride, M. Matteucci, Z. Stabinsky and J.-Y. Tang: Methods in Enzymology *154*, 287 (1987).

103   D.A. Campbell and J.C. Bermak: J. Amer. Chem. Soc. *116*, 6039 (1994).

104   G.B. Fields and R.L. Noble: Int. J. Pept. Protein Res. *35*, 161 (1990).

105   S. Kobayashi, I. Hachiya, S. Suzuki and M. Moriwaki: Tet. Lett. *37*, 2809 (1996).

106   J.M.J. Frechet: Tetrahedron *37*, 663 (1981).

107   H.N. Weller, M.G. Young, S.J. Michalczyk, G.H. Reitnauer, R.S. Cooley, P.C. Rahn, D.J. Loyd, D. Fiore and S.J. Fischman: Mol. Div. 3, 61 (1997).

108   L. Schultz, C.D. Garr, L.M. Cameron, J. Bukowski: Bioorg. Med. Chem. Lett. *8*, 2409 (1998).

109   B.A. Dressman, L.A. Spangle, S.W. Kaldor: Tet. Lett. *37*, 937 (1996).

110   G.C. Look, C.P. Holmes, J.P. Chin and M.A. Gallop: J. Org. Chem. *59*, 7588 (1994).

111   M.M. Murphy, J.R. Schullek, E.M. Gordon and M.A. Gallop: J. Am. Chem. Soc. *117*, 7029 (1995).

112   C.P. Holmes, J.P. Chinn, G.C. Look, E.M. Gordon and N.A. Gallop: J. Org. Chem. *60*, 7328 (1995).

113   C.R. Johnson and B. Zhang: Tet. Lett. *36*, 9253 (1995).

114   W.L. Fitch, G. Detre, C.P. Holmes, J.N. Shoalery and P.A. Keefer: J. Org. Chem. *59*, 7955 (1994).

115   R.C. Anderson, M.A. Jarema, M.J. Shapiro, J.P. Stakes and M. Zilox: J. Org. Chem. *59*, 7955 (1995).

116   K.D. Moeller, C.E. Hanau and A. Darignon: Tet. Lett. *35*, 825 (1994).

117   R.C. Anderson, J.P. Stakes and M.J. Shapiro: Tet. Lett. *36*, 5311 (1995).

118   A. Svensson, K.E. Bergquist, T. Fex and J. Kihlberg: Tet. Lett. *39*, 7193 (1998).

119   M.J. Shapiro and J.R. Wareing: Curr. Opin. Chem. Biol. *2*, 372 (1998).

120   C.L. Brummel, J.C. Vickerman, S.A. Carr, M.E. Hemling, G.D. Roberts, W. Johnson, J. Weinstock, D. Gaitanopoulos, S.J. Benkovic and N. Winograd: Anal. Chem. *68*, 273 (1996).

121   N.J. Haskins, D.J. Huntr, A.J. Organ, S.S. Rahman and C. Thom: Rapid Commun. Mass Spectrom. *9*, 1437 (1995).

122   B.J. Egner, G.J. Langley and M. Bradley: J. Org. Chem. *60*, 2652 (1995).

123   B.J. Egner, M. Cardeno and M. Bradley: J. Chem. Soc. Chem. Comm. 2163 (1995).

124   R.A. Zambias, D.A. Boulton and P.R. Griffin: Tet. Lett. *35*, 4283 (1994).

125   C.X. Chen, L.A.A. Randall, R.B. Miller, A.D. Jones and M.J. Kurth: J. Am. Chem. Soc. *116*, 2661 (1994).

126   D.W. Gordon and J. Stelle: Bioorg. Med. Chem. Lett. *5*, 47 (1995).

127   M. Stankova, S. Wade, K.S. Lam and N. Lebl: Peptide Res. *7*, 292 (1994).

128   T. Wang, L. Zeng, T. Strader, L. Burton and D.B. Kassel: Rapid Commun. Mass Spectrom. *12*, 1123 (1998).

129   D.C. Tutko, K.D. Henry, B.E. Winger, H. Stout and M. Hemling: Rapid Commun. Mass Spectrom. *12*, 335 (1998).

130   R.A. Houghten, J.R. Appel, S.E. Blandelle, J.H. Cuervo, C.T. Dooley and C. Pinilla: Biotechniques *13*, 412 (1992).

131   R.A. Houghten and C.T. Dooley: Bioorg. Med. Chem. Lett. *3*, 405 (1992).

132   J. Eichler and R.A. Houghten: Biochemistry *32*, 11035 (1993).

133   R.A. Houghten and C.T. Dooley: Bioorg. Med. Chem. Lett. *3*, 405 (1993).

134   J. Eichler, J.R. Appel, S.E. Blondelle, C.T. Dooley, B. Doerner, J.M. Estresh, E. Perez-Paya, C. Pinilla and R.A. Houghten: Med. Res. Rev. *15*, 481 (1995).

135   J. Eicher and R.A. Houghten: Mol. Med. Today *7*, 174 (1995).

136   S.E. Blondelle, E. Perez-Paya, C.T. Dooley, C. Pinilla and R.A. Houghten: Trends Anal. Chem. *14*, 83 (1995).

137   S.E. Blondelle, L.R. Simpkins, R.A. Houghten: in: C.H. Schneider and A.N. Eberle (eds): Proc. of the 22nd European Peptide Symposium, Escom Leiden 1993, 761.

138   R.A.P. Lutzke, N.A. Eppens, P.A. Weber, R.A. Houghten and R.H.A. Plasterk: Proc. Natl. Acad. Sci. USA *92*, 11456 (1995).

139   C.T. Dooley, N.N. Chung, B.C. Wilkes, P.W. Scheller, J.M. Bidlack, G.W. Pasternak and R.A. Houghten: Science *266*, 2019 (1994).

140   G. Ferry, J.A. Boutin, G. Atassi, J-L. Fauchere and G.C. Tucker: Mol. Div. *2*, 135 (1996).

141   J. Jiracek, A. Yiotakis, B. Vincent, A. Lecoq, A. Nicolaou, F. Checler and V. Dive: J. Biol. Chem. *270*, 21701 (1995).

142   S.E. Blondelle, E. Takahashi, P.A. Weber and R.A. Houghten: Antimicrob. Agents Chemother. *38*, 2280 (1994).

143   R.A. Owens, P.D. Gesellchen, B.J. Houchins and R.D. DiMarchi: Biochem. Biophys. Res. Comm. *181*, 402 (1991).

144   G. Kapel, C. Dodds, B. Houchins, D. Hunden, D. Johnson, R. Owens, M. Chaney, T. Usden, B. Hoffman and M. Brownstein: *Chem. Biol.* 2, 483 (1995).

145   C.L. Chen, P. Strop, M. Lebl, K.S. Lam: Combinatorial Chem. *267*, 211 (1996).

146   K.H. Wiesmuller, S. Feiertag, B. Fleckenstein, S. Kienle, D. Stall, M. Herrman and G. Jung, in: G. Jung (ed.): Combinatorial Peptides and Nonpeptide Libraries. VCH Weinheim, Germany 1996, 204.

147   B. Kundu, M. Bauser, J, Betschinger, W. Kraas and G. Jung: Bioorg. Med. Chem. Lett. *8*, 1669 (1998).

148   S. Sasaki, M. Takagi, Y. Tanaka and M. Maeda: Tet. Lett. *37*, 85 (1996).

149   X. Zang, Z. Yu and Y-H Chu: Bioorg. Med. Chem. Lett. *8*, 2327 (1998).

150   M. Davies, M. Bonnat, F. Guillier, J.D. Kilburn and M. Bradley: J. Org. Chem. *63*, 8696 (1998).

151   C.G. Bradshaw, A.R. Chollet and T.N.C. Wells, in: C.H. Schneider and A.N. Eberle (eds):

Peptides: Proc of the 22nd Eur. Peptide Symposium, ESOM, Leiden, The Netherlands 1993, 318.

152   A. Krammer, A. Schuster, U. Reincke, R. Malin, R. Volkmer-Engert, C. Landgraf and J. Schneider-Mergner: Methods of Enzymol 6, 338 (1994).

153   C. Darlak, P. Romanovskis and A.F. Aspatola, in: R.S. Hodges and J.A. Smith (eds.): Peptide: Chemistry, Structure and Biology, ESCOM, Leiden, The Netherlands 1994, 981–983.

154   J.D. McBride, N. Freeman, G.J. Domingo and R.I. Leatherbarrow: J. Mol. Div. 2, 819 (1996).

155   A.F. Spatola and P. Romanovskis, in: G. Jung (ed.): Combinatorial Peptide and Nonpeptide Libraries. VCH, Weinheim, Germany 1996, 327–347.

156   S.E. Salmon, K.S. Lam, M. Lebl, A. Kandola, P.S. Khattri, S. Wade, M. Patek, P. Kocis, V. Krchnak, D. Thrope et al: Proc. Natl. Acad. Sci. USA 90, 11708 (1993).

157   J. Eichler, A.W. Lucka, C. Pinilla and R.A. Hoghten: Mol. Div. 1, 233 (1995).

158   N.K. Terrett, D. Bojanic, D. Brown, P.J. Bungay, M. Gardner, D.W. Gordon, C.J. Mayers and J. Steele: Bioorg. Med. Chem. Lett. 5, 917 (1995).

159   D.A. Campell, J.C. Bermak, T.S. Burkath and D.V. Patel: J. Am. Chem. Soc. 177, 5381 (1995).

160   A.P. Combs, T.H. Kapoor, S. Feng, J.K. Chen, L.F. Daudeshaw and S.L. Schreiber: J. Am. Chem. Soc. 118, 287 (1996).

161   P.W. Davis, T.A. Vickers, L. Wilson-Lingardo, J.R. Wyatt, C.J. Guinosso, Y.S. Sanghvi, E.A. DeBae, O.L. Acevedo, P.D. Coak and D.J. Ecker: J. Med. Chem. 38, 4363 (1996).

162   A.A. Virgillo and J.A. Ellman: J. Am. Chem. Soc. 116, 11580 (1994).

163   R.J. Simon, R.S. Kania, R.N. Zuckermann, V.D. Haebner, D.A. Jewell, S. Banville, S. Ng, L. Wang, S. Rosenberg, C.K. Harlowe et al: Proc. Natl. Acad. Sci. USA 89, 9367 (1992).

164   R.N. Zuckerman, J.M. Kerr, S.B.H. Kent and W.H. Moos: J. Am. Chem. Soc. 114, 10646 (1992).

165   R.N. Zuckerman, E.J. Martin, D.C. Spellmeyer, G.B. Stauber, K.R. Shoemaker, J.M. Kerr, G.M. Figlirzzi, D.A. Goff, M.A. Saini, R.J. Simon et al: J. Med. Chem. 37, 2678 (1994).

166   D.A. Campbell, J.C. Bermak: J. Org. Chem. 59, 658 (1994).

167   L. Revesz, F. Bonne, U. Manning and J-F. Zuber: Bioorg. Med. Chem. Lett. 8, 405 (1998).

168   K. Burgess, D.S. Linthicum and H. Shen: Angew. Chem. Int. Ed. 34, 907 (1995).

169   J.M. Kim, Y. Bi, S.J. Paikoff and P.G. Schultz: Tet. Lett. 37, 5305 (1997).

170   B.A. Bunin and J.A. Ellman: J. Am. Chem. Soc. 114, 10997 (1996).

171   B.A. Bunin, J.A. Ellman and N.J. Plunkett: Proc. Natl. Acad. Sci. USA 91, 4708 (1994).

172   N.J. Plunkett and J.A. Ellman: J. Am. Chem. Soc. 117, 3306 (1995).

173   S.H. Dewitt, J.S. Kiely, J.S. Stankovic, M.C. Schroeder, D.M.R. Cody and M.R. Pavia: Proc. Natl. Acad. Sci. USA 90, 6909 (1993).

174   C.G. Boojamra, K.M. Burow and J.A. Ellman: J. Org. Chem. 50, 5742 (1995).

175   G.Bhalay, P. Blaney, V.H. Palmer and A.D. Baxter: Tet. Lett. 38, 8375 (1997).

176   S.H. Dewitt, J.S. Kiley, C.J. Stankovic, Schrredar, D.M.R. Cody and M.R. Pavia: Proc. Natl. Acad. Sci. USA 90, 6909 (1993).

177   B.Dressman, L. Spangle and S. Kalder: Tet. Lett. 37, 937 (1996).

178   S.W. Kim, S.Y. Ahn, J.S. Kah, J.H. Lee, S. Ro and H.Y. Cho: Tet. Lett. 38, 4603 (1997).

179   A.K. Szardenings and T.S. Burkoth: Tetrahedron 53, 6573 (1997).

180   D. Gordon and J. Stelle: Bioorg. Med. Chem. Lett. 5, 47 (1995).

181   J. Kowalski and M. Lipton: Tet. Lett. 37, 5839 (1996).

182   V. Krchnak, A.S. Weichsel, D. Cabel and M. Lebl, in: I.M.Chaiken and K.D. Janda (eds):

Molecular Diversity and Combinatorial Chemistry: Libraries and Drug Discovery. American Chemical Soc., Washington, DC 1996, 99–117.

183 B.O. Scatt, A.C. Siegmund, C.K. Marlowe, Y. Pci and K.L. Spear: Mol Diversity *1*, 125 (1995).

184 A.K. Szardenings, T.S. Burkoth, H.H. Lu, D.W. Tein and D.A. Campbell: Tetrahedron *53*, 6573, 1997.

185 S.N. Dankwardt, R.N. Sherry and J.L. Krstenansky: Tet. Lett. *36*, 4923 (1995).

186 G.A. Morales, J.W. Corbett and W.F. Degrado: J. Org. Chem. *63*, 1172 (1998).

187 T. Vojkovsky, A. Weichsel and M. Patek: J. Org. Chem. *63*, 3162 (1998).

188 D.Gaff and R. Zuckerman: Tet. Lett. *37*, 6247 (1996).

189 M.F. Gordecv, D.V. Patel and E.M. Gordon: J. Org. Chem. *61*, 924 (1996).

190 M.F. Gordecv, D.V. Patel, J. Wu and E.M. Gordon: Tet. Lett. *37*, 4643 (1996).

191 T. Godfraind, R. Miller and M. Wibo: Pharmaceut. Rev. *38*, 321 (1986).

192 P.Wipf and A. Cunningham: Tet. Lett. *36*, 7819 (1996).

193 S.A. Kolodziej and B.C. Hamper: Tet. Lett. *37*, 5277, (1996).

194 C.L. Hetet, M. David, F. Correaux, B. Carboni and A. Sauleau: Tet. Lett. *38*, 5153 (1997).

195 K.M. Short and A.M.M. Majalli: Tet. Lett. *38*, 359 (1997).

196 B.O. Scott, A.C. Siegmund, C.K. Marlowe, Y. Pei and K.L. Spear: Mol. Div. *1*, 125, (1995).

197 A.K. Sardenings, T.S. Burkoth, H.H. Lu, D.W. Tien and D.A. Campbell: Tetrahedron *53*, 6573 (1997).

198 K. Kaljuste and A. Cenden: Tet. Lett. *36*, 9211 (1995).

199 J.P. Mayer, D. Bankitis-Davis, J. Zhang, G. Beaton, K. Bjergarde, C.H. Anderson, B.A. Goodman and C.J. Herrea: Tet. Lett. *37*, 5633 (1996).

200 L. Yang and L. Guo: Tet. Lett. *37*, 5041 (1996).

201 M.C. Griffith, C.T. Dooley, R.A. Houghton and J.S. Kiely, in: I.M.Chaiken and K.D. Janda (eds.): Molecular Diversity and Combinatorial Chemistry: Libraries and Drug Discovery. American Chemical Soc., Washington, DC 1996, 50–57.

202 W.D.F. Meutormans and P.F. Alewood: Tet. Lett. *36*, 7769 (1995).

203 A.A. Mac, S.H. Dewitt, E.M. Hogan and R. Ramage: Tet. Lett. *37*, 4815 (1996).

204 D.A. Gaff and R.N. Zukcermann: J. Org. Chem. *60*, 5748 (1995).

205 A. Gopalsamy and P.V. Pallai: Tet. Lett. *38*, 907, 1997.

206 O. Doebner: Chem. Ber. *16*, 2357 (1983).

207 Y. Pei, R.A. Houghten and J.S. Kiely: Tet. Lett. *38*, 3349 (1997).

208 M.F. Gordeev, H.C. Hui, E.M. Gordon and D.V. Patel: Tet. Lett. *38*, 1729 (1997).

209 A.L. Marzinzik and E. R. Felder: Tet. Lett. *37*, 1003 (1996).

210 S. Sarshar, D. Diev and A.M.M. Mjalli: Tet. Lett. *37*, 1003 (1996).

211 M.T. Blodeau and A.M. Cunningham: J. Org. Chem. *63*, 2000 (1998).

212 B. Ruhland, A. Bhandari, E.M. Gordon and M.A. Gallop: J. Am. Chem. Soc. *118*, 253 (1996).

213 W. Yun and R. Mohan: Tet. Lett. *37*, 7189 (1996).

214 H.C. Zang, K.K. Brumfield and B.E. Maryanoff: Tet. Lett. *38*, 2439, (1997).

215 I.R. Marsh, H. Smith, C.L. Lablanc and M. Bradley: Mol. Div. *2*, 165 (1996).

216 P. Page, S. Burrage, L. Baldock and M. Bradley: Bioorg. Med. Chem. Lett. *8*, 1751 (1998).

217 C.S. Rooney, W.C. Randall, K.B. Streeter, C. Ziegler, E.J. Cragoe, H. Schwam, S.R. Michelson: J. Med. Chem. *26*, 700 (1983).

218 M. Mathews, H.W.R. Williams, E. Eichler, D.E. Duggan, E.H. Ulm and R.M. Noll: J. Org. Chem. *63*, 4308 (1998).

219   M.M. Murphy, J.R. Schullek, E.M. Gordon and M.A. Gallop: J. Am. Chem. Soc. *117*, 7029 (1995).

220   R. Williard, V. Jammalamadaka, D. Zava, C.C. Benz, C.A. Hunt, P.J. Kushner, T.S. Scanlan: Chem. Biol. *2*, 45 (1995).

221   J. Green: J. Org. Chem. *60*, 4287 (1995).

222   H.V. Meyers, G.J. Dilley, T.L. Durgen, J.S. Powers, N.A. Winssinger, H. Zhu and M.R. Pavia: Mol. Div. *1*, 13 (1995).

223   G.C. Look, J.R. Schullek, C.P. Holmes, J.P. Chennn, E.M. Gordon and M.A. Gallop: Bioorg. Med. Chem. Lett. *6*, 707 (1996).

224   N.S. Gray, S. Kwon and P.G. Schultz: Tet. Lett. *38*, 1161 (1997).

225   K.J. Shaw, W.J. Guilford, J.L. Dallas, S.K. Koovakaat, A. Liang, D.R. Light and M.M. Morrissey: J. Med. Chem., in press.

226   R. Mohan, W. Yun, B.O. Buckman, A. Liang, L. Trinh and M.M. Morrissey: Bioorg. Med. Chem. Lett. *8*, 1877 (1998).

227   R. Albert, H. Knecht, E. Andersen, V. Hungerford, M.H. Schreier and C. Papageorgiou: Bioorg. Med. Chem. Lett. *8*, 2203 (1998).

228   H.C. Zang and B.E. Maryanoff: J. Org. Chem. *62*, 1804 (1997).

229   A.L. Marzinzik and E.R. Felder: J. Org. Chem. *63*, 723 (1998).

230   D. Tumelty, M.K. Schwarz and M.C. Needels: Tet. Lett. *39*, 7467 (1998).

231   A. Bhandari, D.G. Jones, J.R. Schullek, K. Vo, C.A. Schunk, L.L. Tamanaha, D. Chen, Z.Yuvan, M.C. Needels, M.A. Gallop: Bioorg. Med. Chem. Lett. *8*, 2303 (1998)

232   V. Krchnak, A.S. Weichesel, D. Cabel, Z. Flegelova and M. Lebl: Mol. Div. *1*, 149 (1995)

233   M.J. Sofia, R. Hunter, T.Y. Chan, A. Vaughan, R. Dulina, H. Wang and D. Gange: J. Org. Chem. *63*, 2802 (1998).

234   J.M. Ostresh, G.M. Husar, S.E. Blondelle, B. Dorner, P.A. Weber and R.A. Houghten: Proc. Natl. Acad. Sci. USA *91*, 11138 (1994).

235   A. Nefzi, J.M. Ostresh, J.P. Meyer, R.A. Houghten: Tet. Lett. *38*, 931 (1997).

236   A. Nefzi, C. Dooley, J.M. Ostresh, R.A. Houghten: Bioorg. Med. Chem. Lett. *8*, 2273 (1998).

237   J.M. Ostresh, C.C. Schoner, V.T. Hamashim, A. Nefzi, J.P. Meyer, R.A. Houghten: J. Org. Chem. *63*, 8622 (1998).

238   T.C. Norman, N.S. Gray, J.T. Koh and P.G. Schultz: J. Am. Chem. Soc. *118*, 7430 (1996).

239   J.J. Baldwin, J.J. BurBaum, I. Henderson and M.H. Ohlmeyer: J. Am. Chem. Soc. *117*, 5588 (1995).

240   M.J. Kurth, L.A.A. Randall, C. Chen, C. Melander, R.B. Miller: J. Org. Chem. *59*, 5862 (1994).

241   K. McAlister, G. Reitz, R. Kang, T. Nakatsu, C. Green: Bioorg. Med. Chem. Lett. *5*, 2953 (1995).

242   M.C. Pirrung and J.H.-L Chan, J. Chen: Curr. Biol. *2*, 621 (1995).

243   X. Cao, E.J. Moran, D. Siev, A. Lio, C. Ohashi and A.M.M. Mjalli: Bioorg. Med. Chem Lett. *8*, 2321 (1998).

244   P.H.H. Hermkens, H.C.J. Ottenheijm and D. Rees: Tetrahedron *52*, 4527 (1996).

245   S. Booth, P.H.H. Hermkens, H.C.J. Ottenheijm and D. Rees: Tetrahedron *54*, 15385 (1998).

246   R. Brown: Contemp. Org. Syn. *216* (1998).

247   C.C. Zikos and N.G. Ferdengos: Tet. Lett. *36*, 3741 (1995).

248   A.B. Dyatkin and R.A. Rivero: Tet. Lett. *39*, 3647 (1998).

249   M.F. Gordeev: Tet. Lett. *37*, 4643 (1996).
250   A.A. MacDonald, S.H. DeWitt, E.M. Hogan and R. Ramage Tet. Lett. *37*, 4815 (1996).
251   N.D. Hone, S.G. Davies, N.J. Devereux, S.L. Taylor and A.D. Baxter: Tet. Lett. *39*, 897 (1998).
252   M.J. Kurth, L.A.A. Randall, C. Chen, C. Melander, R.B. Miller, K. McAlister, G. Reitz, R. Kang, T. Nakatsu and C. Green: J. Org. Chem. *59*, 5862 (1994).
253   S.P. Hollinshead: Tet. Lett.: *37*, 9157 (1996).
254   F. Zaragoza and S.V. Peterson: Tetrahedron *52*, 10823 (1996).
255   B.C. Hamper, S.A. Kolodziej and A.M.Scates: Tet. Lett. *39*, 2047 (1998).
256   J.S. Panek and B. Zhu: Tet. Lett. *37*, 8151 (1996).
257   T.T. Romoff, L. Ma, Y. Wang and D.A. Campbell: Synlet 1341 (1998).
258   N.M. Khan, V. Araumugam and S. Balasubramanian: Tet. Lett. *37*, 4819 (1996).
259   L. Weber: Drug Dis. Today *3*, 379 (1998).
260   E.K. Wilson: Chem. Engg. News *31* (1998).
261   S. Borman: Chem. Engg. News *47* (1998).

Progress in Drug Research, Vol. 53 (E. Jucker, Ed.)
©1999 Birkhäuser Verlag, Basel (Switzerland)

From genome to drug – optimising the drug discovery process

By Paul Spence

G.D. Searle, 700 Chesterfield Parkway North, St. Louis, MO 63198, USA

Paul Spence

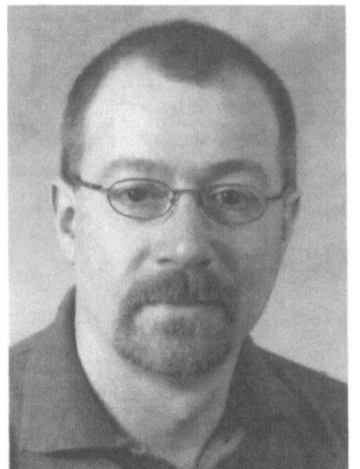

graduated in 1984 from the University of Oxford with a D.Phil. in molecular virology. He worked as a post-doctoral fellow at the Imperial Cancer Research Fund in London, studying the role of human papillomavirus in the development of cervical cancer. He moved to Wellcome in the UK in 1986, and spent several years working in both diagnostics and oncology programs. After a short spell at Xenova, where he headed their oncology programs, he moved to Wyeth-Ayerst Research in the UK to establish a new molecular biology department. In 1995, he moved the department to the Wyeth-Ayerst Research facility in Princeton as part of their reorganization after the merger with American Cyanamid. In Princeton, one of his major responsibilities was the discovery and validation of novel molecular targets for drug discovery, which was carried out in association with Millennium Pharmaceuticals in Cambridge, MA. In June of 1998, he moved to Monsanto Company to take up the position of co-head of genomics research and head of biotechnology for G.D. Searle.

Summary

Current drug discovery and development practices are technologically sophisticated and highly efficient. At the same time the failure rate of compounds in both preclinical and clinical development is high. These failures can be attributed to many factors. Two predominant causes of failure are lack of efficacy and toxicity. Often lack of efficacy is only determined late in the clinical trial process and can be difficult if not impossible to explain, as well as being expensive. Toxicity accounts for many failures during preclinical development, which are less costly, but it also occurs in the clinic. Often the underlying cause of clinical toxicity is never identified. Studies of the structure and activity of the human and other genomes has over the last decade lead to a revolution in biological and medical research. Disease associated genes can now be identified through the application of human genetics, whole genomes have been sequenced and tools have been developed that allow the complete characterization of an organism's gene expression profile in a single experiment. These tools are now being applied to pharmaceutical research and development with the aim to increase the efficiency of the process and the quality of the product.

Contents

Keywords

genome, genes, model organism, human genome project, genetic marker, SNP, EST, transcriptional profiling, pharmacogenetics, polymorphism, homologue

Glossary of abbreviations

BLAST, basic local alignment search tool; *C. elegans, Caenorhabditis elegans*; cDNA, copy deoxyribosenucleic acid; cM, centimorgan; DNA, deoxyribosenucleic acid; *D. melanogaster, Drosophila melanogaster*; EST, expressed sequence tag; IL, interleukin; Mb, megabase; mRNA, messenger ribosenucleic acid; ORF, open reading frame; QTL, quantitative trait loci; RNA, ribosenucleic acid; *S. cerevisiae, Saccharomyces cerevisiae*; SNP, single nucleotide polymorphism; STS, sequence tagged site

1   Introduction

A major factor in the success of modern pharmacological agents is the fundamental improvement in the way they are discovered, developed and tested in the clinic. It has been estimated that over the past 50 years medications have lead to the saving of more than 1.5 million lives and the saving of $ 140 billion in the treatment of coronary artery disease, cerebrovascular disease, poliomyelitis and tuberculosis alone [1]. At the same time the rigorous requirements for safety and efficacy placed on a new therapeutic by government agencies have driven the increasing quality and cost of development of new therapeutics.

The drug discovery and development process can be divided into several phases (Fig. 1). In the discovery phase lead compounds are identified by the use of high throughput screening against chemical libraries, rational design based on knowledge of the three-dimensional structure of the target, modification of known chemical structures or the production of therapeutic proteins. These are then screened through a series of increasingly complex assays, eventually leading to a demonstration of efficacy in an animal model representing the relevant disorder. The concerns that exercise the minds of scientists involved in this process often centre around the choice of target and the drug candidate specificity. Ideally one would select the molecular target based on its intimate involvement in the disorder to be targeted and its limited involvement in other biological processes that might, if disturbed, lead to unwanted side-effects. In addition, even when the appropriate target is chosen and lead compounds identified, concerns will remain as to whether other gene products will be inhibited or activated by these compounds. Selectivity can be addressed experimentally if these other genes and their products are characterised. However, these questions often remain unanswered until later in the development process or even in the clinic.

Preclinical safety and toxicity testing begins immediately following the drug discovery process, although some of these activities often take place concurrently with the final stages of drug discovery. Safety and toxicity testing comprises acute and chronic toxicity tests, mutagenicity assays, reproductive toxicity and drug disposition studies. They are normally carried out in rats and one to two additional mammalian species, although the scientists involved in these safety assessments are acutely aware that these species do not necessarily respond to drugs in the same manner as humans. Com-

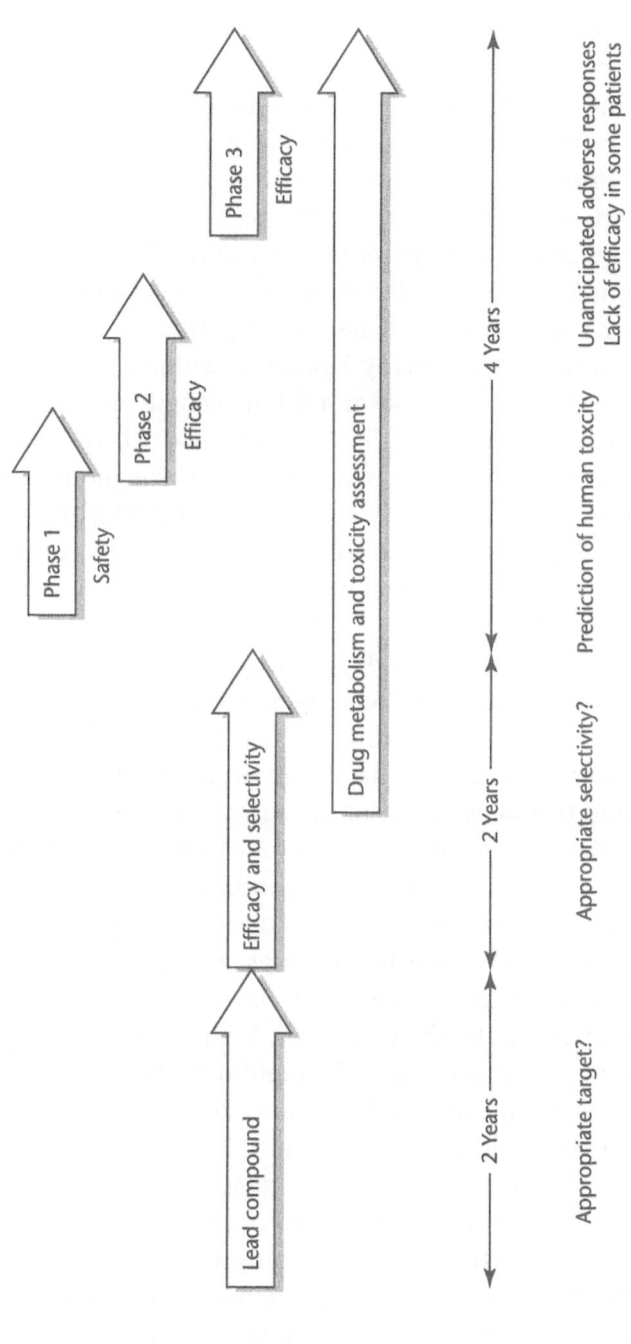

Fig. 1
The phases of drug discovery and development. Throughout the process there are issues which can have significant implications for the success of the drug.

pounds that pass the safety hurdles and are suitable for commercial production enter clinical trials. However, even after these efforts, only about 10-30% of compounds entering clinical trials reach the marketplace. Unlike the controlled environment of the laboratory, the human population can be highly variable in its response to therapeutic compounds. Such variations can include the presence of additional, unidentified disorders or even variations in lifestyle. Furthermore, differences in the pathobiology of a disorder, the underlying cause, might lead to very similar clinical manifestations. This would be of significant concern for those disorders for which no clear biochemical marker can be used to measure the pathological process such as behavioural disorders. Unlike many laboratory animal species the human population is highly heterogeneous in both its genetic makeup and behaviour. Clinical trials are designed with care to generate data that is statistically sound. Care is taken to select and observe patients throughout a clinical trial so that all drug effects can be observed. However, it is a fact that isolated or systematic unanticipated responses (or non-responses) occur. Even drugs that have been marketed for several years can elicit unanticipated and life-threatening responses [2].

Drug discovery development today is a highly efficient process, however as outlined above, there are many areas where improvements in our knowledge and the ability to predict outcomes would be advantageous. One of the most recent revolutions in biology has begun to generate both the knowledge base and the tools to address many of the current concerns of pharmaceutical researchers. This revolution comprises the ability to explore and characterise the structure and activity of whole genomes in a high throughput or massively parallel manner and as such has been called genomics. However, in addition to the scientific benefits it brings, genomics also brings with it concerns from both an ethical and legal point of view as individuals are defined, to a great extent, by their genomes. From a commercial perspective one of the current major concerns is the rapid patenting of human genes to protect their use as therapeutics and more importantly as therapeutic targets. Drews and Ryser have calculated that some 413 gene products can be identified as human therapeutic targets and 56 gene products for infectious and parasitic diseases [3]. The human genome contains from 50 000 to 100 000 genes [4, 5]. Therefore, in their estimation only about 0.5–1% of the genome has been targeted by therapeutics. Obviously not all genes will encode viable therapeutic targets but it is likely that a significant number of genes will, and they remain undiscovered or, as yet, unrecognised. Using an estimate of 100 disease entities with an average contribution from 10 genes, each of which might communicate biochemically with three to 10 genes, Drews and Ryser proposed that there might be between 3000 and 10 000 human drug targets available for exploitation. Genomics activities such as high throughput sequencing are already reducing this number (as available targets) through new gene discovery and patenting [6]. It is also clear that, in the not too distant future, every human gene will be identified and characterized, at least by its sequence. In order to remain competitive the modern pharmaceutical company must recognize the fact that it must not only continually increase the efficiency of its drug discovery efforts but, in addition, must ensure its freedom to operate by creating its own intellectual property rights for the new therapeutic targets in its pipeline. The tools of genomics will contribute significantly to both of these activities.

In this review I will survey the current state of the art in genomic sciences, focusing on those technologies having direct pharmaceutical application.

2   Genomic and expressed gene sequencing

2.1   The human genome project

The advent of automated DNA sequencing about a decade ago coupled with the increasing capacity of computer systems, not only to store but to analyse data, has made exceptionally large sequencing projects feasible. The most recent milestone in whole genome sequencing was the completion of the entire sequence of *C. elegans* last year [7–11]. Presently the human genome sequencing project is reported to be about 6% completed and is projected to be fully complete in about 2003 [12]. One of the most valuable contributions that the human genome project will make to biomedical research is the ability to study natural genetic variations in humans (this is discussed below in section 4). The scale of effort required to fully characterize a genome comprising 23 pairs of chromosomes made up of 3×10^9 base pairs of DNA is immense. For this reason numerous research centres are collaborating in the effort. The list of these centres and the status of their activities can be found on the website of the National Center for Biotechnology Information (NCBI) at http://www.ncbi.nlm.nih.gov. In order to sequence large genomes one has to structure the work with great care, initially through the creating of a high quality genetic map, using genetic markers (see section 4) followed by a physical map using sequence tagged sites (a sequence that can be assigned to a specific chromosomal location and which represents a critical link between genetic and physical maps). Once these maps have been created, the high throughput sequencing data from genomic clones can be assigned to their appropriate chromosomal locations [13]. The computing resource required to support these programs is not insignificant, not only does the sequence data require aligning, or "contiging", so contiguous clones can be placed next to each other, but the information content of the genome (gene coding regions and control regions) can be extracted. The requirement for specific computer programs and databases to handle these tasks has given rise to a new science known as bioinformatics. In addition to generating a complete sequence of the human genome, the Human Genome Project has other objectives: (i) to further develop sequencing technology towards higher throughput and reduced cost, (ii) to develop functional genomics technologies through establishing full length cDNA resources, developing the tools for the study of non protein-coding regions of genes, advancing gene expression analysis (see section below), improving methods for genome wide mutagenesis, developing the technology for global protein analysis, (iii) to advance comparitive genomics through the sequencing the genomes of other organisms such as *C. elegans*, Drosophila and the mouse, (iv) to address the ethical, legal and social implications of the data, especially the data on human genetic variation, (v) to advance the science of bioinformatics and computational biology through improving database utility, better tools for data capture and annotation, better tools for analysing and representing data similarity and the creation of mechanisms to support the production of widely used software, and (vi) to train scientists in the new specialties created by this and related efforts [12]. In parallel with the above activities efforts are underway to map expressed sequences to their chromosomal locations [14]. It is clear that, with access to the entire human genome sequence including the assignments of expressed genes to their chromosomal locations, the way one thinks about biology will be very different. For the pharmaceutical industry it will mean that every potential pharmaceutical target will be known (at least by its nucleic acid and protein sequence) and mapped. All homologues (paralogues) will immediately be known for a new target gene so a high degree of drug specificity can be designed in the very early stages of a development program and mechanism based adverse effects will be avoidable, or at the very least explainable. The possibility also exists that, as our understanding of the complexities of gene control increases, a whole new category of drug targets will become available based on the targeting of promoter and enhancer elements, transcription factors and sequences involved in mRNA turnover. In keeping with these hopes the potential commercial value of human genomic sequence data has spawned alternative sequencing efforts [15].

2.2 EST sequencing and database mining

The data coming out of the Human Genome Project will have a significant impact on the way pharmaceutical research is carried out, however the competitive pressures in the industry have driven an additional approach to accessing data on gene sequences through sequencing of snippets of expressed genes in order to create a database of expressed sequence tags or ESTs [16–20]. The human genome probably contains over 100 000 genes. However, only a subset of these will be expressed in a specific cell or tissue at any time. By sequencing cDNA clones from libraries made from specific cell or tissue types one can create a database of expressed gene sequences. Furthermore, by comparing the sequences found in one cell or tissue type with other tissues one can build a picture of tissue specific gene expression. ESTs comprise short sequences (100–500 base pairs) from either the 3' or 5' end of a cloned cDNA. EST sequencing can be automated so databases of EST sequences can be rapidly produced. For a pharmaceutical or biotechnology company the value of EST sequences is that they are concentrated datasets of sequences coding for the proteins expressed in a particular cell or tissue type. EST databases can be searched or "mined" for sequences showing similarity to known genes. Various search tools have been developed for this purpose. Perhaps the most widely used tool is the BLAST program developed by Altschul et al. [21] and routinely refined [22–24]; it is based on a statistical model that greatly increases search speed (critical for very large databases). As a tool for identifying new genes by homology to known ones EST sequences benefit by being as long as possible, however, as an alternative to STSs, ESTs need to be short to ensure that the two ends of the sequence are contiguous in the genome (they contain no intron). An alternative use of EST databases is the comparison of ESTs from normal and diseased tissue. This method is widely used in biotechnology and pharmaceutical research to identify new genes that might be associated with the disease. Unlike homology searching one does not have to know anything about the gene sequence but only know its relative abundance. This is determined by comparing how many times the sequence occurred in one cDNA library versus another. These methods allow one to identify a sequence of interest but generally supply no further information about that sequence. More recently efforts have been made to pre-analyse sequence data in order to give some annotation to each sequence, even if it is just a record of sequences to which it shows homology. A major challenge for bioinformatics will be to incorporate more annotation from diverse sources into sequence databases. In addition to EST sequences public databases also contain many full length cDNA sequences which clearly supplement the EST data greatly. One exceptionally powerful attribute of sequence comparisons is the ability to compare genes across species. Clearly the mouse and rat are evolutionarily very similar to humans and for this reason they have made valuable models for both the understanding and therapy of human disorders. However, the similarities are less obvious when one considers more distantly related organisms. The genome sequencing programs for the baker's yeast (*Saccharomyces cerevisiae*) [25, 26], the nematode worm (*Caenorhabditis elegans*) [27] and the fruit fly (*Drosophila melanogaster*) [28] have informed us how very similar their genes are to human genes. Botstein and co-workers compared all yeast protein sequences to the mammalian sequences in GenBank and found a robust homology between 31% of the yeast open reading frames or ORFs with the mammalian protein sequences [29]. Chervitz and co-workers compared all the *C. elegans* ORFs with the yeast ORFs and showed that many of the core biological functions of the two organisms were shared [27]. It is worthy of note that the dataset generated in this study was too large to be included in the original publication. However, this data is available on a website (http://genome-www.stanford.edu/Saccharomyces/worm/). Due to the very large volume of data now available it has become standard practise to make these available on the Web and there are now many public domain databases available on the Web. Some, such as GenBank, contain nucleic acid and protein sequences from many species [30] while others focus on specific species or are organised by biochemical pathway. A list of these databases can be found in Nucleic Acids Research [31].

The phenotypic divergence of species over time is the result of accumulated changes in their gene sequences. When searching for orthologous genes from different species one relies on the sequence similarity being great enough to be able to make distinctions between true orthologues and coincidental sequence similarities. The algorithms developed for making sequence comparisons make a trade between sensitivity (the ability to detect distantly related sequences) and selectivity (the avoidance of false positives). At some point one might expect very distantly related sequences to become lost in a sea of false positives. It is possible to detect protein sequences sharing a common ancestor more than one billion years ago [32]. However, gene duplication rearrangements can result in complex gene families. It is now becoming apparent that many proteins are comprised of shorter protein modules that have themselves evolved in complex ways. This clearly complicates gene or protein taxonomy. Methods are now being developed to make comparisons between proteins based on their structure rather than primary sequence. It is hoped that these approaches will allow the identification of distantly related proteins based on the structural constraints required to retain function [33]. The gross anatomies of animals and plants are used to guide biologists in assigning evolutionary relationships [34]. It has long been known in this field that anatomical structures that look similar are not necessarily derived from the same archaic structures. Obvious examples are the fins of whales and fish which are analogous structures and the wings of birds and bats which are simultaneously homologous (as forelimbs) and analogous (as functional wings). In a similar way it is probable that protein structures might converge through evolutionary processes, especially as there is probably a limited number of protein substructures that are energetically possible [35, 36]. The value of such "deep mining" for pharmaceutical companies is that it should enable them to identify structural similarities between novel genes and known genes that might be drug targets, thereby preventing unwanted cross reactivity, or identifying by novel targets having structures compatible with established small molecule libraries.

3   The analysis of gene expression

The human genome is not a static entity. In all living cells the genome is continually being transcribed into messenger RNA which, after translation into protein, carries out the cell's many biological functions. Eukaryotic cells have evolved highly complex, multi-layered mechanisms to control the expression of specific genes in response to specific environmental stimuli, whether it be hypoxia, osmotic shock or stimulation by a hormone. Although it has been known for a long time that modulation of gene expression is a critical component of a cell's response to environmental changes, technological limitations tended to focus researchers' attention on the expression changes of a limited number of genes within a single experiment. As the sequence databases became larger and biological research became automated, with high throughput and miniaturisation, the tools became available to analyse the expression of large numbers of genes in parallel. Currently one of the most widely used tools for parallel gene expression analysis is the DNA chip or microarray [37–39]. Figure 2 illustrates the general principle of microarray technology. It is possible to create arrays containing thousands of genes allowing one to survey expression changes for whole genomes within a single experiment. Microarrays have been used to profile gene expression patterns in alveolar rhabdomyosarcoma (ARMS) cell lines [40]. In this study 37 genes were found to be highly expressed in four or more of the seven ARMS cell lines when compared to the control cell line and eight were highly expressed in all seven cell lines. It is likely that expression profiling of tumours will not only supplement standard diagnosis and prognosis procedures but may lead to the identification of novel therapeutic targets. A comparative study of the inflammation process in rheumatoid arthritis (RA) and inflammatory bowel disease using a customised 96 element microarray [41]. Both cultured cells and tissue samples were used to determine the expression changes in genes known to be or postulated to be involved in the inflammatory process. The data from these studies supported the major role that TNF is thought to play in RA as it was upregulated in advance of other genes such as IL-1α, IL-β, IL-6 and granolocyte colony stimulating factor. Both syn-

Fig. 2

Oligonucleotides or cDNAs are arrayed onto glass slides. The array here shows 12×13 spots but arrays of thousands of genes are possible. The probes for the arrays come from experimental RNA samples and are fluorescently labeled during first strand cDNA synthesis. The probes are then hybridized to the arrays. Differentially expressed mRNAs are identified by the difference in flourescence at equivalent sequences on the array. In the diagram above the white spots represent genes whose expression is not changed between the samples. The black spots represent genes that are differentially expressed (either up or down). Alternative methods make use of different coloured fluorescent probes hybridized together against the same array, the differential expression being determined ratiometrically.

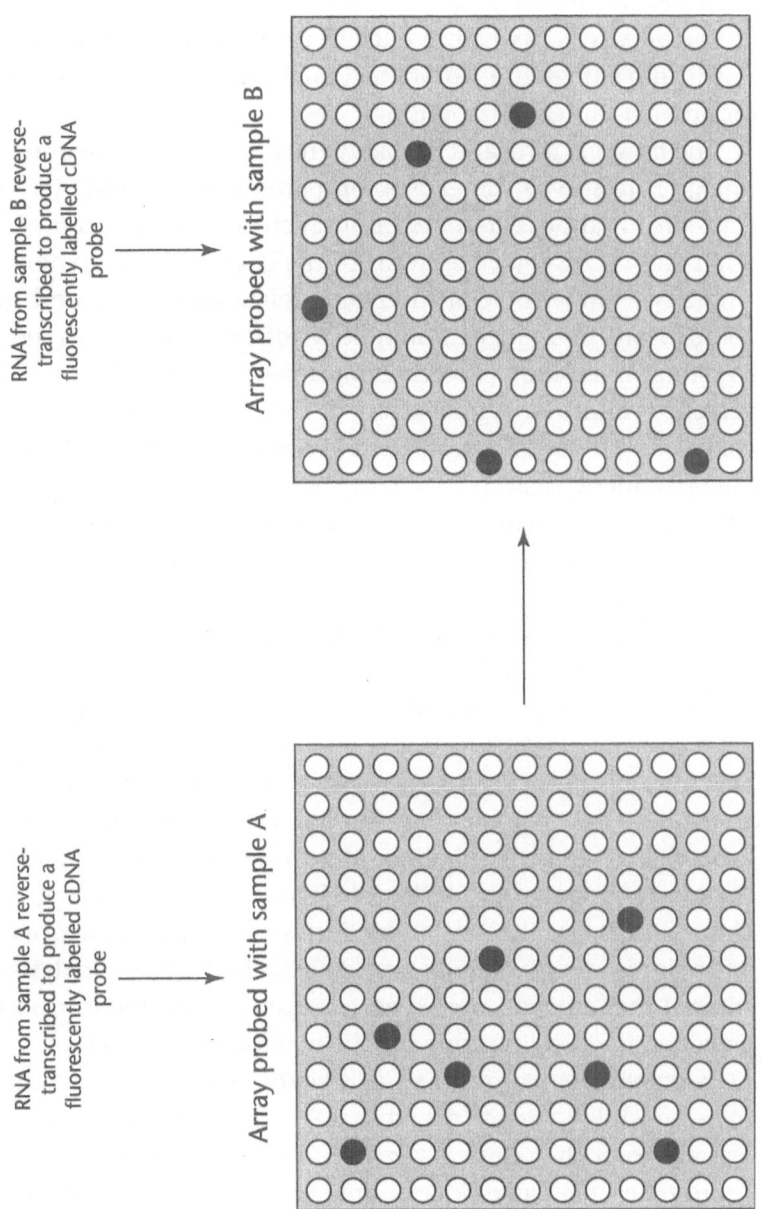

RNA from sample B reverse-transcribed to produce a fluorescently labelled cDNA probe

Array probed with sample B

RNA from sample A reverse-transcribed to produce a fluorescently labelled cDNA probe

Array probed with sample A

ovial fibroblasts and articular chondrocytes had very similar gene expression profiles with the matrix metalloproteinases being most prominently expressed. Human matrix metallo-elastase expression was observed in chondrosarcoma cells. As its presence in RA tissue could lead to destruction of elastin and basement membrane it might therefore become a valuable target for pharmaceutical intervention.

The most exciting and probably the most fruitful use of microarray technology is to survey the expression patterns of all genes in a genome after exposure to various external stimuli. Such experiments, carried out with thorough and sophisticated analysis of the data, have the potential to create a whole new dimension of inter-gene relationships, beyond that seen with comparisons by sequence homology (direct evolutionary relationships) or structural homology (distant evolutionary relationships and possibly convergent evolution). A microarray of over 1000 human cDNAs was used to study transcriptional modulation brought about by heat shock or phorbol ester treatment. Heat shock treatment caused expression changes of 17 genes with some of those induced being heat shock genes. Phorbol ester treatment caused the induction of six genes including PAC-1 and NF-κB1 which are known to be responsive to phorbol esters. In addition they identified four novel genes (about 0.4% of their gene sample) that were modulated by these treatments even though these response pathways have been well studied. Further studies by this group focused on *S. cerevisiae* and the control of whole genome gene expression under various physiological conditions [42, 43]. DeRisi and colleagues grew yeast in glucose depleted media to explore the changes in gene expression at several time points during the change from anaerobic to aerobic respiration. At steady state exponential growth they only observed changes in expression of 19 genes, however, after glucose depletion changes of at least twofold induction were seen in approximately 710 genes and a similar degree of reduction in about 1030 genes. Analysis of these genes showed that changes were seen in genes responsible for specific metabolic activities involved in supplying the tricarboxylic acid (TCA) cycle (for example aldehyde dehydrogenase, and acytyl-coenzyme A synthase expression increase while pyruvate decarboxylase expression decreased). In addition it was apparent that classes of genes involved in coordinated activities were coordinately regulated (for example genes involved in protein synthesis were down regulated). As samples from various time points were taken distinct temporal patterns of expression could be recognised as well. It is worthy of note that more than 400 of the differentially expressed genes have no apparent homology to genes of known function. This data would indicate that they are probably involved in the metabolic changes in some way. These studies were extended to the analysis of sequential induction of genes during sporulation in budding yeast [43]. Seven temporal expression profiles were identified although it was clear that genes showed clear relationships to associated profiles. Genes with related functions tended to be expressed with similar temporal patterns. Genes of unknown function having the same expression profile can therefore be functionally associated and tested for these specific functions by deletion. Chu and colleagues [43] used microarray to study the transcription of 97% of yeast genes during sporulation, which consists of meiosis and spore morphogenesis. They were able to show that 500 genes were induced during this process (50 had been previously described) and 500 suppressed. In addition their data supported the view that sporulation could be divided into two major stages, meiotic prophase followed by meiotic division and gamete morphogenesis. Since several genes seen to be induced during this process had vertebrate homologues they speculated the existence of similar processes operating in spermatogenesis and oogenesis. The significance of these yeast studies is their focus of temporal data to generate gene expression profiles leading to new insights into gene function and biological pathways.

Recently the use of microarrays to analyse the response of human fibroblasts to serum stimulation has been reported [44]. The temporal program of gene expression was derived using 8613 different human genes at 12 time points over 24 h after serum stimulation. The changing expression pattern was analysed using novel clustering and display algorithms [45]. Clustering was carried out based on no prior model of the pattern of gene expression using the hierarchical clustering approach of pairwise average-linkage cluster analysis. This method is also used to create dendrograms to denote sequence similarities by homology. The results of these analyses for the entire gene set at all time points was displayed graphically with gene clusters plotted against time with no expression change displayed black, increased expression in red (intensity proportional to magnitude of increased expression) and decreased expression in green (intensity proportional to magnitude of decreased expression). The plots can be seen in [44] and at http://genome-www.stanford.edu/serum/figures.html. The data showed a coordinated regulation of groups of genes whose products were associated with common

171

processes. Over 200 uncharacterised genes were found in the various clusters, which might give an indication of their biological function. An added benefit from these experiments was the observation that many genes involved in the wound healing process were modulated. The authors noted that serum stimulation *in vitro* might be analogous to fibroblast exposure to serum during the wound healing process.

In the not too distant future all human genes (and genes of model organisms) will be characterised and their sequences available on microarrays. This will allow many experiments to be carried out *in vitro* and *in vivo* that can address entire genome responses to biological and pathological processes. Coupled to our increasing understanding of gene expression clusters and the sophisticated data analysis being developed to extract and display the information transcriptional profiling will become an enormously powerful tool in drug discovery, not only in the identification of new targets but in the detailed analysis of the specific (and non-specific) activity of drug candidates.

4   Genetics and pharmacogenetics

Genetic variation within a population is the base upon which evolution operates. It is clear from even the most cursory observations that a great deal of genetic variation exists within human populations and one would expect that variations will be found within the genes that are involved in both disease processes and those involved in drug responses. Indeed, it has been accepted for some considerable time that polymorphisms within the genes involved in drug metabolism can play a critical role in the variable responses to drugs within patient populations [46, 47]. For simplicity, I will divide the application of genetics to pharmaceutical discovery and development into two broad categories. Firstly, I will discuss the application of genetics to the discovery of disease genes and describe some of the tools available for these analyses. In addition, I will outline some of the criteria required for such studies and address the issues they create. The second category, which I will define as pharmacogenetics, addresses the application of human genetics in understanding drug response. It will become apparent that many of the tools required for both these applications are the same. However, there are some significant differences in how they might be applied which will have a bearing on the organization of these efforts.

4.1.1 Identifying disease gene through human genetics

It has been known for many years that some diseases have a genetic basis. Two classic genetic disorders are sickle cell anaemia and phenylketonuria. These were identified due to their mode of inheritance and the significant clinical and biochemical phenotypes they display [48]. In sickle cell anaemia the erythorocytes sickle at low oxygen tensions and have a shorter lifespan, which leads to anaemia, they also clump together when deoxygenated, leading to clinical crisis. These clear clinical features are the result of a single amino acid change in haemoglobin β-chain (valine replacing glutamine at position 6). Heterozygotes having one normal and one altered β-chain possess sickle cell trait and live fairly normal lives. Phenylketonuria is due to the absence of phenylalanine 4-monooxygenase leading to the production of phenylpyruvic acid which, in childhood, can cause mental retardation through its accumulation in the blood. As expected, this disorder is recessive as it is due to the loss of a gene. Both these cases illustrate an important point, these disorders are the result of a single gene defect and display a clear biochemical phenotype. Many human disorders are not so simple, either displaying a complex phenotype, giving no biochemical clues, or being the result of defects or polymorphisms in more than one gene. Duchenne muscular dystrophy (DMD) is an example of a single gene disorder displaying a relatively complex phenotype, it is also one of the most common and devastating genetic diseases of childhood [49]. DMD is an X-linked disease affecting about 0.03% of live male births each year. Those affected have severe muscle weakness, the muscle being replaced by fat or connective tissue, and high levels of muscle enzymes in the blood. Most patients die in their early 20s. The gene responsible for DMD was identified using positional cloning as nothing was known regarding its function [50, 51]. Due to the X-linked nature of the disorder the search was restricted to the X-chromosome and was further localised to Xp21 by linkage analysis, using polymorphic DNA markers, by the observation of gross structural X-chromosome mutations in rare female DMD involving the Xp21 region and the identification of microdeletions in a subset of DMD patients localized to Xp21. Part of the coding sequence for the DMD gene was identified through the comparison of DNA from normal and affected individuals and this was used to clone the remainder of the expressed gene from muscle cDNA libraries. The DMD gene encodes a protein called dystrophin which is abundant in skeletal muscle and probably plays a role in the mechanical reinforcement of muscle fibers. Although DMD is a single gene defect with a clear phenotype, the identification of the gene responsible required the application of molecular genetics, since the nature of the disorder gave no clear biochemical insight into the underlying mechanism.

Type 2 diabetes, or non-insulin dependent diabetes mellitus, appears to have a genetic component [52, 53]. The pathological progression of type 2 diabetes is well understood, as is the physiology of the disorder, so one might expect that predisposing genetic polymorphisms would be found. However the genetics of type 2 diabetes is complex, probably involving multiple genes, and to date there are no clear gene leads for the most common forms of this disease, even amongst those genes closely associated with insulin regulation and glucose metabolism [52]. Recently the use of animal models and their more facile genetics has led to the identification of a candidate gene for type 2 diabetes [54]. I will discuss animal genetic models in more detail below. However, it is clear that even with a significant understanding of the biochemistry of a disorder, the identification of predisposing genetic polymorphisms in humans is not trivial. Therefore, is it possible or practical to identify the genes responsible for the most common human disorders, where only a limited knowledge of the physiology and biochemistry is available, coupled with the presence of more than one predisposing gene? The expectation of many working in the field of human genetics is that linkage studies using the tools now available will be capable of identifying the genes that play a role in disorders having complex genetics [55].

Linkage analysis requires an understanding of the structure of the human genome and the availability of reagents that simultaneously identify polymorphisms and map them onto their position in the genome. I will summarize the principles of linkage studies below as detailed descriptions of linkage analysis and the markers used can be found in Strachan and Read [56] and Pawlowitzki et al. [57]. Over the last few years genetic markers have become available in ever increasing numbers. These reagents are used for linkage studies, the aim of which is to determine how often two loci are separated by meiotic recombination. If two loci are on different chromosomes they will segregate independently at meiosis. However if they are present on the same chromosome they have a greater chance of segregating together, this chance being inversely proportional to their distance apart on the chromosome (assuming recombination is randomly distributed along chromosomes). In order to identify a disease loci in humans one needs to make use of genetic markers. These are Mendelian characters having sufficient polymorphism such that randomly selected individuals are heterozygous. In practice genetic markers need to be spaced throughout the genome at intervals no greater than 20 cM (a centimorgan is approximately 1 Mb) for initial mapping purposes, with spacing down to 1 cM for gene cloning. The genetic markers presently in use are DNA polymorphisms which can be typed by the same techniques and can be mapped directly onto their chromosomal location through physical mapping [56]. DNA polymorphisms, such as microsatellites, are mostly comprised of (CA)n repeats, commonly observed in the 15–30 repeat range and are found throughout the genome. There may be as many as 50 000 microsatellites in the human genome. The advantage of these markers is that they are highly polymorphic and therefore highly informative. More recently an alternative set of markers have been developed, based to a large extent on the data coming out of the human genome project. The single nucleotide polymorphisms or SNPs represent single base variations in the genomic DNA sequence at defined positions that are found at a frequency of over 1% in the human population [58]. SNPs represent the most common type of human genetic variation. It is anticipated that SNPs will aid in the identification of disease genes by family linkage studies, linkage disequilibrium studies in isolated populations [59] and even association studies of patients and control healthy subjects [55]. As SNPs can only have two alleles, they are less informative than microsatellite markers, however they are more abundant and lend themselves to automation (SNPs can be analysed through direct hybridization). In a recent study SNPs were used to design genotyping microarray chips to demonstrate the feasibility for high throughput genotyping [58]. We can now consider the possibility of screening entire human genomes, at high resolution, for the detection of disease associated genes or other important traits, such as differential drug response. However, we still need to proceed with caution as some recent reports have suggested the use of SNPs is not going to be as straight forward as originally hoped, and the final density of SNPs required to map disease genes may need to be greater than anticipated [60]. For example, high levels of recombination within certain regions of the genome may thwart efforts in association mapping [61].

The powerful tools now available for the genetic analysis of complex disease need to be applied appropriately in order to fully realize their value.

When setting out to identify the gene or genes responsible for a human disorder one needs to plan appropriately. Below are some questions that need to be asked (and answered) before embarking on such a study:

1. Does the disease under study have a genetic component? One of the most valuable indicators of genetic disease is its predominance in certain families. However, genes are not the only thing shared in families!
2. Is it possible to determine the disease status as well as collect DNA from living individuals?
3. Is the population one intends to study large enough to give a statistically significant result? Linkage studies rely on the presence of informative meioses and a minimum of 10 is required.
4. Is it likely one is studying a multigene effect? One cannot sum the Lod scores from different families (Lod scores are the statistical measure for the evidence for linkage) [56].

In many cases it will not be possible to find a family large enough to give a statistically sound result. However, population geneticists have recognised that isolated populations derived from a small number of individuals (founder populations) can be very powerful in population association studies. Founder populations should have greater genetic homogeneity thereby reducing the "noise" in association studies. Unless carefully controlled, association studies can give meaningless results [62]. With care on population selection, study design and analysis, complex disorders are beginning to reveal their genetic secrets [59, 63, 64]. With significant efforts underway to map expressed genes to their chromosomal locations the task of positional cloning is made easier [14]. One will be able to select candidate genes from the region of interest, based on their likely function and a knowledge of the disease under study, for further study and possibly a short-cut in the final cloning steps (Fig. 3).

It is likely that population genetics will contribute to the identification of new disease genes and that these will lead, directly or indirectly, to the development of disease modifying therapeutics. It is important to remember, when using population genetics to identify disease genes, that nothing will be known about the structure or function of the gene until it is cloned so a significant amount of analysis will still be required. These activities are discussed elsewhere in this review.

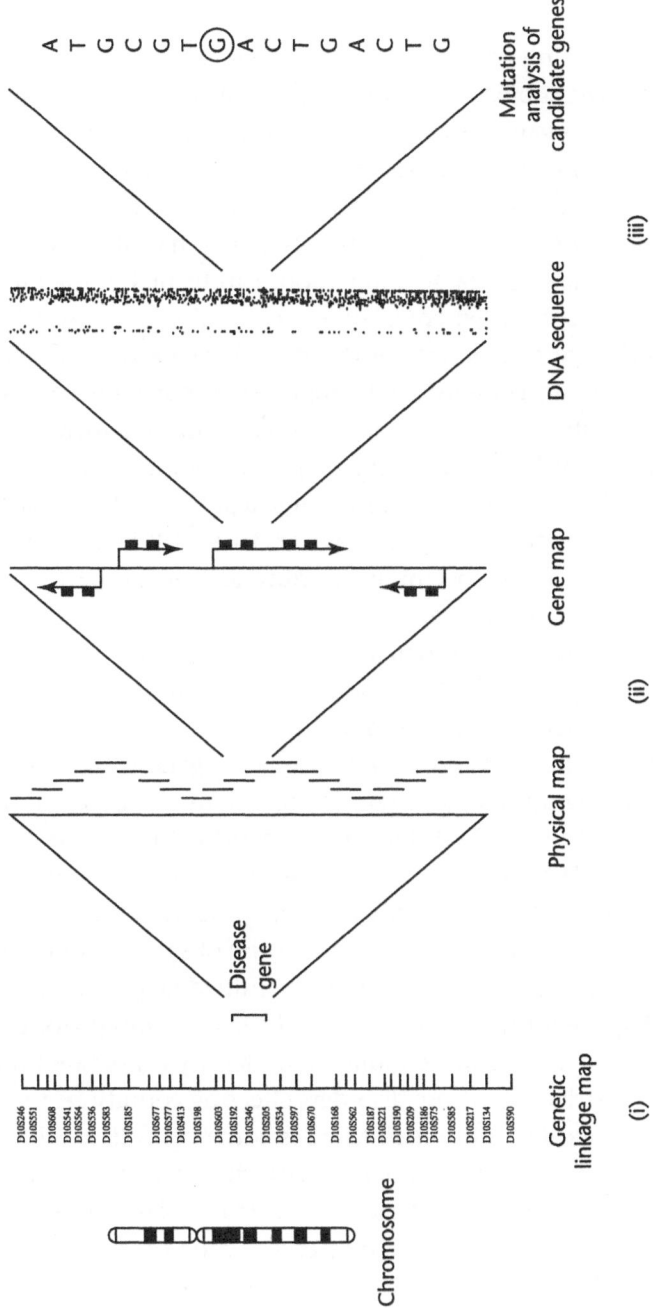

Fig. 3

Association and positional cloning studies. (i) Genetic markers are used to identify disease loci. (ii) Genomic DNA clones, typically yeast artificial chromosomes (YACS) or bacterial artificial chromosomes (BACS) representing these loci are used to determine the specific region more accurately. (iii) Once the region is narrowed down to a suitable size the disease gene can be identified through mutation analysis and/or the study of the candidate genes within the region.

177

4.1.2 Identifying disease genes using animal models

The major advantage in using an animal model for genetic studies is the ability to selectively breed the subjects (a luxury unavailable in the human population). Of all the model organisms available the mouse is probably the most suited for disease-driven studies. As a mammal it is closely related to humans, it has been used as a genetic tool for many years so a large number of mutants are available, it has a relatively short generation time and has high fecundity. In addition, due to its small size, large populations can be maintained in the laboratory under tightly controlled environmental conditions. Mouse mutations resembling human disorders, such as dwarfism have been used to identify the orthologous human gene [65, 66]. Single gene trait mouse mutants have been used to identify the genes involved in biochemical pathways relevant to human diseases such as obesity [67–71]. The identification of these genes and the further elucidation of their biochemical pathways has generated a number of potential therapeutic targets. However, there still remains a question as to the relevance of the specific gene mutations to human obesity, although it is likely that the human and mouse are similar in their control of energy balance and that the discoveries made in mouse have identified the critical biochemical pathways on which we need to focus. In parallel with the expanding number of genetic markers in humans, markers for the analysis of mouse traits have been generated and used to dissect the genetic loci involved in multigenic traits. Using inbred mouse strain combinations several of these loci, or quantitative trait loci (QTLs), have been identified in the control of energy balance [72, 73]. The challenge still remains to clone the genes which represent each QTL. This is not necessarily a simple process as the individual genes may interact epistatically, such that the isolation of each does not affect the phenotype, or the phenotype penetrance with individual genes is too low to be detected (perhaps requiring identification of a subphenotype for detection). It is likely that the use of mouse mutants to identify candidate human disease genes will be restricted to those disorders effecting conditions that are easily assayed physiologically and where there is some confidence that the human and mouse phenotype are fundamentally similar at the molecular level. However, with the advent of SNPs for mouse studies and the ability to do high throughput genotyping, the day may come when the mouse is used as the genetic background to elucidate the biology of human disease genes in a manner similar to studies using *C. elegans* and *Drosophila*.

4.2   Pharmacogenetics

Pharmacogenetics is the study of gene polymorphisms that effect the response of a patient to a drug. The knowledge that genetic variability impacts drug response has been with us for some time [74]. One could imagine three ways pharmacogenetic studies might be undertaken. (1) As we know a great deal about the enzymes involved in drug metabolism, which includes some knowledge of polymorphisms in the genes that code for them, screens could be established to identify these polymorphisms in clinical trial and patient populations. (2) Most modern drug discovery efforts are focused at specific gene products which are well characterized. It would be of significant value to determine the genetic polymorphism of specific drug targets within the population at large as well as clinical trial and patient populations. This activity might also be taken a step further by identifying the polymorphisms that are present within the genes involved in the biochemical or signal transduction pathways associated with the target gene. (3) One might also consider carrying out genome scans of a population receiving a specific drug in order to identify any genetic linkages with adverse responses not associated with known drug metabolising systems or variations in the target gene. All of the above activities require the availability of DNA samples and the technology to carry out high throughput genotyping. In the previous section the potential of SNPs to be adapted to high throughput analyses was discussed so it is anticipated that SNPs will become the major tool for pharmacogenetic studies.

4.2.1   The genetics of drug metabolism

The xenobiotic or drug metabolizing enzymes comprise several superfamilies of enzymes which are responsible for metabolizing the vast majority of chemicals to which humans are exposed [75]. Both subtle and gross polymorphisms in the genes encoding these enzymes have been identified associated with significant changes in enzyme activity. Since these enzymes can have opposing activities it emphasises the importance in understanding the full genetic complement of these enzymes when analysing drug responses. It is likely that the response of an individual to a drug will be quite unique and vary from the average in minor (inconsequential) or major (problematic) ways. These variations might affect efficacy through excessive metabolism or toxicity through poor metabolism or the creation of active metabolites. A catalogue of variations in drug metabolizing enzymes is described in detail in Puga et al. [75]. The majority of marketed drugs are metabolised by members of the cytochrome P450 family (CYP450) of which there are at least eight major isoforms. Several different P450 isoforms have been identified and characterized [76–80]. It is known that subtle changes in the amino acid sequences can have dramatic effects on enzyme activity. The alteration of a single amino acid residue has been shown to alter the substrate specificity of murine CYP2a-5 [81]. It would be of significant value to identify the variations in P450 isoforms that occur naturally in the population and then use these both in genotyping studies in clinical trials as well as determine the functional implication of the variations *in vitro*. A more complete understanding of the genetics of P450 enzymes should have a positive impact on the analysis of human drug responses. Interestingly, one of the best illustrations of pharmacogenetic benefits does not involve the P450 enzyme family. It is known that the apolipoprotein E genotype (APOE) is a predisposing factor for Alzheimer's disease. Poirer and colleagues [82, 83] stratified Alzheimer's patients on undergoing tacrine therapy according to their APOE allotype. They demonstrated that APOE allotype was a good predictor for tacrine response. Those patients homozygous for the APOE e4 allele responded much more poorly than those possessing the other APOE alleles. Furthermore, studies on another Alzheimer's experimental drug, S12024, demonstrated a clear benefit for patients having the APOE ε4 allele [84]. This shows that alleles that are associated with a relevant clinical outcome can be used to select the appropriate subgroup of patients for further clinical studies. It is important to note that the association is with clinical outcome rather than variations in the drug target (tacrine is a cholinesterase inhibitor and S12024 modulates noradrenalin and vasopressin). This emphasises the need to study the genetics of drug response more broadly.

4.2.2 The genetics of therapeutic targets

It would be reasonable to assume, based on the variations identified in drug metabolizing systems, that many other human genes display polymorphisms. An argument can be made that the maintenance of polymorphisms

in biological systems responsible for dealing with a wide variety of exoge-
nous chemicals is advantageous while functional variations in other systems
might be less advantageous. However, pharmaceutical products have been
designed not only to mimic natural ligand activity but to antagonize them
and to modulate them allosterically. Therefore, polymorphisms existing in
genes in a functionally neutral manner under normal circumstances may
have significant implications for the activity of pharmaceuticals. Furthermore, functionally modified variants in drug target genes might themselves
play a role in specific disorders. The population variation for many genes was
first noticed by comparing the sequences of these genes isolated from different samples. However, only a limited number of studies have been carried out to systematically survey populations for variations in potential target genes. The receptors for serotonin and dopamine have been surveyed due
to their importance as targets in the treatment of psychiatric disorders [47].
The $5HT_{1A}$ receptor has been show to display natural variants at two positions near the amino-terminus [85, 86] which do not appear to affect binding of agonists or antagonists [87]. Variations in the $5HT_{1D\beta}$ receptor have
been described [88] although the functional consequences of this change (a
phenylalanine substitution of cysteine at position 124), which is sited within
the third transmembrane domain, have not been explored. The dopamine
receptor family members also display polymorphisms. For example, the
dopamine D3 receptor contains a polymorphism (a serine substitution for
glycine) at position 9, but this does not appear to predict for any psychiatric
disorder [89, 90]. The dopamine D4 receptor appears to be highly polymorphic [47] and some polymorphisms might affect ligand binding [91] while
others lead to null mutations [92]. Interestingly the atypical neuroleptic
clozapine binds to the D4 receptor and a combination of studies have shown
that predictions can be made, with a reasonable degree of confidence, and
that combinations of certain variants can predict response to the drug
[93–95]. There exists tantalizing evidence from a limited number of studies
that drug response can be affected by polmorphisms in target genes. It
would also be a valuable exercise to explore variations in genes falling downstream of the drug target to determine whether these would impact drug
response or indeed predict for the disorder. Finally it must be remembered
that polymorphisms may not only affect the sequence of target genes but
also their expression level through altering their level of transcription or
message stability.

4.2.3 Genome scans for non-specific effects

In addition to surveying clinical trial populations to score specific variations in drug metabolizing and drug target genes and pathways it might also be of value to carry out genome scans of these populations. These scans would use DNA markers, ideally SNPs to generate association data on outcome and adverse response. If successful this approach would give the clinician another parameter for patient stratification that would be of value in clinical trial optimization. The specific gene need not be isolated, the response being considered a type of QTL. In order to be achievable the method of genome scanning must be high throughput and relatively cheap.

The application of molecular genetics to drug development can therefore be considered initially as a highly focused effort, identifying polymorphisms in populations for the specific genes of interest (drug targets and genes known to be involved in drug disposition) and using these as probes in clinical studies. SNPs have an added advantage here in that they should be found within gene coding regions and so can target amino acid variations. Once a drug candidate enters the clinic genome scans would be carried out in parallel with the specific gene probes to generate associations with clinical responses. Depending on the number of specific gene polymorphisms and complexity of their biology functional data might also be generated allowing for the selection of "preferred" patient populations. Finally, a knowledge of the nature of variations in target genes might also guide medicinal chemistry efforts away from compounds with allele specific activities.

5   Model organisms and genomics

The gene approaches described above represent only the first steps in the process of identifying the best new drug targets. In order to fully validate a new target (as much as it is possible to do so before entering the clinic) one needs to be able to determine the biochemical function of the gene product, identify the biochemical pathway in which it sits and the significance of the pathway to the biology and pathobiology of the whole organism. In the clinic the whole organism will be human, however the sequencing of other organisms, that superficially appear to be very dissimilar to humans, has led to the realization that many complex processes are conserved through significant evolutionary distances. In this section I will summarise the properties of some well established invertebrate model organisms and emphasise their value as tools in target validation studies.

5.1   Yeast

The genome of the baker's yeast, *Saccharomyces cerevisiae*, was the first eukaryotic genome to be fully sequenced [96]. Although it had been clear to researchers that many genes in mammals and yeast showed significant homology [25] it was only after the entire yeast genome was sequenced that a reasonable estimate could be made as to how many genes had mammalian homologues. Botstein and colleagues compared all the yeast protein sequences to the mammalian sequences present in GenBank and demonstrated that over 30% of yeast protein sequences showed statistically strong homology to mammalian protein sequences [29]. Of the approximately 60% of yeast genes for which no function has been assigned most contain sequence motifs that would serve as some guide to function. Only 25% of yeast genes cannot be assigned any putative function. This situation could change rapidly if one now considers the functional "binning" that can be made based on temporal transcription profiling experiments and the focused expermentation that can follow [42, 43]. The functional similarity between yeast and human genes is clearly illustrated by the observation that at least 71 human genes are capable of complementing yeast mutations (see http://www.ncbi.nlm.nih.gov/Bassett/cerevisiae /ComplementNew.html).

   S. cerevisiae is a very well studied organism and has been used for many years as a model for functional studies on higher eukaryotes. Yeast are very easy to manipulate in the laboratory making them economical in comparison with mammalian models and even mammalian cell culture. The yeast life cycle is admirably suited for genetic studies as it exists in both haploid and diploid states and undergoes meiosis. In addition yeast undergo mitotic recombination allowing the rapid production of targeted gene knockouts in the laboratory. As yeast can be cultured in a similar manner to bacteria and have a rapid life cycle, experiments can be carried out in weeks rather than months or years in comparison to mouse genetics. As a single cell organism yeast would not be the organism of choice for studies focused on cell differentiation or many aspects of intercellular signalling, although yeast does possess the capability to signal through G-protein coupled receptors [97, 98]. Yeast would contribute to a target validation program by enabling a very rapid understanding of the basic biochemistry of a novel gene sequence, by overexpression and knockout studies, provided that sequence has a yeast homologue.

5.2   Caenorhabditis elegans

C. elegans is the most thoroughly characterised multicellular organism. It has been used as a model organism for the study of developmental genetics since its utility was first recognised in the early 1960s by Sidney Brenner. Meticulous work by John Sulston and colleagues led to the developmental description of every one of the worm's 959 cells [99]. In 1998, virtually the entire sequence of *C. elegans* was reported, making it the first multicellular organism to be characterized at a genomic level [7–11, 27, 100]. To be of value in pharmaceutical research the genes of *C. elegans* need to show significant homology to those of humans. Previous sequencing efforts had indicated that in many cases this would be true but now it is possible to compare every *C. elegans* gene with those available for humans. Pairwise comparisons were made between *C. elegans* and two other fully characterised organisms (*S. cerevisiae* and *E. coli*) as well as about 5000 human genes. There were substantially more protein sequence matches between *C. elegans* and humans than between *C. elegans* and the other organisms. This would have been expected on evolutionary grounds. As has already been described above, yeast shows substantial similarity to humans in many genes. The closer relationship of *C. elegans* to humans illustrates the value this organism may have in determining the function of novel human genes. *C. elegans* is a facile laboratory organism with a wealth of associated genetic data. It has been used to dissect biochemical processes, such as programmed cell death, which has clinical significance in humans. Programmed cell death or apoptosis is a tightly regulated process under normal circumstances and is used to remove unwanted or damaged cells. It is thought to play a role in various pathological processes leading to disorders such as Parkinson's and Alzheimer's disease [101]. Three *C. elegans* genes, ced-3, ced-4 and ced-9 are involved in the apoptotic death of all cells. Ced-3 and ced-4 are pro-apoptotic while ced-9 is anti-apoptotic. Ced-3 shows homology to the cysteine protease genes which are known to be pro-apoptotic in mammalian cells while ced-9 shows homology to the anti-apoptotic Bcl-2 gene [102]. Until recently no mammalian homologue for ced-4 had been identified. Genetic studies in *C. elegans* had demonstrated that ced-4 acted downstream of ced-9. As the *C. elegans* data supported its existence, a significant effort was focused on the identification of a ced-4 functional homologue in mammalian cells. The existence of a ced-4 homologue was eventually demonstrated confirming the value of *C. elegans* genetics in understanding mammalian cell biology [103]. Although *C. elegans* will become a valuable tool in the elucidation of gene function it is probably too far removed from humans to become a routine model for pathological processes.

5.3 *Drosophila melanogaster*

The fruit fly has a long history in classical genetics and an extensive knowledge base exists on its natural and induced mutations. *Drosophila* is substantially more complex than *C. elegans* but can still be subjected to genetic manipulations that require large populations (a mated female lays between 700–1000 eggs in a lifetime) and short generation times (about 10 days) to analyse. The fruit fly only has four chromosomes and a genome size of about 1.65×10^8 base pairs comprising between 8000–20000 genes. A unique feature of flies is that the salivary gland chromosomes of the developing larva are comprised of many parallel chromosome threads having a characteristic banding pattern. These bands are visible by light microscopy and can be used to track genetic recombination events and the location of gene insertions. Of all the invertebrate model organisms the fruit fly genome shows the highest degree of structural homology to mammals. In addition many biochemical and signal transduction pathways are well conserved between fly and humans [104, 105]. Early in 1998, it was announced that a collaboration between academic and commercial groups will deliver the entire sequence of *D. melanogaster* by the end of 1999 [106]. The availability of this data will allow researchers to identify fly homologues of mammalian genes and to explore their function in genetic models leading to the identification of biochemically linked genes whose homologues can then be identified in mammalian databases. It is therefore likely that experimental approaches that identify novel genes with limited or no associated biological data (such as positional cloning or transcriptional profiling) will be well complemented by *Drosophila* genetics.

6   Conclusion

At the beginning of this review several concerns facing scientists involved in drug discovery and development activities were outlined and these are listed in Table 1 together with the genomics tools that can be employed to increase the likelihood of success and quality of the drug product. Success in the marketplace will require new drugs to have significant advantages over current therapies or address current unmet medical needs. Both these requirements will drive the search for new drug targets. Competition within the industry means it is likely that pharmaceutical research and development in the future will include significant efforts in new target discovery. Therefore, for every therapeutic indication being addressed it is important to define clearly the properties of a new target that make it well suited for pharmaceutical intervention. These might be defined generically as a protein (or nucleic acid), the activity of which can be modulated to bring about the desired therapeutic effect, while producing no undesired biological consequences. Therefore the protein should mediate a (single) specific process that is directly associated with the mechanism causing the disorder (or its pathology). In addition, as a result of the increasingly competitive intellectual property environment the target should be free of legal obligations. Although it is unclear what the eventual value of EST patents will be, it is clear that patent applications on full length genes, accompanied with data associating the gene function with specific pathologies, will be allowed, and should at the very least ensure a freedom to operate for the holder. It is therefore critical to generate as much functional data as one can on all the candidate genes one has identified. Tools such as transcriptional profiling coupled to advanced bioinformatic analysis and the astute application of model organisms should lead rapidly to the elucidation of gene function. In order to associate new genes with human disease it is likely that one would need to make use of mammalian models. These might be mouse genetic models, as discussed in section 4.1.2, or transgenic and knockout models. The availability of mouse expressed gene and genomic sequences will facilitate the rapid design and generation of transgenic mouse models. These models will be further enhanced by the application of tran-

Table 1.

R&D issues	Application of genomic tools
Selection of appropriate target	Human and mouse genetics, transcriptional profiling
Selectivity of lead compounds	Access to gene sequence databases
Safety and use of non-human models	Transcriptional profiling, drug disposition gene comparisons
Clinical response	Human genetics, high throughput mapping tools
Clinical safety	Human genetics, high throughput mapping tools

scriptional profiling to identify genes with defined temporal and tissue expression patterns. These genes can be used to create refined expression cassettes for transgenic models. In addition the use of high throughput mapping tools such as SNPs will allow one to determine whether genetic polymorphisms within the gene, or its pathway partners, associate with the disorder under study. Obviously, if the gene was identified through human genetics, these polymorphisms would have already been identified. Perhaps one of the most exciting areas of genomics research is the use of SNPs to rapidly scan the entire genome for polymorphisms. As described above SNPs should enable high resolution genome wide scans on many individuals. Apart from facilitating association studies to discover new therapeutic targets, SNPs should become cost effective tools in clinical trials (and even in the market) that will firstly associate genotype with response and subsequently allow patient selection for further trials and drug selection in the clinic. Once a genotype has been obtained for a patient it is possible to imagine that this can be used by the clinician in deciding on numerous therapeutics (having genotype/response data) for a whole range of disorders.

Our understanding of the structure and function of the human genome has, within the last ten years, increased beyond the most optimistic of predictions. It is likely that, over the next ten years, our insights into genome function in development, health and disease will develop in many obvious and unexpected ways. Presently our increased knowledge and the application of genomics tools are poised to optimise drug discovery and development activities as well as add value to the resulting drugs. It is likely that, in the future, these tools as well as tools and technologies yet to be developed, will significantly change the way we perform drug discovery.

References

1   S. A. Billstein: Antimicrob. Agents Chemother. *38*, 2679–2682 (1994).
2   J. Lazarou, B. H. Pomeranz and P. N. Corey: JAMA *279*, 1200–1205 (1998).
3   J. Drews: Nature Biotechnology *14*, 1516–1517 (1996).
4   F. Antequera and A. Bird: Nature Genetics *8*, 114 (1994).
5   C. Fields, M. D. Adams, O. White and J. C. Venter: Nature Genetics *7*, 345–346 (1994).
6   S. M. Thomas: Drug Discovery Today *4*, 134–138 (1999).
7   Science *282*, 2012–2018 (1998) (for authors see http://www.sanger.ac.uk/Projects/C_ele-gans/ and http://genome.wustl.edu/gsc/C_elegans/).
8   N. D. Clarke and J. M. Berg: Science *282*, 2018–2022 (1998).
9   C. I. Bargmann: Science *282*, 2028–2033 (1998).
10   M. Blaxter: Science *282*, 2041–2046 (1998).
11   G. Ruvkun and O. Hobert: Science *282*, 2033–2041 (1998).
12   F. S. Collins, A. Patrinos, E. Jordan, A. Chakravarti, R. Gesteland and L. Walters: Science *282*, 682–689 (1998).
13   F. S. Collins: Hospital Practice (Office Edition) *32*, 35–43, 46–9, 53–4 (1997).
14   P. Deloukas, G. D. Schuler, G. Gyapay, E. M. Beasley, C. Soderlund, P. Rodriguez-Tome, L. Hui, T. C. Matise, K. B. McKusick, J. S. Beckmann et al.: Science *282*, 744–746 (1998).
15   J. C. Venter, M. D. Adams, G. G. Sutton, A. R. Kerlavage, H. O. Smith and M. Hunkapiller: Science *280*, 1540–1542 (1998).
16   M. D. Adams, M. Dubnick, A. R. Kerlavage, R. Moreno, J. M. Kelley, T. R. Utterback, J. W. Nagle, C. Fields and J. C. Venter: Nature *355*, 632–634 (1992).
17   M. D. Adams, M. B. Soares, A. R. Kerlavage, C. Fields and J. C. Venter: Nat. Genet. *4*, 373–380 (1993).
18   M. D. Adams, A. R. Kerlavage, C. Fields and J. C. Venter: Nat. Genet. *4*, 256–267 (1993).
19   W. R. McCombie, M. D. Adams, J. M. Kelley, M. G. FitzGerald, T. R. Utterback, M. Khan, M. Dubnick, A. R. Kerlavage, J. C. Venter and C. Fields: Nat. Genet. *1*, 124–131 (1992).
20   J. C. Venter: J. Pharm. Pharmacol. *45* (Suppl. 1), 355–360 (1993).
21   S. F. Altschul, W. Gish, W. Miller, E. W. Myers and D. J. Lipman: J. Mol. Biol. *215*, 403–410 (1990).
22   S. F. Altschul, T. L. Madden, A. A. Schaffer, J. Zhang, Z. Zhang, W. Miller and D. J. Lipman: Nucleic Acids Res. *25*, 3389–402 (1997).
23   S. F. Altschul and E. V. Koonin: Trends Biochem. Sci. *23*, 444–447 (1998).
24   Z. Zhang, A. A. Schaffer, W. Miller, T. L. Madden, D. J. Lipman, E. V. Koonin and S. F. Altschul: Nucleic Acids Res. *26*, 3986–3990 (1998).
25   S. Tugendreich, D. E. Bassett, Jr., V. A. McKusick, M. S. Boguski and P. Hieter: Human Mol. Gen. *3*, 1509–1517 (1994).
26   H. W. Mewes, K. Albermann, M. Bahr, D. Frishman, A. Gleissner, J. Hani, K. Heumann, K. Kleine, A. Maierl, S. G. Oliver et al.: Nature *387*, 7–65 (1997).
27   S. A. Chervitz, L. Aravind, G. Sherlock, C. A. Ball, E. V. Koonin, S. S. Dwight, M. A. Harris, K. Dolinski, S. Mohr, T. Smith et al.: Science *282*, 2022–8 (1998).
28   S. Banfi, G. Borsani, E. Rossi, L. Bernard, A. Guffanti, F. Rubboli, A. Marchitiello, S. Giglio, E. Coluccia, M. Zollo et al.: Nature Genetics *13*, 167–74 (1996).
29   D. Botstein, S. A. Chervitz and J. M. Cherry: Science *277*, 1259–60 (1997).

30   D. A. Benson, M. S. Boguski, D. J. Lipman, J. Ostell, B. F. F. Ouellette, B. A. Rapp and D. L. Wheeler: Nucleic Acids Res. *27*, 12–17 (1999).

31   C. Burks: Nucleic Acids Res. *27*, 1–19 (1999).

32   W. R. Pearson: Methods in Enzymology *266*, 227–258 (1996).

33   M. B. Swindells, C. A. Orengo, D. T. Jones, E. G. Hutchinson and J. M. Thornton: Bioessays *20*, 884–891 (1998).

34   R. Lewin: *Patterns in Evolution: The New Molecular View*, W.H. Freeman and Company, New York 1996.

35   M. Y. Galperin, D. R. Walker and E. V. Koonin: Genome Res. *8*, 779–790 (1998).

36   C. A. Orengo, D. T. Jones and J. M. Thornton: Nature *372*, 631–634 (1994).

37   D. J. Duggan, M. Bittner, Y. Chen, P. Meltzer and J. M. Trent: Nat. Genet. *21*, 10–14 (1999).

38   R. J. Lipshutz, S. P. Fodor, T. R. Gingeras and D. J. Lockhart: Nat. Genet. *21*, 20–24 (1999).

39   M. Schena, D. Shalon, R. W. Davis and P. O. Brown: Science *270*, 467–470 (1995).

40   J. Khan, R. Simon, M. Bittner, Y. Chen, S. B. Leighton, T. Pohida, P. D. Smith, Y. Jiang, G. C. Gooden, J. M. Trent et al.: Cancer Res. *58*, 5009–5013 (1998).

41   R. A. Heller, M. Schena, A. Chai, D. Shalon, T. Bedilion, J. Gilmore, D. E. Woolley and R. W. Davis: Proc. Nat. Acad. Sci. USA *94*, 2150–2155 (1997).

42   J. L. DeRisi, V. R. Iyer and P. O. Brown: Science *278*, 680–686 (1997).

43   S. Chu, J. DeRisi, M. Eisen, J. Mulholland, D. Botstein, P. O. Brown and I. Herskowitz: Science *282*, 699–705 (1998).

44   V. R. Iyer, M. B. Eisen, D. T. Ross, G. Schuler, T. Moore, J. C. F. Lee, J. M. Trent, L. M. Staudt, J. Hudson Jr., M. S. Boguski et al.: Science *283*, 83–87 (1999).

45   M. B. Eisen, P. T. Spellman, P. O. Brown and D. Botstein: Proc. Nat. Acad. Sci. USA *95*, 14863–14868 (1998).

46   S. Ball and N. Borman: Nat. Biotechnol. *15*, 925–926 (1997).

47   P. Propping and M. M. Nothen: Pharmacogenetics *5*, 318–325 (1995).

48   S. J. Kendrew: *The Encyclopedia of Molecular Biology*, Blackwell Science Ltd., Oxford 1994.

49   A. E. H. Emery, in: P. Harper and M. Bobrow (eds): *Duchenne Muscular Dystrophy*, Oxford University Press, Oxford 1987.

50   D. R. Love and K. E. Davies: Mol. Biol. Med. *6*, 7–17 (1989).

51   M. Koenig, E. P. Hoffman, C. J. Bertelson, A. P. Monaco, C. Feener and L. M. Kunkel: Cell *50*, 509–517 (1987).

52   C. R. Kahn, D. Vicent and A. Doria: Annu. Rev. Med. *47*, 509–531 (1996).

53   M. A. Permutt, K. Chiu, J. Ferrer, B. Glaser, H. Inoue, A. Nestorowicz, C. A. Stanley and Y. Tanizawa: Recent Prog. Horm. Res. *53*, 201–216 (1998).

54   T. J. Aitman, A. M. Glazier, C. A. Wallace, L. D. Cooper, P. J. Norsworthy, F. N. Wahid, K. M. Al-Majali, P. M. Trembling, C. J. Mann, C. C. Shoulders et al.: Nat. Genet. *21*, 76–83 [MEDLINE record in process] (1999).

55   E. S. Lander: Science *274*, 536–539 (1996).

56   T. Strachan and A. P. Read: *Human Molecular Genetics*, BIOS Scientific Publishers Ltd., Oxford 1996.

57   I.-H. Pawlowitzki, J. H. Edwards and E. A. Thompson: *Genetic Mapping of Disease Genes*, Academic Press, London 1997.

58   D. G. Wang, J. B. Fan, C. J. Siao, A. Berno, P. Young, R. Sapolsky, G. Ghandour, N. Perkins, E. Winchester, J. Spencer et al.: Science *280*, 1077–1082 (1998).

59   C. Ober, N. J. Cox, M. Abney, A. Di Rienzo, E. S. Lander, B. Changyaleket, H. Gidley, B. Kurtz, J. Lee, M. Nance et al.: Hum. Mol. Genet. *7*, 1393–1398 (1998).

60   E. Pennisi: Science *281*, 1787–1789 (1998).

61   A. G. Clark, K. M. Weiss, D. A. Nickerson, S. L. Taylor, A. Buchanan, J. Stengard, V. Salomaa, E. Vartiainen, M. Perola, E. Boerwinkle et al.: Am. J. Hum. Genet. *63*, 595–612 (1998).

62   E. S. Lander and N. J. Schork: Science *265*, 2037–2048 (1994).

63   Freimer, N. B., Reus, V. I., Escamilla, M., Spesny, M., Smith, L., Service, S., Gallegos, A., Meza, L., Batki, S., Vinogradov, S. et al.: Am. J. Med. Genet. *67*, 254–263 (1996)

64   N. B. Freimer, V. I. Reus, M. A. Escamilla, L. A. McInnes, M. Spesny, P. Leon, S. K. Service, L. B. Smith, S. Silva, E. Rojas et al.: Nature Genetics *12*, 436–441 (1996).

65   W. Wu, J. D. Cogan, R. W. Pfaffle, J. S. Dasen, H. Frisch, S. M. O'Connell, S. E. Flynn, M. R. Brown, P. E. Mullis, J. S. Parks et al.: Nat. Genet. *18*, 147–149 (1998).

66   M. W. Sornson, W. Wu, J. S. Dasen, S. E. Flynn, D. J. Norman, S. M. O'Connell, I. Gukovsky, C. Carriere, A. K. Ryan, A. P. Miller et al.: Nature *384*, 327–333 (1996).

67   J. K. Naggert, L. D. Fricker, O. Varlamov, P. M. Nishina, Y. Rouille, D. F, Steiner, R. J. Carroll, B. J. Paigen and E. H. Leiter: Nat. Genet. *10*, 135–142 (1995).

68   K. Noben-Trauth, J. K. Naggert, M. A. North and P. M. Nishina: Nature *380*, 534–538 (1996).

69   L. A. Tartaglia, M. Dembski, X. Weng, N. Deng, J. Culpepper, R. Devos, G. J. Richards, L. A. Campfield, F. T. Clark, J. Deeds et al.: Cell *83*, 1263–1271 (1995).

70   Y. Zhang, R. Proenca, M. Maffei, M. Barone, L. Leopold and J. M. Friedman: Nature *372*, 425–432 (1994).

71   P. W. Kleyn, W. Fan, S. G. Kovats, J. J. Lee, J. C. Pulido, Y. Wu, L. R. Berkemeier, D. J. Misumi, L. Holmgren, O. Charlat et al.: Cell *85*, 281–290 (1996).

72   Y. C. Chagnon, L. Perusse and C. Bouchard: Obes. Res. *6*, 76–92 (1998).

73   J. Suto, S. Matsuura, K. Imamura, H. Yamanaka and K. Sekikawa: Mamm. Genome *9*, 506–510 (1998).

74   A. G. Motulsky: J. Am. Med. Assoc. *165*, 835–837 (1957).

75   A. Puga, D. W. Nebert, R. A. McKinnon and A. G. Menon: Crit. Rev. Toxicol. *27*, 199–222 (1997).

76   A. K. Daly, J. Brockmoller, F. Broly, M. Eichelbaum, W. E. Evans, F. J. Gonzalez, J. D. Huang, J. R. Idle, M. Ingelman-Sundberg, T. Ishizaki et al.: Pharmacogenetics *6*, 193–201 (1996).

77   A. K. Daly, K. S. Fairbrother, O. A. Andreassen, S. J. London, J. R. Idle and V. M. Steen: Pharmacogenetics *6*, 319–328 (1996).

78   D. Marez, M. Legrand, N. Sabbagh, J. M. Guidice, C. Spire, J. J. Lafitte, U. A. Meyer and F. Broly: Pharmacogenetics *7*, 193–202 (1997).

79   Y. Hu, M. Oscarson, I. Johansson, Q. Y. Yue, M. L. Dahl, M. Tabone, S. Arinco, E. Albano and M. Ingelman-Sundberg: Mol. Pharmacol. *51*, 370–6 (1997).

80   M. J. Stubbins, L. W. Harries, G. Smith, M. H. Tarbit and C. R. Wolf: Pharmacogenetics *6*, 429–439 (1996).

81   R. L. Lindberg and M. Negishi: Nature *339*, 632–634 (1989).

82   J. Poirier, M. C. Delisle, R. Quirion, I. Aubert, M. Farlow, D. Lahiri, S. Hui, P. Bertrand, J. Nalbantoglu, B. M. Gilfix et al.: Proc. Nat. Acad. Sci. USA *92*, 12260–12264 (1995).

83   M. R. Farlow, D. K. Lahiri, J. Poirier, J. Davignon, L. Schneider and S. L. Hui: Neurology *50*, 669–677 (1998).

84   F. Richard, N. Helbecque, E. Neuman, D. Guez, R. Levy and P. Amouyel: Lancet *349*, 539 (1997).

85   B. Nakhai, D. A. Nielsen, M. Linnoila and D. Goldman: Biochem. Biophys. Res. Com-
      mun. *210*, 530–536 (1995).
86   J. Erdmann, D. Shimron-Abarbanell, M. Rietschel, M. Albus, W. Maier, J. Korner, B.
      Bondy, K. Chen, J. C. Shih, M. Knapp et al.: Hum. Genet. *97*, 614–619 (1996).
87   M. Bruss, M. Buhlen, J. Erdmann, M. Gothert and H. Bonisch: Naunyn Schmiedebergs
      Arch. Pharmacol. *352*, 455–458 (1995).
88   N. M. Nothen, J. Erdmann, D. Shimron-Abarbanell and P. Propping: Biochem. Biophys.
      Res. Commun. *205*, 1194–1200 (1994).
89   L. Yang, T. Li, C. Wiese, L. Lannfelt, P. Sokoloff, C. T. Xu, Z. Zeng, J. C. Schwartz, X. Liu
      and H. W. Moises: Am. J. Med. Genet. *48*, 83–86 (1993).
90   E. Jonsson, L. Lannfelt, P. Sokoloff, J. C. Schwartz and G. Sedvall: Acta Psychiatr. Scand.
      87, 345–349 (1993).
91   J. B. Lichter, C. L. Barr, J. L. Kennedy, H. H. Van Tol, K. K. Kidd and K. J. Livak: Hum. Mol.
      Genet. *2*, 767–773 (1993).
92   S. Cichon, M. M. Nothen, M. Catalano, D. Di Bella, W. Maier, D. Lichtermann, J. Minges,
      M. Albus, M. Borrmann, E. Franzek et al.: Psychiatr. Genet. *5*, 97–103 (1995).
93   S. Shaikh, D. Collier, R. W. Kerwin, L. S. Pilowsky, M. Gill, W. M. Xu and A. Thornton:
      Lancet *341*, 116 (1993).
94   P. A. Rao, D. Pickar, P. V. Gejman, A. Ram, E. S. Gershon and J. Gelernter: Arch. Gen. Psy-
      chiatry *51*, 912–917 (1994).
95   J. L. Kennedy, A. Petronis, J. Gao, F. M. Macciardi, H. M. M. Van Tol, P. Cola and H. Y.
      Meltzer: Am. J. Hum. Genet. *55* (Suppl.), A190 (1994).
96   A. Goffeau, B. G. Barrell, H. Bussey, R. W. Davis, B. Dujon, H. Feldmann, F. Galibert, J.
      D. Hoheisel, C. Jacq, M. Johnston et al.: Science *274*, 546, 563–567 (1996).
97   H. Reilander and H. M. Weiss: Curr. Opin. Biotechnol. *9*, 510–517 (1998).
98   M. H. Pausch: Trends Biotechnol. *15*, 487–494 (1997).
99   J. E. Sulston, E. Schierenberg, J. G. White and J. N. Thomson: Developmental Biology
      100, 64–119 (1983).
100   J. Hodgkin, H. R. Horvitz, B. R. Jasny and J. Kimble: Science *282*, 2011 (1998).
101   P. Spence, A. Wood, J. Moyer and R. Franco: Expert Opinion in Therapeutic Patents *6*,
      345–366 (1996).
102   H. Steller: Science *267*, 1445–1449 (1995).
103   M. D. Jacobson: Trends in Cell Biology *7*, 467–469 (1997).
104   R. Derynck and Y. Zhang: Curr. Biol. *6*, 1226–1229 (1996).
105   E. Pennisi: Science *281*, 1438–1439, 1441 (1998).
106   E. Pennisi: Science *283*, 767 (1999).

Progress in Drug Research, Vol. 53 (E. Jucker, Ed.)
©1999 Birkhäuser Verlag, Basel (Switzerland)

Phosphodiesterase 4 (PDE4) inhibitors in asthma and chronic obstructive pulmonary disease (COPD)

By Mary S. Barnette

Pulmonary Pharmacology, SmithKline Beecham Pharmaceuticals, 709 Swedeland Road, King of Prussia, PA 19406-0939, USA

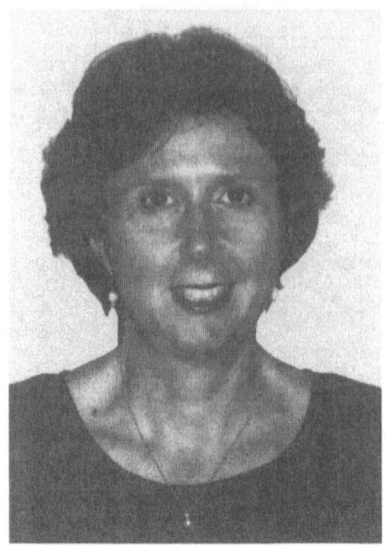

Mary S. Barnette

is currently an Associate Director in the Pulmonary Pharmacology, SmithKline Beecham Pharmaceuticals. She received her doctoral degree in Pharmacology from the University of Pennsylvania. Mary is married with two children and in her spare time enjoys reading and ice dancing.

Summary

Phosphodiesterases (PDE) are a family of enzymes responsible for the metabolism of the intracellular second messengers cyclic AMP and cyclic GMP. PDE4 is a cyclic AMP specific PDE that is the major if not sole cyclic AMP metabolizing enzymes found in inflammatory and immune cells, and contributes significantly to cyclic AMP metabolism in smooth muscles. Based on its cellular and tissue distribution and the demonstration that selective inhibitors of this isozyme reduce bronchoconstriction in animals and suppress the activation of inflammatory cells, PDE4 has become an important molecular target for the development of novel therapies for asthma and COPD. This chapter will review the evidence demonstrating the ability of PDE4 inhibitors to modify airway obstruction, airway inflammation and airway remodelling and hyperreactivity, will present some preliminary findings obtained with theses compounds in clinical trials and and will discuss experimental approaches designed to identify novel compounds that maintain the beneficial activity of the initial selective PDE4 inhibitors but with a reduced tendency to elicit the gastrointestinal side effects observed with this class of compounds.

Contents

Keywords

Airway, airway obstruction, asthma, basophils, bronchoconstriction, edema, eosinophils, inflammation, macrophages, monocytes, neutrophils, phosphodiesterase, T cells

Glossary of abbreviations

BAL, bronchoalveolar lavage; CNS, central nervous system; COPD, chronic obstructive pulmonary disease; cyclic AMP, $3'5'$ cyclic adenosine monophosphate; cyclic GMP, $3'5'$ cyclic guanosine monophosphate; FEV_1, forced expiratory volume in one second; fMLP, formyl methionine leucine phenylalanine; GM-CSF, granulocyte macrophage colony stimulating factor; 5-HT, 5-hydroxytryptamine; HPDE4, high affinity phosphodiesterase 4; IL, interleukin; LPS, lipopolysaccharide; LPDE4, low affinity phosphodiesterase 4; LTB_4, leukotriene B_4; LTD_4, leukotriene D_4; NANC, non-cholinergic, non adrenergic; NO, nitric oxide; PAF, platelet activating factor; PGE_2, prostaglandin E_2; PDE, phosphodiesterase; RNA ribonucleic acid; TNF, tumor necrosis factor

Mary S. Barnette

1   Introduction

The cyclic nucleotide phosphodiesterases (PDE) comprise a superfamily of proteins with 10 individual families whose function is to inactivate cyclic AMP or cyclic GMP, two critical intracellular second messengers [1, 2]. The individual families are defined by their substrate preference and catalytic activity, their sensitivity to endogenous activators and inhibitors and their distinct genes [1–3]. Moreover, each family of PDE exhibits varying patterns of tissue and cellular distribution as well as functional roles [1–3]. Because of the importance of cyclic nucleotides in regulating cellular function and the ability to identify selective inhibitors of individual families, this superfamily of proteins have been the focus of intensive drug discovery efforts [2, 3]. This chapter will review the family of PDEs known as PDE4.

PDE4 has emerged as important drug discovery target for the identification of novel anti-asthmatic and anti-inflammatory agents based on the results of studies demonstrating that: (1) cyclic AMP is an important intracellular regulator of inflammatory cell activation, airway and vascular smooth cell contractility and proliferation, and pulmonary neuronal responsiveness; (2) PDE4 represents the major, if not sole, cAMP metabolizing activity in these cells; (3) prototypical PDE4 or first generation inhibitors such as rolipram have demonstrated impressive activity in in vivo models of airway disease [1].

The PDE4 family of enzymes is comprised of four genes with the subtypes designated by the letters, A, B, C, and D [4] and each gene has a unique chromosomal location [5, 6]. The PDE4 genes encode for multiple proteins that vary in size due to alternate splicing of the genes. Two main divisions exist for all of the PDE4 splice variants, referred to as the "long and short" forms of PDE4. Numerical numbers, e.g. PDE4A4, refers to the splice variants within each subtype. These proteins consist of a conserved catalytic core and the absence (short) or presence (long) of two additional regions of homology within the N-terminal domain of the protein. These additional regions of sequence homology found in the PDE4 genes are known as UCR1 (upstream conserved region) and UCR2 [7, 8]. These regions appear to be important for subcellular distribution, potential post-translational regulation and the potency of some but not all structural classes of selective PDE4 inhibitors [8]. All subtypes of PDE4 selectively catalyze the hydrolysis of cAMP with a Km of 1–4 μM [1, 2] and several structural classes of selective inhibitors of PDE4 have been identified [2, 9–12]. A greater discussion of the molecular biology of this family of proteins is beyond the scope of this review, and moreover, this topic has been the subject of several comprehensive publications [8, 13].

This review will be divided into three main parts. The first section will describe briefly the pathophysiology or asthma and chronic obstructive pulmonary disease (COPD). The second section will outline the ability of PDE4 inhibitors to modify these processes and present the results obtained in the initial clinical trials with select compounds. The final section will discuss the potential challenges and strategies in the search for novel PDE4 inhibitors with improved profiles compared to current compounds.

2 Pathophysiology of asthma and COPD

2.1 Airways obstruction

Asthma is defined as a disease of reversible airway obstruction characterized by a decrease in FEV_1 and peak expiratory flow that can be reversed with spasmolytics such as β-adrenergic agonists [14, 15]. Airways obtained from individuals who died from asthma have a lumen filled with thick mucus, an increased collagen deposition beneath the basement membrane of the epithelium and a thickened bronchial wall due to edema and vascular congestion within the wall as well as smooth muscle cell contraction [16]. Biopsy samples obtained from individuals with milder forms of asthma also show similar features of airway obstruction [15, 16] emphasizing the clinical importance of these observations. Thus, a key goal in asthma treatment is the ability to reduce or eliminate the intermittent obstruction that occurs with this disease.

Chronic obstructive pulmonary disease is an umbrella term covering a spectrum of diseases with the two ends represented by emphysema and chronic bronchitis [17]. Both diseases are characterized by airway obstruction that is poorly reversible and progressive [17]. COPD is considered to be a disease of the small airways and alveoli [17]. In chronic bronchitis, airflow obstruction arises from increased mucus secretion due to mucus gland hyperplasia and metaplasia, in addition to peribronchiolar inflammation and fibrosis of the small airways. In contrast, in emphysema, airway obstruction primarily results from the loss of elastic recoil due to the destruction of alveolar walls and enlargement of the airspaces [17].

2.2 Airways inflammation

Asthma is recognized as an inflammatory disease of both the large and small airways [15, 18–20]. Indeed, chronic asthma is characterized by a cell-mediated immune response irrespective of the presence of atopy [21]. The inflammatory reaction seen in asthmatic airways consists of an increased number of degranulated mast cells [15] and their products, such as histamine and the cystienyl leukotrienes measured in bronchoalveolar lavage fluid [22]. These mediators contribute to the immediate bronchoconstrictive response and airway edema upon antigen challenge [15, 22]. In addition, mast cells release cytokines such as TNFα, IL-4 and IL-5 that recruit and activate additional inflammatory cells such as eosinophils and T lymphocytes [23]. Both the number and the activation state of eosinophils and T lymphocytes are increased in asthmatic airways [15, 19, 24]. Eosinophils, by virtue of their ability to release reactive oxygen intermediates and toxic granule products such as major basic protein (MBP), have been implicated in the epithelium cell damage and denudation characteristically seen in biopsy samples from asthmatic airways [15]. Also the degree of airway reactivity appears to be correlated with the level of airway eosinophils [15, 18]. The majority of T cells found in asthmatic biopsies are CD4+ T cells expressing the Th2 phenotype, i.e. producing mainly the cytokines IL-4 and IL-5 upon activation [25]. These cytokines, in addition to recruiting and activating additional inflammatory cells (e.g. IL-5 recruits eosinophils) may play a role in the airway remodeling characteristic of chronic asthma [26]. Furthermore, there appears to be a correlation between the number of CD4+ T cells and the degree of airway reactivity [18]. Indeed it has been postulated that the hyperreactivity seen in asthma is secondary to the airway inflammation [15, 19].

The inflammatory reaction in COPD is distinct from that seen in asthma. In COPD, the neutrophil is a key inflammatory cell in causing the pathophysiology [17, 27]. Neutrophils numbers are increased in the bronchioalveolar lavage (BAL) fluid obtained from individuals with COPD [28–

30]. These leukocytes are found in the epithelial layer and bronchial mucous glands [28, 30]. Increases in both neutrophil chemoattractants, such as IL-8, and neutrophil degranulation products, such as myeloperoxidase and elastase, in BAL fluid also are found in COPD [27–29]. Genetic studies demonstrating the increased risk of developing emphysema associated with the lack of several serine protease inhibitors lend further credence to the emerging role of neutrophils in the pathophysiology of COPD [17, 31]. An increased number of subepithelial T cells, especially CD8[+] T cells and macrophages has been recently observed in chronic bronchitis, especially in those individuals who demonstrate airflow obstruction [28, 32, 33]. These T cells are found in the lamina propria and epithelium along with an increased number of B cells in the adventitia [34]. In concert, these findings argue strongly that COPD like asthma is an inflammatory disease of the airways.

2.3 Airway reactivity and remodeling

The exact causes of airways hyperreactivity found in asthma are currently unknown, although a correlation with epithelial damage has been demonstrated and there is evidence for a relationship with inflammation [18]. Damage to the epithelium may reduce the production of epithelium-derived relaxing factors such as PGE_2 or nitrous oxide (NO) [35]. The loss of the epithelial barrier could expose the non-myelinated sensory C fibers to the environmental stimuli increasing the probability of their activation. Also, the release of inflammatory mediators has been shown to sensitize the sensory neurons to stimuli [36]. Once stimulated, these sensory neurons elicit a reflex bronchoconstriction, with increases in vascular permeability and mucus secretion [37]. These fibers innervate the parasympathetic ganglion as well and activation of this path could modulate both the cholinergic input to the airways as well as the inhibitory non-cholinergic non adrenergic pathway [36, 37]. Both the changes in neuronal control of the airways with inflammation and the regulatory role of the epithelium on inflammation and airways responsiveness are emerging areas of investigation.

Airway remodeling occurs in both asthma and COPD. In asthmatic airways there is a thickening of the airway wall with subepithelial fibrosis and hyperplasia and hypertrophy of medial smooth muscle layer [38, 39]. In addition, there is an increase in the number of goblet cells in the epithelial layer and a hypertrophy of the subepithelial mucus glands [17, 40]. Changes in the extracellular matrix occur in asthma with increased levels of collagen, types I, III, and V but not type VI [26].

Airways hyperresponsiveness is also a characteristic of COPD; two-thirds of individuals with early stages of COPD demonstrate hyperresponsiveness and its presence predicts a faster decline in FEV_1 [28]. The cellular and physiological changes that are responsible for airways hyperresponsiveness in this disease are less understood than those that occur in asthma. One potential mechanism is airway remodeling [41]. The thickness of the airway wall increases in COPD due to an enhanced amount of submucosal and advential tissue. Several factors contribute to this change. Firstly, enhanced edema and proteoglycan deposition occurs. Secondly, chronic inflammation of the airways produces an irreversible augmentation in collagen deposition and fibrosis. Thirdly, there is an increased number of bronchial capillaries and hypertrophy or hyperplasia of airway smooth muscle [41]. Finally, there is a striking increase in the number of goblet cells present in the mucosal layer of the small bronchioles (< 2 mm in diameter); this is not found in asthma [42].

This brief overview demonstrates that COPD and asthma share common features of airway obstruction, airway inflammation and airway hyperresponsiveness and remodeling. The mechanism responsible for these changes have both common and unique aspects and an ideal therapy for chronic airway disease would modify all of these changes.

3   Ability of selective PDE4 inhibitors to modify pathophysiology of asthma and COPD

3.1   Airway obstruction

3.1.1 Airway smooth muscle tone

Airway smooth muscle contains multiple forms of PDE [1, 2]. The major cyclic AMP metabolizing activities found in tracheal and bronchial smooth muscle are PDE3 and PDE4 [43–47]. Functionally both isozymes contribute to the regulation of airway smooth muscle tone. Selective inhibitors of either PDE3 or PDE4 reduce spontaneous tone of airway smooth muscle *in vitro* and partially relax pre-contracted tissues [43, 45, 46]. In general, selective PDE3 inhibitors produce a greater magnitude of relaxation than selective PDE4 inhibitors [44, 46, 48]. Addition of a combination of a PDE3 and a PDE4 inhibitor or a combined PDE3/4 inhibitors such as benzafentrine or zardarverine causes greater relaxation of airway smooth muscle tone than elicited by the selective inhibitor alone [43, 48–50]. As expected PDE3 and PDE4 inhibitors elevate cyclic AMP content of isolated airway smooth muscles and enhance both the relaxant effects of β-adrenergic receptor agonists or prostaglandins in these tissues and their ability to elevate smooth muscle cyclic AMP content [1, 2].

There are initial reports to suggest that the functional importance PDE4 varies in controlling airway smooth muscle tone among species and the region of the airway [45, 51]. For example, in human bronchial tissue, it appears that PDE4 rather than PDE 3 regulates tone in the smaller airways (2–3 mm) [45]. Both the biochemical and functional data provide compelling evidence that by blocking the activity of PDE4, especially in the smaller airways, selective PDE4 inhibitors could substantially reduce the airway obstruction seen in both asthma and COPD.

Selective PDE4 inhibitors produce bronchodilation *in vivo* in several species. For example, PDE4 inhibitors, such as rolipram, have been reported to reduce the bronchoconstriction elicited by histamine, LTD_4, 5-HT, bombesin or endothelin [43, 52–55]. Although selective PDE3 inhibitors also produce bronchodilation, the effect is usually accompanied by alterations in the cardiovascular parameters. This latter effect is not apparent with PDE4 inhibitors [54]. Especially relevant to the proposed therapeutic use of PDE4 inhibitors in asthma is the observation that these compounds prevent antigen-induced airway smooth muscle contraction and bronchoconstriction in the guinea pig [1, 52]. It has been speculated that this pharmacological activity of this class of compounds resides more in their ability to suppress mediator release from tissue mast cells than from a direct effect on airway smooth muscle since rolipram was less effective at inhibiting histamine- or LTD4-induced bronchospasm [56]. Unlike the results obtained in the guinea pig, rolipram did not prevent the immediate bronchoconstrictive response to antigen in ascaris-sensitized monkeys, neonatally sensitized rabbits or sensitized rats [57–59]. The mechanisms behind these species differences have not been extensively studied; however, they could reflect a differential sensitivity of lung mast cells to the suppressive effects of PDE4 inhibition. A key question, currently under study in a number of clinical trials, is what is the sensitivity of antigen-induced bronchospasm in humans to PDE4 inhibitors.

3.1.2 Vascular endothelial cells and airway edema

Airway edema contributes to airflow obstruction by increasing the size of the airway wall. Biochemical studies indicate that PDE4 is present in vascular endothelial cells [60–63]. It has been difficult to precisely define the PDE isozyme profile in these cells since the length of time in culture changes the relative proportion of each PDE isozyme [64]. Functionally, selective PDE4 inhibitors attenuate increased endothelial cell permeability induced by certain stimuli such as H_2O_2 [62], thrombin [63] or hemolysin A of *E. coli* [63], but not to others such as the pore forming protein, *S. aureus* toxin or botulinum toxin [62]. In endothelial cells, as seen in airway smooth muscle cells, addition of a PDE3 inhibitor augments the inhibitory effects of the selective PDE4 inhibitor [62, 63] and stimulation of adenylate cyclase by PGE2 or isoproterenol will potentiate the inhibitory effects of both PDE4 and PDE3 inhibitors [62, 63]. In general, *in vivo* studies show that PDE4 inhibitors but not PDE3 inhibitors reduce vascular leakage in the airways to diverse proinflammatory stimuli such as PAF [53, 65, 66] LPS [67, 68], antigen [68, 69], and to ischemic reperfusion injury [70] but not to histamine or substance P [69]. With regard to selective PDE3 inhibitors there are a few studies that demonstrate a reduction in vascular permeability [71, 72]. However, most of the data indicate that PDE4 is the functionally important isozyme in endothelial cells, suggesting that selective inhibitors may limit airway obstruction by reducing airway edema.

3.1.3 Airway epithelium and mucus secretion

An emerging area of investigation is the role of airway epithelium in regulating both airway smooth muscle tone and airway inflammation. Airway epithelial cells produce bronchorelaxant substances such as NO and PGE_2 [35,

73, 74]. These cells also release cytokines which augment the recruitment and activation of inflammatory cells, and contribute to the airway remodeling that occurs in chronic disease [35, 73, 74]. Airway epithelial cells express several PDE isozymes including PDE1, PDE3, PDE4 , PDE5 and some PDE7 [75–77]. At the RNA level, primary human airway epithelial cells express PDE4A, PDE4C and PDE4D but little PDE4B [77]. PDE4 appears to be the predominant isozyme in regulating cyclic AMP content of these cells and in enhancing the release of PGE_2 [77], whereas PDE3 may be more important in suppressing IL-1β-induced release of GM-CSF [76]. PDE4 inhibitors may enhance the barrier function of the epithelium, since rolipram exhibited a protective effect against microbial adherence and damage in cultured nasal explants [78].

The contribution of the various PDE isozyme to mucus secretion is only beginning to be defined. In an initial report, PDE4 inhibitors, but not selective PDE3 or PDE5 inhibitors, increased mucus secretion in isolated rat trachea [79]. How these agents modify the hyperplasia of mucus glands seen in COPD or the enhanced mucus production in asthma is unknown.

By relaxing airway smooth muscles, limiting edema formation, and enhancing the release of endogenous bronchorelaxants, PDE4 inhibitors offer the potential for reducing substantially airway obstruction in both asthma and COPD.

3.2 Airway inflammation

3.2.1 Introduction

The inflammatory cells considered most important in asthma are mast cells T lymphocytes, eosinophils, macrophages and basophils, whereas in COPD, it is believed that macrophages, neutrophils and T cells are the important cells. Elevation of cyclic AMP in these cells suppresses the release of inflammatory mediators, reactive oxygen free radicals and cytokines and chemokines [1, 2, 80, 81]. Analysis of the biochemical profiles of PDE isozymes in inflammatory cells indicate that PDE4 is a major cyclic AMP metabolizing isozyme in most leukocytes [1, 80, 82, 83]. The following sections will describe the ability of selective PDE4 inhibitors to modify the activation of these cells both *in vitro* and *in vivo*.

3.2.2 Mast cells and basophils

Purified human basophils, isolated lung mast cells and bone marrow derived murine mast cells contain both PDE3 and PDE4 [84–86]. In both basophils and mast cells elevation of cyclic AMP content inhibits release of histamine, leukotrienes and cytokines [84, 85, 87–90]. However, the sensitivity of these two cells types to selective PDE4 inhibitors differs. In basophils, treatment with PDE4 inhibitors alone suppresses antigen-induced histamine and leukotriene release as well as IL-4/IL-13 release [84, 86–90]; whereas, PDE4 inhibitors by themselves do not attenuate antigen induced mediator release from mast cells from several species [85, 86, 91–93]. The guinea pig lung mast cell appears to be an exception since rolipram reduced the antigen-induced release of histamine and prostaglandins [56]. An explanation for these species differences may be a variation in the basal level of adenylate cyclase activity. It was initially observed in airway smooth muscle that the pharmacological activity of PDE4 inhibitors can be dramatically enhanced in the presence of a low level of adenylate cyclase activation [1]. A similar phenomenon occurs for murine bone marrow derived mast cells since rolipram inhibits antigen-induced LTC_4 release in the presence of a threshold concentration of forskolin [85]. However, the level of adenylate cyclase activation does not explain the inability of PDE4 inhibitors to suppress mediator release from activated human lung mast cells since these compounds were ineffective at inhibiting IgE-mediated histamine or leuktriene release in the absence or presence of forskolin [86]. Furthermore, although PDE4 inhibitors blocked antigen-induced histamine release from guinea pig tissues [56] they did not reduce its release from isolated human lung fragments [92, 94] suggesting a species difference in the sensitivity to PDE4 inhibitors. These observations may explain the lack of effect of PDE4 inhibitors on the initial bronchoconstriction produced by antigen challenge that has been observed in several species as described previously.

3.2.3 Monocytes and macrophages

Macrophages are important for both the initiation and suppression of immune responses in the lung [21, 95]. These tissue-based cells are believed to be derived from the emigration and differentiation of peripheral blood monocytes. Although in many situations monocytes and macrophages behave similarly, each cell type has a distinct phenotype. For example, human blood monocytes contain predominately PDE4 [85, 96–99], whereas alveolar macrophages express substantial amounts of PDE3 along with PDE4 [101–103]. Indeed, differentiation of monocytes in culture to macrophages decreases the expression of PDE4 [102] while increasing the expression of PDE3, a profile which resembles that found in alveolar macrophage [100]. Differentiation of monocytes into macrophages also changes the expression of PDE4 subtypes. Thus, peripheral blood monocytes express PDE4, PDE4B and PDE4D subtypes [99, 104–106], whereas, human monocyte derived macrophages express only the PDE4A subtype [102].

Selective PDE4 inhibitors potently inhibit LPS-induced TNFα formation in peripheral blood monocytes [98, 107–112] while not markedly attenuating LPS-induced IL-1β or IL-6 production [107, 108, 110]. Moreover, the majority of studies demonstrate little or no effect of selective PDE3 inhibitors on cytokine production in these cells [107, 110]; although some reports demonstrate a modest suppression of IL-1β production [107, 113]. PDE4 inhibitors increase the release of the anti-inflammatory cytokine IL-10 [114, 115] and block the release of arachidonic acid release [116, 117]. Finally, PDE4 inhibitors synergize with endogenous activators of adenylate cyclase to inhibit the activation of monocytes [118, 119].

In macrophages, the functional role of PDE4 is not as clear and may depend on the species, tissue localization, or activation stimuli. For example, neither PDE4 nor PDE3 inhibitors alone were particularly effective in reducing LPS-induced TNFα formation in human macrophages [102] whereas added in combination, these inhibitors reduced TNFα formation by approximately 40–50% [102]. In contrast, PDE4 inhibitors but not PDE3 potently suppressed TNFα production in murine peritoneal and alveolar macrophages [120, 121]. The dependence of the effectiveness of PDE4 inhibitors on the activation stimuli can be exemplified by the observations that PDE4 inhibitors decreased superoxide production in response to fMLP and PAF but were ineffective in reducing PMA or opsonized zymosan induced supreoxide production in macrophages [122, 123]. These findings demonstrate that pharmacological effects of PDE4 inhibitors on macrophages are more complex than initially observed in monocytes.

Changes in cyclic AMP content regulate PDE4 activity at both the transcriptional and post-translational levels [124–126]. In monocytes, it was initially observed that stimulation of monocytes by histamine, PGE_2 or isoproterenol increased a RO 20-1724 sensitive PDE activity (suggestive of PDE4) [127]. Using monocytic cell lines, several groups demonstrated that elevation of cyclic AMP upregulates both the expression and activity of PDE4 [105, 128]. The increase in PDE4 content was produced by an elevation in the expression of PDE4 proteins especially PDE4A and PDE4 B subtypes [129]. A similar change in PDE4 expression has been observed in peripheral blood monocytes [99, 105]. The functional consequence of this change in PDE4 content was a reduction in the potency of cyclic AMP mediated stimuli to suppress monocyte activation which could be restored in the presence of selective PDE4 inhibitors [99, 129]. In addition to an enhanced expression of PDE4 proteins, PDE4 activity, particularly PDE4D can be regulated by protein kinase A mediated phosphorylation [130–134]. Treatment of the monocytic cell line, U937 with PGE_2 produced a rapid increase in PDE4 activity that was independent of protein synthesis [135, 136]. Immunoprecipitation of PDE4 proteins with subtype selective antibodies demonstrated that enhanced enzyme activity was the results of phosphorylation of PDE4D subtype by protein kinase A. Moreover phosphorylation of PDE4D but not PDE4B [137] increased the potency of some but not all PDE4 inhibitors [135].

The ability of inflammatory cells, like the monocyte, to regulate both the level and activity of PDE4 raises the possibility that a disease process might also change the cellular complement of these proteins. It was initially reported by Hanifin that peripheral blood mononuclear cells isolated from atopic donors contained more PDE activity than found in cells isolated from normal individuals. This increased PDE activity had the characteristics PDE4 [138, 139]. More recently, a direct comparison of PDE4 expression and activity in monocytes obtained from normal and atopic donors did not demonstrate any significant differences in total PDE4 activity or in the expression of the PDE4 subtypes [140]. Moreover, monocytes from either type of donor were equally sensitive to two different structural classes of PDE4 inhibitors [140]. Although not eliminating the possibility that disease processes in asthma or COPD, might influence PDE4 expression, these results do demonstrate that atopy *per se* does not.

3.2.4 Eosinophils

Eosinophils are considered a pivotal inflammatory cell in causing epithelial cell damage and airway hyperreactivity observed in asthma [1, 2, 141, 142]. Identification of novel therapeutics that prevent the recruitment or activation of these cells is a key goal of drug discovery efforts. Experiments using human and animal eosinophils indicate that PDE4 is the predominant PDE enzyme in these cells [143–148]. Information on the subcellular localization of PDE4 is equivocal, perhaps due to differences in the method of cell lysis or species. In guinea pig eosinophils, PDE4 activity is predominately membrane bound [143–146], whereas in human eosinphils the majority of PDE4 activity is found in the cytosolic fraction [147, 148]. Like most inflammatory cells, eosinophils express multiple subtypes of PDE4. Human eosinophils express PDE4A, PDE4B and PDE4D [13, 104, 140] whereas guinea pig eosinophils only express the PDE4D subtype [149]. Neither the amount nor the distribution of subtypes of PDE4 appears to change between eosinophils isolated from normal or atopic donors [140].

Selective PDE4 inhibitors influence the function of eosinophils at mutiple levels. These compounds inhibit the production and release of IL-5, a key cytokine in the generation, maturation and survival of eosinophils [150, 151]. PDE4 inhibitors prevent the chemotaxis of animal and human eosinophils to a variety of pro-inflammatory mediators such as LTB_4, C5a and PAF and the chemokine, eotaxin [152–156]. These compounds also suppress the activation of eosinophils as determined by a reduction in the release of superoxide free radicals [143, 144, 147, 157, 158] and arachidonic acid metabolites [154, 159]. Although potent at reducing the release of newly synthesized mediators, such as leukotrienes, PDE4 inhibitors by themselves are not very effective at preventing the degranulation of human eosinophils [148, 158]. However, in combination with an activator of adenylate cyclase, the suppressive action of these compounds is enhanced [148, 159]. Finally, PDE4 inhibitors have been reported to reduce the expression of the adhesion molecule, CD11/CD18 which is important for eosinophil trafficking *in vivo* [155, 160, 161].

Based on the results obtained with purified cells, it is not surprising that one of the most striking *in vivo* effects of selective PDE4 inhibitors is their ability to prevent eosinophil recruitment into tissues in response to multiple stimuli. For example, it has been demonstrated that selective PDE4 but not selective PDE3 or PDE5 inhibitors reduce or eliminate eosinophil recruitment in the guinea pig induced by PAF [162], IL-5 [163, 164], histamine [165] and LTD_4 [166]. Furthermore, this class of compounds reduces the antigen-induced elevation of eosinophil numbers in the lung or BAL fluid obtained from guinea pigs [52, 53, 59, 162, 164, 167–171], rabbits [172] and primates [57, 173] with an efficacy stimilar to corticosteriods [68, 164, 171]. Certain studies suggest that this is a preferential effect on eosinophil recruitment since the numbers of neutrophils were not changed [59, 172], however, other studies have demonstrated a reduction in antigen-induced neutrophil recruitment [57, 168]. Finally, PDE4 inhibitors, but not PDE3 inhibitors, reduce eosinophil recruitment into the skin elicited by PAF, antigen or zymosan [174]. These preclinical findings offer the exciting possibility that PDE4 inhibitors will also reduce eosinophil activation and trafficking in individuals with asthma; a hypothesis is currently under study in clinical trials.

3.2.5 Neutrophils

PDE4 appears to be the predominant cyclic AMP hydrolyzing enzyme in neutrophils [175–178]. PDE4 activity is found both in cytosolic and membrane fractions [177–179]. Neutrophils express predominately PDE4B [13, 104] with lower amounts of message for PDE4A or PDE4D [13]. However, using monoclonal antibodies, all three subtypes are found with a similar subcellular distribution [179].

Selective PDE4 inhibitors modify the pro-inflammatory activity of neutrophils at multiple levels. These compounds inhibit the production and release of chemokines [180], superoxide free radicals [177, 181–183], leukotrienes [112, 184] and proteolytic and toxic granular enzymes [111, 177, 181], as well as reducing neutrophil adherence to endothelial cells [185] and the activation-induced increase in adhension molecule expression [185–187]. The magnitude of these inhibitory actions is dramatically increased in the presence of PGE_2 or adenosine [181–183, 188, 189], confirming previously observations in other granulocytes, that PDE4 inhibitors are particularly effective in the presence of endogenous activators of adenylate cyclase.

In animal models, the ability of PDE4 inhibitors to decrease neutrophil recruitment is not as consistent as that seen with eosinophil migration. For example, using the tissue levels of myeloperoxidase as a marker for neutrophil influx, rolipram inhibited neutrophil influx elicited by arachidonic acid challenge to the ear [190]. Furthermore, selective PDE4 inhibitors abolished the LTB_4-induced neutropenia observed in a rabbit model [191] and prevented the LPS-induced increase in neutrophils in BAL fluid from guinea pigs [68, 192]. In contrast, PDE4 inhibitors did not reduce the number of neutrophils present in the skin after a passive cutaneous antigen challenge in guinea pigs [174], zymosan-induced neutrophil influx into an air pouch in mice [193] or the elevated number of cells seen after carregeenan-induced pleurisy in rats [164]. PDE4 inhibitors attenuated antigen-induced increases in lung neutrophils in primates [57, 173, 194] and rats [58], but not rabbits [59, 172]. There are data to suggest that PDE4 inhibitors decrease the activation of neutrophils even after they have migrated into tissues. For example, in the LPS challenged guinea pigs PDE4 inhibitors reduced neutrophil mediated lung edema without decreasing the absolute number of cells [72] and prevented the zymosan-induced enhancement of lung permeability in mice after LPS-induced neutrophil migration [195]. Thus, PDE4 inhibitors decrease neutrophil migration and attentuate their activation. These pharmacological effects should provide significant benefit in chronic lung diseases.

3.2.6 Lymphocytes

Both $CD4^+$ and $CD8^+$ T lymphocytes have been implicated in the pathophysiology of asthma and COPD [25, 28, 32, 33]. Both types of T cells can be further subdivided in Th1 and Th2 cells ($CD4^+$ cells) and Tc1 and Tc2 cells ($CD8^+$) cells based on their cytokine production [25, 196]. Th2 cells contribute significantly to the pathophysiology of asthma and allergic diseases [25]. The role of $CD8^+$ cells in COPD is just emerging [28, 32, 33].

T cells contain significant amounts of both PDE3 and PDE4 [197–200]. PDE4 activity accounts for approximately 60–70% of the total soluble cyclic AMP activity [199, 201] whereas PDE3 is primarily membrane-bound [198, 201, 202]. The total amount of PDE4 activity or the expression the different subtypes of PDE4 does not differ between $CD4^+$ and $CD8^+$ cells [201, 202]. Both subsets of T cells express PDE4A, PDE4B and PDE4D. No consistent differences in the amount of PDE3 and PDE4 activity have been found between Th1 and Th2 cells [203]. Initial studies examining the PDE4 subtype expression between Th1 and Th2 cells demonstrated that Th1 cells expressed PDE4A and PDE4B; whereas Th2 cells also expressed PDE4D [204].

Activation of T cells by mitogens increases cyclic AMP PDE activity [205–209] as does treatment with IL-2 and antigen [203]. There are probably two mechanisms resposible for this increase. One, activation of lymphocytes releases phosphatidic acid [210] which stimulates PDE4 activity [210–213], particularly the long forms of PDE4A, PDE4B and PDE4D [213–214]. Secondly, activation of T cells increases the expression of PDE4A, PDE4B and PDE4D3 [208, 215]. PDE4 activity in T cells is also up regulated by elevation of the cyclic AMP content [216] with increases the expression of PDE4A and PDE4D subytpes [208, 216, 217]. Even though T cells regulate the expression of PDE4, there have been no reported differences in the amount or subtype expression between T cells obtained from normal donors or those with atopic disease [140, 218].

The PDE profile of B lymphocytes has not been as extensively characterized as that of T cells. However, like T cells, B cells contain both PDE3 and PDE4 [219]. The PDE4 subtypes found in B cells are similar to those of T cells and include PDE4A, PDE4B and PDE4D [13, 104, 219].

A common theme with the in vitro anti-inflammatory effects of selective PDE4 inhibitors is that they modify the activation of cells at multiple levels and T cells are no exception. Selective PDE4 inhibitors attenuate proliferation induced by mitogens [198, 201, 220, 221] antigens [199, 203], and anti CD3+ antibodies [222] but not that induced by PMA plus ionomycin [201]. PDE4 inhibitors synergize with PDE3 inhibitors to block T cell proliferation by mitogens [198, 201] and certain antigens such as tetanus toxoid and myelin basic protein [150, 199, 203], but not others such as ragweed [150, 199]. Also, antigen-induced proliferation of Th1 and Th2 clones is blocked by selective PDE4 inhibitors [203, 204].

Another marker of T cell activation is cytokine production. Interestingly, PDE4 inhibitors but not PDE3 inhibitors suppress the production of Th1 and Th2 cytokines induced by antigen [150, 204, 223, 224], anti CD3 plus PMA [222], mitogens [201, 224–226] and PMA plus ionomycin [201]. When comparing the ability of PDE4 inhibitors to reduce Th1 versus Th2 cytokine production, the magnitude of the suppression is greater for the Th1 cytokines, IL-2 and IFNγ than for IL-4 or IL-5 hinting at a greater sensitivity of the Th1 cells [226]. Selective PDE4 inhibitors also reduce the production of IL-13 in both Th1 and Th2 cells [227]. This observation takes on added significance given the recently published data suggesting an important role for IL-13 in asthma [228, 229]. Finally, PDE4 inhibitors decrease transendothelial cell migration of activated human T cells [230].

Given the broad actions of PDE4 inhibitors on T cell function, it is not unexpected to see an impressive activity of these compounds in models of T cell-mediated disease. For example, PDE4 inhibitors are effective in number of rodent and primate animal models of EAE [231–233]. PDE4 inhibitors, admininstered orally or topically, reduce delayed type hypersensitivity responses in the skin after oxazolone challenge [234, 235] and diminish local cytokine production [235, 236]. This class of PDE inhibitors also reduces the disease severity score in a rodent models of arthritis [237–239], decreases both IFNγ production by the regional lymph nodes [238] and attenuates the number of TNFα-positive cells recovered from the affected joints [239]. Finally, rolipram was protective against the development of diabetes in the NOD mouse [240].

3.2.7 Potential interaction of selective PDE4 inhibitor with endogenous anti-inflammatory substances

In view of the common demonstration that the most dramatic anti-inflammatory effects of PDE4 inhibitors are observed after activation of adenylate cyclase, the question arises as to the importance of these substances in the in vivo anti-inflammatory actions of PDE4 inhibitors. A few studies have begun to shed light on this issue. Endogenous catecholamines, but not prostaglandins, appear essential for the bronchoprotective effects of PDE4 inhibitors in the antigen challenge guinea pig and for the suppression of arachidonic acid ear edema since nadolol, a β-adrenergic antagonist, or adrenalectomy, but not indomethacin or naproxen abolished the activity of rolipram [190, 241]. In contrast, neither removal of the adrenal medulla nor administration of nadolol nor indomethacin reduced the ability of rolipram to decrease antigen-induced eosinophil influx in the guinea pig [241]. PDE4-mediated suppression of LPS-induced TNFα production *in vivo* is the most characterized of the cytokine suppressive effects of selective PDE4 inhibitors [235, 237, 242–245] and neither propranolol treatment nor adrenalectomy prevents the suppressive effects of selective PDE4 inhibitors [245, 246]. These findings suggest that although activators of adenylate cyclase can potentiate the pharmacological effects of PDE4 inhibitors that do not appear essential for many of the *in vivo* anti-inflammatory effects.

Another potential mechanism for the anti-inflammatory actions of PDE4 is elevation of corticosteroid levels. In rodents, PDE4 inhibitors from several structural classes increased serum levels of glucocorticosteroids [247, 248]; however, these steroids do not appear essential for the cytokine suppressive actions of PDE4 inhibitors since neither adrenalectomy [245] nor administration of the steriod antagonist, RU486 [246] changed the ability of rolipram to reduce the LPS-induced elevation of serum TNFα. These preliminary results suggest that while PDE4 inhibitors may increase glucocorticoid levels in some species, this does not appear to play an important role in the anti-inflammatory effects of this class of compounds.

3.3   Airways hyperreactivity and remodeling

3.3.1 Hyperreactivity

A key feature of both asthma and COPD is the enhanced bronchoconstrictive response of individuals to a variety of stimuli [28]. The physiological mechanisms behind this hyperreactivity are still not well defined but probably include components of inflammation, tissue remodeling and increased neuronal reflexes. In a number of animal models, selective PDE4 inhibitors reduce hyperresponsiveness seen after challenge with PAF [53], antigen [57, 59, 168, 171], ozone [249], or LPS [192, 250]. This reduction in hyperresponsiveness was observed even in the absence of a direct effect on the initial bronchoconstrictive response to antigen challenge [59, 171, 249, 251] or the influx of neutrophils produced by LPS [250]. PDE4 inhibitors have been reported to decrease the elevation of citric acid-induced cough induced by antigen challenge [252].

Modulation by PDE4 inhibitors of pulmonary neuronal activity may be a mechanism contributing to the observed effects on airway reactivity. For example, in the isolated guinea pig bronchus, rolipram and RO 20-1724 blocked the non-cholinergic non-adrenergic (NANC) contractions produced by electrical field stimulation or vagal stimulation [253, 254]. Furthermore, PDE4 inhibitors enhanced NANC induced relaxations in cat bronchial smooth muscle [255], guinea trachea [256] and human bronchi [257]. These initial observations support the exciting possibility that in addition to their broad anti-inflammatory actions selective PDE4 inhibitor can modulate neuronal input into the lung.

3.3.2 Airway remodeling

A relatively unexplored area is the ability of phosphodiesterase inhibitors to modify or prevent the airway remodeling seen in chronic lung diseases. Although the presence of PDE4 activity in airway smooth muscle is well established, little is known about the distribution and regulation of the PDE4 subtypes. In vascular smooth muscle, the predominate subtype of PDE4 appears to be PDE4D [149, 258] and elevation of cyclic AMP content increases both PDE4 and PDE3 activity [259]. No similar studies have been reported using airway smooth muscle nor is there any information available describing changes in PDE4 activity occurring after inflammatory insult.

Increases in cyclic AMP content of airway smooth muscle by activation of adenylate cyclase or non-selective blockade of PDE activity inhibit proliferation induced by thrombin [260], histamine [261] or serum [262, 263]. Both PDE4 and PDE 3 inhibitors attenuate the proliferation of human [264], rat [265] and pig [266] vascular smooth muscle and inhibit the proliferation of human airway smooth muscle to PDGF-bb [267]. Finally selective PDE3 and PDE4 inhibitors can modify the PDGF-induced migration of smooth muscle cells [258]. These initial observations suggest that PDE4 inhibitors have the potential to modify airway remodeling by reducing smooth muscle cell proliferation and migration.

Equally important in airway remodeling is the function and phenotype of the fibroblast. Currently, there is a paucity of information regarding the distribution of PDE isozymes in lung fibroblasts and the ability of selective PDE inhibitors to modulate their function. In an initial study, human lung fibroblasts were shown to contain a high affinity form of cAMP PDE activity reminiscent of PDE3 or PDE4 although no further biochemical characterization was reported [268]. One could speculate that selective PDE3 or PDE4 inhibitors would reduce proliferation, cytokine and production of extracellular matrix proteins since increases in cyclic AMP content of lung fibroblasts attenuates these functions [269–271]. These findings suggest that PDE inhibitors might attenuate the progressive fibrosis and airway stenosis seen in COPD. Indeed, the non selective PDE inhibitor, aminophylline, reduced bleomycin-induced pulmonary fibrosis in a hamster model [272].

Secondary pulmonary hypertension develops in a significant proportion of individuals with COPD. The ability of selective PDE inhibitors to prevent or attenuate this pathophysiological consequence is largely unexplored. Recently it was demonstrated that selective PDE4 inhibitors attenuated the contraction of pulmonary arterial smooth muscle to thromboxane analog, U46619 in preparations obtained from hypoxic rats [273].

3.4   Clinical experience with selective PDE inhibitors in asthma and COPD

The marked anti-inflammatory, bronchodilatory and neural modulatory activities demonstrated by selective PDE4 inhibitors in animal models suggest that this class of compounds could provide significant therapeutic benefit in both asthma and COPD. Indeed the non-selective PDE inhibitor theophylline is used to treat both disorders [34, 274, 275]. Unfortunately there are limited number of reported clinical trials with selective PDE4 inhibitors. Tibenilast, a weak PDE4 inhibitor, produced a small but not statistically significant increase in FEV_1 in asthmatic subjects [1]. Two mixed PDE3/PDE4 inhibitors have been evaluated in normal and asthmatic subjects. Benzafentrine when administered by inhalation, but not when given orally or intravenously, produced a small but significant reduction in a methacholine-induced bronchoconstriction [276] in normal individuals. Another mixed PDE3/4 inhibitor, zardaverine, when given by the inhaled route, produced a modest bronchodilation in individuals with asthma [277] but was ineffective in patients with COPD [278]. Of particular interest are the results obtained with two more recent second generation PDE4 inhibitors, CDP840 and SB 207499. Oral administration of CDP840 for 9 days produced a significant reduction in the late response to antigen challenge in asthmatic individuals without inhibiting the immediate bronchoconstriction to antigen or histamine [279]; this effect is reminiscent of its action in the antigen-challenged primate model [280]. Furthermore, these results support the hypothesis that selective PDE4 inhibitors suppress the late response by inhibiting the inflammatory reaction and not by direct bronchodilation. SB 207499 (Ariflo™), an orally active PDE4 inhibitor, attenuated the decline in

FEV_1 in individuals with exercise-induced asthma [281] at doses that were well tolerated and produced minimal side-effects [282]. Furthermore, SB 207499 improved FEV_1 in asthmatic individuals who symptoms were poorly controlled on inhaled steriods [283]. Most exciting were the findings that after 6 weeks of therapy SB 207499 produced a significant improvement in FEV_1 concommitant with significant improvements in quality of life measurements, in individuals with COPD who were poorly reversible [284–286]. This is the first demonstration that selective PDE4 inhibitors are effective in the treatment of COPD.

4   Future challenges to drug discovery

Notwithstanding the recent exciting results obtained with CDP840 and SB 207499, side-effects have limited the clinical utility of PDE4 inhibitors. These side-effects are extensions of the pharmacology of this class of compounds, i.e. produced by inhibiting PDE4 in non-target tissues. The signature side-effects observed for PDE4 inhibitors are for the most part gastrointestinal including nausea, vomiting and increased gastric acid secretion [82, 284, 287, 288]. Based on results obtained in animals, the nausea and vomiting are produced through an action on the central nervous system [289–291] although there may be a contribution from direct effects on the gastrointestinal system, [292–296]. The key challenge to drug discovery efforts has been the identification of novel compounds that maintain the desirable effects on the earliest or first generation PDE4 inhibitors, such as rolipram, but demonstrate a reduced propensity to produce gastrointestinal effects.

There are two main experimental approaches to identify novel second and third generation PDE4 inhibitors. One is directed to selectively inhibiting one of the two unique conformers of PDE4 [82, 83, 285, 287] and the other on targeting one of the subtypes of PDE4 [1, 13, 82]. The first approach is based on the observation that rolipram bound to rat brain membranes with an affinity in the nM range but inhibited partially purified PDE4 from brain with a K_i in the μM range [297]. Later work with recombinant PDE4A showed that the high affinity binding site for ^{3}H-rolipram was on the PDE4 protein [97, 298, 299]. Intriguingly, there was a poor correlation between the ability of compounds to inhibit the catalytic activity of rhPDE4A and their ability to compete with ^{3}H-rolipram binding to this protein [97]. Studies using recombinant protein suggest that one of these conformers binds rolipram at the catalytic site with high affinity and the other binds rolipram with a much lower affinity also at the catalytic site [287, 298, 299]. These conformers have been termed "HPDE4" or "high affinity rolipram binding PDE4" and "LDPE4" or "low affinity rolipram binding PDE4" [1, 82].

The significant ramifications of this finding, at least for drug discovery efforts, are twofold. Firstly, each subtype of PDE4 can exist in either the low or high affinity conformation [97, 135, 299], and secondly that the relative proportion of PDE4 existing in the HPDE4 conformation varies among tissues and cell types [1, 82]. For example, the CNS appears to contain a high proportion of PDE4 in the HPDE4 conformation as determined by ^{3}H-rolipram binding [297, 300], whereas in the majority of immune and inflammatory cells PDE4 assumes the LPDE4 conformation [111, 146, 157]. This leads to the hypothesis that perhaps certain functional actions of PDE4 inhibitors are caused by inhibition of HPDE4 versus inhibition of LPDE4. Indeed, many, but not all, of the anti-inflammatory actions of selective PDE4 inhibitors are associated with inhibition of LPDE4 and not HPDE4 [1, 82, 285, 287, 301]. In contrast, certain of the gastrointestinal side effects such as enhanced acid secretion [82], reduction in gut transit [293] and nausea and vomiting [82, 302] as well as the psychotropic effects [82, 303] are associated with inhibition of HPDE4 and not LPDE4. There is evidence that certain therapeutic effects of PDE4 inhibitor appeared to be mediated through inhibition of HPDE4 among these are suppression of neutrophil activation [111] inhibition of guinea pig peritoneal macrophage activation [101] and antagonism of histamine induced bronchoconstriction [43, 283]. Nevertheless, these observations led to the idea that an improved therapeutic index for PDE4 inhibitors could be achieved by increasing the selectivity for LPDE4 conformer of PDE4. Indeed, results obtained in animal model indicates that this approach is successful in identifying selective PDE4 inhibitors with an improved therapeutic index [82, 194, 235, 304, 305]. Furthemore, as discussed previously, results from recent clinical trials indicates that this improvement is maintained in man. Final validation of this approach awaits the results of the larger clinical studies with these compounds.

An alternative, more recent approach toward improving the therapeutic index of PDE4 inhibitors involves targeting an individual PDE4 subtype over the other three [13, 82]. This approach is based on the differential distribution of PDE4 subtypes among tissues and cells [8, 13, 82]. Most immune or inflammatory cells express one or more gene products of the PDE4A, PDE4B and PDE4D genes [97, 99, 104, 105, 140, 150, 306, 307] but not PDE4C. Airway epithelial cells express PDE4A, PDE4D and uniquely PDE4C [76, 77]. Unfortunately, there are no published reports on the PDE4 subtype distribution in airway smooth muscle cells or airway nerves. PDE4 subtypes show regional differences in expression within the central nervous system [306, 308–310] although the brain expresses all four subtypes of PDE4. A preliminary finding is that PDE4D expression is increased in those regions of the brain, e.g. area postrema, implicated in the emetic reflex [309], whereas PDE4A expression is lower in this and other brainstem nuclei [308, 309]. This suggests that one could achieve an improvement in therapeutic index by targeting the PDE4 subtype important for inflammatory cell regulation while avoiding those subtypes implicated in producing the side-effects. Unfortunately, this strategy is not without its challenges. One is the high degree of structural homology among the catalytic domains of the PDE4 subtypes [8] implying it might be difficult to synthesize subtype selective PDE4 inhibitors. However, some initial strides have been made in this direction. For example, SB 207499 demonstrates a higher affinity for the PDE4D subtype than for the other subtypes [304]. Second, because PDE4 subtypes are expressed in a variety of tissues, expression patterns alone are not sufficient to identify the relevant subtype important for the beneficial therapeutic effects of PDE4 inhibitors versus their side effects. This will depend on characterizing the functional relevance of each PDE4 subtype in producing the pharmacological actions of these compounds. Third, it is clear that cells regulate both the level and subtype of PDE4 expressed [8, 82, 124–126]. Thus, it is important to determine if disease changes the complement of PDE4 proteins. To date, no major differences in the level of PDE4 activity has been found between T cells (CD4+), B cells, monocytes and eosinophils obtained from normal or atopic donors nor did the percentage of PDE activity found in the soluble or particulate fraction change [140, 218, 219]. Moreover the complement of PDE4 subtypes expressed by these inflammatory cells did not differ between cells obtained from normal or atopic donors. Thus at least on the basis of these initial findings examining PDE4 gene expression, it does not appear that atopic disease produces a different complement of PDE4 proteins. Unfortunately, there are no studies comparing the expression of PDE4 subtypes in patients with COPD and normal individuals to help in identifying the most relevant subtype for COPD.

In conclusion, selective PDE4 inhibitors modify many aspects of the pathophysiology of both asthma and COPD. Preliminary results from on-going clinical trials provide data in support of the hypothesis that this class of compounds produces beneficial effects in both asthma and COPD. However, there are still hurdles to overcome before it is likely that PDE4 inhibitors realize their optimal therapeutic potential. Chief among these is maximizing their therapeutic activity for chronic airways disease while minimizing their gastrointestinal side effects. Fortunately, insights into the diversity, structure and regulation of this family of proteins have shed light on several approaches toward the design of new generations of selective PDE4 inhibitors.

References

1   Torphy T.J.: Am. J. Respir. Crit. Care Med. *157*, 351–370 (1998).
2   Torphy T.J., Murray K.J. and Arch J.R., in: C.P. Page and W.J. Metzger (eds.): *Drugs and the Lung*, Raven Press, New York 1994, 397–447.
3   Burns F., Zhao A.Z. and Beavo J.A.: Adv. Pharmacol. *36*, 29–48 (1996).
4   Beavo J.A., Conti M. and Heaslip R.J.: Mol. Pharmacol. *46*, 399405 (1994).
5   Milatovich A., Bolger G., Michaeli T. and Francke U.: Somat. Cell Mol. Genet. *20*, 75–86 (1994).
6   Szpirer C., Szpirer J., Riviere M., Swinnen J., Vicini E. and Conti M.: Cytogenet. Cell Genet. *69*, 11–14 (1995).
7   Bolger G., Michaeli T., Martins T., St. John T., Steiner B., Rodgers L., Riggs M., Wigler M. and Ferguson K.: Mol. Cell. Biol. *13*, 6558–6571 (1993).
8   Houslay M.D., Sullivan M. and Bolger G.B.: Adv. Pharmacol. *44*, 225–342 (1998).
9   Teixeria M., Gristwood R.W., Cooper N. and Hellewell P.G.: TIPS *18*, 164–170 (1997).
10   Cavalla D. and Frith R.: Curr. Med. Chem. *2*, 561–572 (1995).
11   Stafford J.A. and Feldman P.L.: Ann. Rep. Med. Chem. *31*, 71–80 (1996).
12   Karlsson J.A. and Aldous D.: Exp. Opin. Ther. Patents *7*, 989–1003 (1997).
13   Muller T., Engels P. and Fozard J.R.: TIPS *17*, 294–298 (1996).
14   Morley J.: Immunol. Today *14*, 317–322 (1993).
15   Busse W.W. and, Parry D.E., in: A.P. Fishman, J.A. Elias, J.A. Fishman, M.A. Grippi, L.R. Kaiser and R.M. Senior (eds.): *Fishman's Pulmonary Diseases and Disorders*, McGraw-Hill, New York 1998, 721–733.
16   Beasley R., Burgess C., Crane J., Pearce N. and Roche W.: J. Allergy Clin. Immunol. *93*, 148–154 (199).
17   Senior R.M. and Shapiro S.D., in: A.P. Fishman, J.A. Elias, J.A. Fishman, M.A. Grippi, L.R. Kaiser and R.M. Senior (eds.): *Fishman's Pulmonary Diseases and Disorders*, McGraw-Hill, New York 1998, 659–681.
18   Pueringer R.J. and Hunninghake G.W.: Am. J. Med. *92*, 6A-32S–6A-38S (1992).

19   Hamid Q., Song Y., Kotsimbos T.C., Minshall E., Bai T.R., Hegele R.G. and Hogg J.C.: J. Allergy Clin. Immunol. *100*, 44–51 (1997).
20   Roche W.R.: Am. J. Respir. Crit. Care Med. *15*, S191–S194 (1998).
21   Poulter L.W., Janossy G.J., Power C., Sreenan S. and Burke C.: Immunol. Today *15*, 258–261 (1994).
22   Holgate S.T.: Clin. Rev. Asthma *12*, 65–78 (1994).
23   Church M.K., Okayama Y. and Bradding P.: N.Y. Acad. Sci. *725*, 13–21 (1994).
24   Holgate S.T., Djukanovic R., Howarth P.H., Montefort S. and Roche W.: Chest *103*, 125S–128S (1993).
25   Aebischer I. and Stadler B.M.: Adv. Immunol. *61*, 341–403 (1996).
26   Rennard S.I.: Am. J. Respir. Crit. Care Med. *153*, S14–S15 (1996).
27   Rennard S.I.: Eur. Respir. Rev. 7, 206–210 (1997).
28   Postma D.S. and Kerstjens H.A.M.: Am. J. Respir. Crit. Care Med. *158*, S187–S192 (1998).
29   Hiemstra P.S., van Wetering S. and Stolk J.: Eur. Respir. J. *12*, 1200–1208 (1998).
30   Pesci A., Majori M., Cuomo A., Borciani N., Bertacco S., Cacciani G. and Gabrielli M.: Respir. Med. *92*, 863–870 (1998).
31   Sandford A.J., Weir T.D. and Pare P.D.: Eur. Respir. J. *10*, 1380–1391 (1997).
32   O'Shaoughnessy T.C., Ansari T.W., Barnes N.C. and Jeffery P.K.: Am. J. Respir. Crit. Care Med. *155*, 852–857 (1997).
33   Lams B.E., Sousa A.R., Rees P.J. and Lee T.H.: Am. J. Respir. Crit. Care Med. *158*, 1518–1523 (1998).
34   Peleman R.A., Kips J.C. and Pauwels R.A.: Clin. Exp. Allergy *28* (Suppl. 3), 53–56 (1998).
35   Folkerts G. and Nijkamp F.P.: TIPS *19*, 334–341 (1998).
36   Barnes P.J.: Chest *107*, 119S–125S (1995).
37   Verleden G.M.: Biochem. Pharmacol. *51*, 1247–1257 (1996).
38   Halayko A.J. and Stephens N.L.: Can. J. Physiol. Pharmacol. *72*, 1448–1457 (1994).
39   Halayko A.J., Salari H., Ma X. and Stephens N.L.: Am. J. Physiol. *270*, L1040–L1051 (1996).
40   Laitinen L.A. and Laitinen A.: J. Allergy Clin. Immunol. 97, 153–158 (1996).
41   Pare P.D. and Bai T.R.: Eur. Respir. Rev. *6*, 259–263 (1996).
42   Jeffery P.K.: Am. J. Respir. Crit. Care Med. *150*, S6–S13 (1994).
43   Harris A.L., Connell M.J., Ferguson E.W., Wallace A.M., Gordon R.J., Pagani E.D. and Silver P.J.: J. Pharmacol. Exp. Ther. *251*, 199–206 (1989).
44   Torphy T.J. and Cielinski L.B.: Mol. Pharmacol. *37*, 206–214 (1990).
45   Cortijo J., Bou J., Beleta J., Cardelus I., Llenas J., Morcillo E. and Gristwood R.W.: Br. J. Pharmacol. *108*, 562–568 (1993).
46   Qian Y., Naline E., Karlsson J.-A., Raeburn D. and Advenier C.: Br. J. Pharmacol. *109*, 774–778 (1993).
47   Torphy T.J., Undem B.J., Cieslinski L.B., Luttman M.A., Reeves M.L. and Hay D.W.P.: J. Pharmacol. Exp. Ther. *265*, 1213–1223 (1993).
48   Torphy T.J., Zhou H.-L., Burman M. and Huang B.F.: Mol. Pharmacol. *39*, 376–384 (1991).
49   Small R.C., Boyle J.P., Duty S., Elliott K.R.F., Foster R.W. and Watt A.J.: Br. J. Pharmacol. *97*, 1165–1173 (1989).
50   Small R.C., Berry J.L., Boyle J.P., Chapman I.D., Elliott K.R.F., Foster R.W. and Watt A.J.: Eur. J. Pharmacol. *192*, 417–426 (1991).
51   Tomkinson A., Karlsson J.-A. and Raeburn D.: Br. J. Pharmacol. *108*, 57–61 (1993).

52   Underwood D.C., Osborn R.R., Novak L.B., Matthews J.K., Newsholme S.J., Undem B.J., Hand J.M. and Torphy T.J.: J. Pharmacol. Exp. Ther. 266, 306–313 (1993).

53   Ortiz J.L., Valles J.M., Marti-Cabrera M., Cortijo J. and Morcillo E.J.: Nauyn-Schmiedeberg's Arch. Pharmacol. 353, 200–206 (1996).

54   Heaslip R.J., Buckley S.K., Sickels B.D. and Grimes D.: J. Pharmacol. Exp. Ther. 257, 741–747 (1991).

55   Held H.-D., Wendel A. and Uhlig S.: Biochem. Biophys. Res. Commun. 231, 22–25 (1997).

56   Underwood D.C., Kotzer C.J., Bochnowicz S., Osborn R.R., Luttman M.A., Hay D.W.P. and Torphy T.J.: J. Pharmacol. Exp. Ther. 270, 250–259 (1994).

57   Turner C.R., Andresen C.J., Smith W.B. and Watson J.W.: Am. J. Respir. Crit. Care Med. 149, 1153–1159 (1994).

58   Elwood W., Sun J., Barnes P.J., Giembycz M.A. and Chung K.F.: Inflamm. Res. 44, 83–86 (1995).

59   Gozzard N., Herd C.M., Blake S.M., Holbrook M., Hughes B., Higgs G.A. and Page C.P.: Br. J. Pharmacol. 117, 1405–1412 (1996).

60   Lugnier C. and Schini V.B.: Biochem. Pharmacol. 39, 75–84 (1990).

61   Kishi Y., Ashikaga T. and Numano F.: Adv. Second Messengers Phosphoprotein Res. 25, 201–213 (1992).

62   Suttorp N., Weber U., Welsch T. and Schudt C.: J. Clin. Invest. 91, 1421–1428 (1993).

63   Suttorp N., Ehreiser P., Hippenstiel S., Fuhrmann M., Krull M., Tenor H. and Schudt C.: Lung 174, 181–194 (1996).

64   Ashikaga T., Strada S.J. and Thompson W.J.: Biochem. Pharmacol. 54, 1071–1079 (1997).

65   Ortiz J.L. Cortijo J., Valles J.M., Bou J. and Morcillo E.J.: Fundam. Clin. Pharmacol. 6, 247–249 (1992).

66   Raeburn D. and Karlsson J.-A.: J. Pharmacol. Exp. Ther. 267, 1147–1152 (1993).

67   Turner C.R., Esser K.M. and Wheeldon E.B.: Circulatory Shock 39, 237–245 (1993).

68   Underwood D.C., Osborn R.R., Bochnowicz S., Hay D.W.P. and Torphy T.J.: Am. J. Respir. Crit. Care Med. 157, A827 (abstract) (1998).

69   Planquois J.-M., Mottin G., Artola M., Lagente V., Payne A. and Dahl S.: Eur. J. Pharmacol. 344, 59–66 (1998).

70   Barnard J.W., Seibert A.F., Prasad V.R., Smart D.A., Strada S.J., Taylor A.E. and Thompson W.J.: J. Appl. Physiol. 77, 774–781 (1994).

71   Svensjo E., Andersson K.E., Bouskela E., Cyrino F.Z.G.A. and Lindgren S.: Agents Actions 39, 35–41 (1993).

72   Howell R.E., Jenkins L.P. and Howell D.E.: J. Pharmacol. Exp. Ther. 275, 703–709 (1995).

73   Knight D.A., Stewart G.A. and Thompson P.J.: Clin. Exp. Allergy 24, 698–706 (1994).

74   Polito A.J. and Proud D.: J. Allergy Clin. Immunol. 102, 714–718 (1998).

75   Rousseau E., Gagnon J. and Lugnier C.: Mol. Cell Biochem. 140, 171–175 (1994).

76   Wright L.C., Seybold J., Robichaud A., Adcock I.M. and Barnes P.J.: Am. J. Physiol. 275, L694–L700 (1998).

77   Fuhrmann M., Jahn H.-U., Seybold J., Neurohr C., Barnes P.J., Hippenstiel S., Kraemer J. and Suttorp N.: Am. J. Respir. Cell Mol. Biol. 20, 292–302 (1999).

78   Dowling R.B., Johnson M., Cole P.J. and Wilson R.: J. Pharmacol. Exp. Ther. 282, 1565–1571 (1997).

79   Wagner U., Bredenbroker D., Fehmann H.-C., Schwarz F., Schudt C. and von Wichert P.: Eur. J. Pharmacol. 298, 265–270 (1996).

80   Torphy T.J. and Undem B.J.: Thorax *46*, 512–523 (1991).

81   Giembycz M.A.: Biochem. Pharmacol. *43*, 2041–2051 (1992).

82   Barnette M.S., Christensen S.B., Underwood D.C. and Torphy T.J.: Pharmacol. Rev. Commun. *8*, 65–73 (1996).

83   Torphy T.J., DeWolf W.E., Green D.W. and Livi G.P.: Agents Actions *43S*, 51–71 (1993).

84   Peachell P.T., Undem B.J., Schleimer R.P., MacGlashan D.W., Lichtenstein L.M., Cieslinski L.B. and Torphy T.J.: J. Immunol. *148*, 2503–2510 (1992).

85   Torphy T.J., Livi G.P., Balcarek J.M., White J.R., Chilton F.H. and Undem B.J.: Adv. Second Messengers Phosphoprotein Res. *25*, 289–305 (1992).

86   Weston M.C., Anderson N. and Peachell P.T.: Br. J. Pharmacol. *121*, 287–295 (1997).

87   Kleine-Tebbe J., Wicht L., Gagne H., Friese A., Schunack W., Schudt C. and Kunkel G.: Agents Actions *36*, 200–206 (1992).

88   Louis R., Bury T.H., Corhay J.L. and Radermecker M.: Int. J. Immunopharmac. *14*, 191–194 (1992).

89   Weston M.C. and Peachell P.T.: Gen. Pharmac. *31*, 715–719 (1998).

90   Shichijo M., Shimizu Y., Hiramatsu K., Inagaki N., Tagaki K. and Nagai H.: Int. Arch. Allergy Immunol. *114*, 348–353 (1997).

91   Frossard N., Landry Y., Pauli G. and Ruckstuhl M.: Br. J. Pharmacol. *73*, 933–938 (1981).

92   Banner K.H., Moriggi E., Da Ros B., Schioppacassi G., Semeraro C. and Page C.P.: Br. J. Pharmacol. *119*, 1255–1261 (1996).

93   Shichijo M., Inagaki N., Nakai N., Kimata M., Nakahata T., Serizawa I., Iikura Y., Saito H. and Nagai H.: Clin. Exp. Allergy *28*, 1228–1236 (1998).

94   Nagai H., Takeda H., Iwama T., Yamaguchi S. and Mori H.: Jpn. J. Pharmacol. *67*, 149–156 (1995).

95   Poulter L.W. and Burke C.M.: Immunobiol. *195*, 574–587 (1996).

96   Elliott K.R.F. and Leonard E.J.: FEBS Letters *254*, 94–98 (1989).

97   Torphy T.J., Stadel J.M., Burman M., Cieslinski L.B., McLaughlin M.M., White J.R. and Livi G.P.: J. Biol. Chem. *267*, 1798–1804 (1992).

98   Seldon P.M., Barnes P.J., Meja K. and Giembycz M.A.: Mol. Pharmacol. *48*, 747–757 (1995).

99   Manning C.D., McLaughlin M.M., Livi G.M., Cieslinski L.B., Torphy T.J. and Barnette M.S.: J. Pharmacol. Exp. Ther. *276*, 810–818 (1996).

100   Tenor H., Hatzelmann A., Kupferschmidt R., Stanciu L., Djukanovic R., Schudt C., Wendel A., Church M.K. and Shute J.K.: Clin. Exp. Allergy *25*, 625–633 (1995).

101   Kelly J.J., Barnes P.J. and Giembycz M.A.: Biochem. J. *318*, 425–436 (1996).

102   Ganter F., Kuperschmidt R., Schudt C., Wendel A. and Hatzelmann A.: Br. J. Pharmacol. *121*, 221–231 (1997).

103   Germain N., Bertin B., Legendre A., Martin B., Lagente V., Payne A. and Boichot E.: Eur. Respir. J. *12*, 1334–1339 (1998).

104   Engels P., Fichtel K. and Lubbert H.: FEBS Letters *350*, 291–295 (1994).

105   Verghese M.W., McConnell R.T., Lenhard J.M., Hamacher L., Jin S.-L.C.: Mol. Pharmacol. *47*, 1164–1171 (1995).

106   Souness J.E., Griffin M., Maslen C., Ebsworth K., Scott L.C., Pollock K., Palfreyman M.N. and Karlsson J.-A.: Br. J. Pharmacol. *118*, 649–658 (1996).

107   Molnar-Kimber K.L., Yonno L., Heaslip R.J. and Weichman B.M.: Mediators Inflamm. *1*, 411–417 (1992).

108   Molnar-Kimber K., Yonno L., Heaslip R. and Weichman B.: Agents Actions *39*, C77–C79 (1993).
109   Semmler J., Wachtel. and Endres S.: Int. J. Immunopharmacol. *15*, 409–413 (1993).
110   Prabhakar U., Lipshutz D., O'Leary Bartus J., Slivjak M.J., Smith E.F., Lee J.C. and Esser K.M.: Int. J. Immunopharmacol. *16*, 805–816 (1994).
111   Barnette M.S., O'Leary Bartus J., Burman M., Christensen S.B., Cielslinski L.B., Esser K.M., Prabhakar U.S., Rush J.A. and Torphy T.J.: Biochem. Pharmacol. *51*, 949–956 (1996).
112   Brideau C., van Staden C., Styhler A., Rodger I.W. and Chan C.-C.: Br. J. Pharmacol. *126*, 979–988 (1999).
113   Verghese M.W., McConnell R.T., Strickland A.B., Gooding R.C., Stimpson S.A., Yarnall D.P., Taylor J.D. and Furdon P.J.: J. Pharmacol. Exp. Ther. *272*, 1313–1320 (1995).
114   Kambayashi T., Jacob C.O., Zhou D., Mazurek N., Fong M. and Strassmann G.: J. Immunol. *155*, 4909–4916 (1995).
115   Siegmund B., Eigler A., Moeller J., Greten T.F., Hartmann G. and Endres S.: Eur. J. Pharmacol. *321*, 231–239 (1997).
116   Hichami A., Boichot E., Germain N., Legrand A., Moodley I. and Lagente V.: Eur. J. Pharmacol. *291*, 91–97 (1995).
117   Hichami A., Boichot E., Germain N., Coqueret O. and Lagente V.: Life Sci. *59*, 255–261 (1996).
118   Sinha B., Semmler J., Eisenhut T., Eigler A. and Endres S.: Eur. J. Immunol. *25*, 147–153 (1995).
119   Greten T.F., Sinha B., Haslberger C., Eigler A. and Endres S.: Eur. J. Pharmacol. *299*, 229–233 (1996).
120   Schade U.F. and Schudt C.: Eur. J. Pharmacol. *230*, 9–14 (1993).
121   Gonclaves de Moraes V.L., Singer M., Vargaftig B.B. and Chignard M.: Br. J. Pharmacol. *123*, 631–636 (1998).
122   Turner N.C., Wood L.J., Burns F.M., Gueremy T. and Souness J.E.: Br. J. Pharmacol. *108*, 876–883 (1993).
123   Turner N.C. and Wood L.J.: Cell Signal *6*, 923–931 (1994).
124   Conti M., Jin S.-L.C., Monaco L., Repaske D.R. and Swinnen J.V.: Endocrine Rev. *12*, 218–234 (1991).
125   Sette C., Vicini E. and Conti M.: Mol. Cell Endocrinol. *100*, 75–79 (1994).
126   Conti M., Nemoz G., Sette C. and Vicini E.: Endocrine Rev. 16, 370–389 (1995).
127   Holden C.A., Chan S.C., Norris S. and Hanifin J.M.: Agents Actions *22*, 36–42 (1987).
128   Torphy T.J., Zhou H.-L. and Cieslinski L.B.: J. Pharmacol. Exp. Ther. *263*, 1195–1205 (1992).
129   Torphy T.J., Zhou H.-L., Foley J.J., Sarau H.M., Manning C.D. and Barnette M.S.: J. Biol. Chem. *270*, 23598–23604 (1995).
130   Bates M.D., Olsen C.L., Becker B.N., Alber F.J., Middleton J.P., Mulheron J.G., Jin S.-L.C., Conti M. and Raymond J.R.: J. Biol. Chem. *268*, 14757–14763 (1993).
131   Sette C., Iona S. and Conti M.: J. Biol. Chem. *269*, 9245–9252 (1994).
132   Sette C., Vicini E. and Conti M.: J. Biol. Chem. *269*, 18271–18274 (1994).
133   Nemoz G., Sette C., Hess M., Muca C., Vallar L. and Conti M.: Mol. Endocrinol. *9* 1279–1287 (1995).
134   Sette C. and Conti M.: J. Biol. Chem. *271*, 16526–16534 (1996).
135   Alvarez R., Sette C., Yang D., Eglen R.M., Wilhelm R., Shelton E.R. and Conti M.: Mol. Pharmacol. *48*, 616–622 (1995).

136   Saldou N., Obernolte R., Huber A., Baecker P.A., Wilhem R., Alvarez R., Li B., Xia L., Callan O., Su C. et al.: Cell Signal *10*, 427–440 (1998).
137   Lenhard J.M., Kassel D.B., Rocque W.J., Hamacher L., Holmes W.D., Patel I., Hoffman C. and Luther M.: Biochem. J. *316*, 751–758 (1996).
138   Chan S.C., Reifsnyder D., Beavo J.A. and Hanifin J.M.: J. Allergy Clin. Immunol. *91*, 1179–1188 (1993).
139   Hanifin J.M. and Chan S.C.: J. Invest. Dermatol. *105*, 84S–88S (1995).
140   Gantner F., Tenor H., Gekeler V., Schudt C., Wendel A. and Hatzelmann A.: J. Allergy Clin. Immunol. *100*, 527–535 (1997).
141   Martin L.B., Kita H., Leiferman K.M. and Gleich G.J.: Int. Arch. Allergy Immunol. *109*, 207–215 (1996).
142   Walsh G.M.: Br J. Haematol. *97*, 701–709 (1997).
143   Souness J.E., Carter C.M., Diocee B.K., Hassall G.A., Wood L.J. and Turner N.C.: Biochem. Pharmacol. *42*, 937–945 (1991).
144   Dent G., Giembycz M.A., Rabe K.F. and Barnes P.J.: Br. J. Pharmacol. *103*, 1339–1346 (1991).
145   Souness J.E., Malsen C. and Scott L.C.: FEBS Letters *302*, 181–184 (1992).
146   Souness J.E. and Scott L.C.: Biochem. J. *291*, 389–395 (1993).
147   Dent G., Giembycz M.A., Evans P.M., Rabe K.F. and Barnes P.J.: J. Pharmacol. Exp. Ther. *271*, 1167–1174 (1994).
148   Hatzelmann A., Tenor H. and Schudt C.: Br. J. Pharmacol. *114*, 821–831 (1995).
149   Souness J.E., Malsen C., Webber S., Foster M., Raeburn D., Palfreyman M.N., Ashton M.J. and Karlsson J.-A.: Br. J. Pharmacol. *115*, 39–46 (1995).
150   Essayan D.M., Huang S.-K., Kagey-Sobotka A. and Lichtenstein L.M.: Am. J. Respir. Cell Mol. Biol. *13*, 692–702 (1995).
151   Barnette M.S., Christensen S.B. Essayan D.M., Grous M., Prabhakar U., Rush J.A., Kagey-Sobotka A. and Torphy T.J.: J. Pharmacol. Exp. Ther. *284*, 420–426 (1998).
152   Kaneko T., Alvarez R., Ueki I.F. and Nadel J.A.: Cell Signal *7*, 527–534 (1998).
153   Alves A.C., Pires A.L.A., Cruz H.N., Serra M.F., Diaz B.L., Cordeiro R.S.B., Lagente V., Martins M.A. and Silva P.M.R.: Eur. J. Pharmacol. *312*, 89–96 (1996).
154   Tenor H., Hatzelmann A., Church M.K., Schudt C. and Shute J.K.: Br. J. Pharmacol. *118*, 1727–1735 (1996).
155   Santamaria L.F., Palacios J.M. and Beleta J.: Br. J. Pharmacol. *121*, 1150–1154 (1997).
156   Cohan V.L., Showell H.J., Fisher D.A., Pazoles C.J., Watson J.W., Turner C.R. and Cheng J.B.: J. Pharmacol. Exp. Ther. *278*, 1356–1361 (1996).
157   Barnette M.S., Manning C.D., Cieslinski L.B., Burman M., Christensen S.B. and Torphy T.J.: J. Pharmacol. Exp. Ther. *273*, 674–679 (1995).
158   Ezeamuzie C.I. and Al-Hage M.: Int. Arch. Allergy Immunol. *118*, 162–168 (1998).
159   Souness J.E., Villamil M.E., Scott L.C., Tomkinson A., Giembycz M.A. and Raeburn D.: Br. J. Pharmacol. *111*, 1081–1088 (1994).
160   Teixeira M.M., Rossi A.G., Giembycz M.A. and Hellewell P.G.: Br. J. Pharmacol. *118*, 2099–2106 (1996).
161   Momose T., Okubo Y., Horie S., Suzuki J., Isobe M. and Sekiguchi M.: Int. Arch. Allergy Immunol. *117*, 138–145 (1998).
162   Lagente V., Moodley I., Perrin S., Mottin G., Junien J.-L.: Eur. J. Pharmacol. *255*, 253–256 (1994).

163 Lagente V., Pruniaux M.-P., Junien J.-L. and Moodley I.: Am. J. Respir. Crit. Care Med. *151*, 1720–1724 (1995).

164 Hughes B., Howat D., Lisle H., Holbrook M., James T., Gozzard N., Blease K., Hughes .P, Kingaby R., Warrellow G. et al.: Br. J. Pharmacol. *118*, 1183–1191 (1996).

165 Newsholme S.J. and Schwartz L.: Inflammtion *17*, 25–31 (1993).

166 Underwood D.C., Bochnowicz S., Osborn R.R., Kotzer C.J., Luttmann M.A., Hay D.W.P., Gorycki P.D., Christensen S.B. and Torphy T.J.: J. Pharmacol. Exp. Ther. *287*, 988–995 (1998).

167 Banner K.H. and Page C.P.: Br. J. Pharmacol. *114*, 93–98 (1995).

168 Danahay H. and Broadley K.J.: Br J. Phamacol *120*, 289–297 (1997).

169 Cortijo J., Pons R., Dasi F., Marin N., Martinez-Losa M., Advenier C. and Morcillo E.J.: Naunyn-Schmiedeberg's Arch. Pharmacol. *356*, 806–814 (1997).

170 Kaminuma O., Kikkawa H., Matsubara S. and Ikezawa K.: Int. Arch. Allergy Immunol. *112*, 406–411 (1997).

171 Danahay H. and Broadley K.J.: Clin. Exp. Allergy *28*, 513–522 (1998).

172 Gozzard N-, El-Hashim A., Herd C.M., Blake S.M., Holbrook M., Hughes B., Higgs G.A. and Page C.P.: Br. J. Pharmacol. *118*, 1201–1208 (1996).

173 Turner C.R., Cohan V.L., Cheng, J.B., Showell H.J., Pazoles C.J. and Watson J.W.: J. Pharmacol. Exp. Ther. *278*, 1349–1355 (1996).

174 Teixeira M.M., Rossi A.G., Williams T.J. and Hellewell P.G.: Br. J. Pharmacol.*112*, 332–340 (1994).

175 Smith G.P. and Peter T.J.: Clinica Chimica Acta *103*, 193–201 (1980).

176 Grady P.G. and Thomas L.L.: Biochim. Biophys. Acta *885*, 282–293 (1986).

177 Wright C.D., Kuipers P.J., Kobylarz-Singer D., Devall L.J., Klinkefus B.A. and Weishaar R.E.: Biochem. Pharmacol. *40*, 699–707 (1990).

178 Schudt C., Winder S., Forderkunz S., Hatzelmann A. and Ullrich V.: Naunyn-Schmiedeberg's Arch. Pharmacol. *344*, 682–690 (1991).

179 Pryzwansky K.B., Kidao S. and Merricks E.P.: Cell Biochem. Biophys. *28*, 251–275 (1998).

180 Au B.-T., Teixeira M.M., Collins P.D. and Williams T.J.: Br. J. Pharmacol. *123*, 1260–1266 (1998).

181 Nielson C.P., Vestal R.E., Sturm R.J. and Heaslip R.: J. Allergy Clin. Immunol. *86*, 801–808 (1990).

182 Ottonello L., Morone M.P., Dapino P. and Dallegri F.: Br. J. Haematol. *91*, 566–570 (1995).

183 Sullivan G.W., Carper H.T. and Mandell G.L.: Int. J. Immunopharmacol. *17*, 793–803 (1995).

184 Denis D. and Riendeau D.: Eur. J. Pharmacol. *367*, 343–350 (1999).

185 Derian C., Santulli R.J., Rao P.E., Solomon H.F. and Barrett J.A.: J. Immunol. *154*, 308–317 (1995).

186 Currie M.S., Rao M.K., Padmanabhan J., Jones A., Crawford J. and Cohen H.J.: J. Leukocyte Biol. *47*, 244–250 (1990).

187 Berends C., Dijkhuizen B., de Monchy J.G.R., Dubois A.E.J., Gerritsen J. and Kauffman H.F.: Eur. Respir. J. *10*, 1000–1007 (1997).

188 Ottonello L., Morone M.P., Dapino P. and Dallegri F.: Clin. Exp. Immunol. *101*, 502–506 (1995).

189 Nourshargh S. and Hoult J.R.S.: Eur. J. Pharmacol. *122*, 205–212 (1986).

190 Griswold D.E., Webb E.F., Breton J., White J.R., Marshall P.J. and Torphy T.J.: Inflammation *17*, 333–344 (1993).

191 Griswold D.E., Martin L.D. and Torphy T.J.: Am. J. Respir. Crit. Care Med. *159*, A90 (abstract) (1999).

192 Kips J.C., Joos G.F., Peleman R.A. and Pauwels R.A.: Clin. Exp. Allergy *23*, 518–523 (1993).

193 Klemm P., Harris H.J. and Perretti M.: Eur. J. Pharmacol. *281*, 69–74 (1995).

194 Duplantier A.J., Andresen C.J., Cheng J.B., Cohan V.L., Decker C., DiCapua F.M., Kraus K.G., Johnson K.L., Turner C.R., UmLand J.P. et al.: J. Med. Chem. *41*, 2268–2277 (1998).

195 Miotla J.M., Teixeira M.M. and Hellewell P.G.: Am. J. Respir. Cell Mol. Biol. *18*, 411–420 (1998).

196 Salgame P., Abrams J.S., Clayberger C., Goldstein H., Convit J., Modlin R.L. and Bloom B.R.: Science *254*, 279–282 (1991).

197 Robicsek S.A., Krzanowski J.J., Szentivanyi A. and Polson J.B.: Biochem. Biophys. Res. Commun. *163*, 554–560 (1989).

198 Robicsek S.A., Blanchard D.K., Djeu J.Y., Krzanowski J.J., Szentivanyi A. and Polson J.B.: Biochem. Pharmacol. *42*, 869–877 (1991).

199 Essayan D.M., Huang S.-K., Undem B.J., Kagey-Sobotka A. and Lichtenstein L.M.: J. Immunol. *153*, 3408–3416 (1994).

200 Sheth S.B., Chaganti K., Bastepe M., Ajuria J., Brennan K., Biradavolu R. and Colman R.W.: Br. J. Haematol *99*, 784–789 (1997).

201 Giembycz M.A., Corrigan C.J., Seybold J., Newton R. and Barnes P.J.: Br. J. Pharmacol. *118*, 1945–1958 (1996).

202 Tenor H., Staniciu L., Schudt C., Hatzelmann A., Wendel A., Djukanovic R., Church M.K. and Shute J.K.: Clin. Exp. Allergy *25*, 616–624 (1995).

203 Ekholm D., Hemmer B., Gao G., Vergelli M., Martin R. and Manganiello V.: J. Immunol. 159, 1520–1529 (1997).

204 Essayan D.M., Kagey-Sobotka A., Lichtenstein L.M. and Huang S.-K.: J. Pharmacol. Exp. Ther. *282*, 505–512 (1997).

205 Epstein P.M., Mills J.S., Hersh E.M., Strada S.J. and Thompson W.J.: Cancer Res. *40*, 379–386 (1980).

206 Valette L., Prigent A.F., Nemoz G., Anker G., Macovschi O. and Lagarde M.: Biochem. Biophys. Res. Commun. *169*, 864–872 (1990).

207 Meskini N., Hosni M., Nemoz G., Lagarde M. and Prigent A.-F.: J. Cell Physiol. *150*, 140–148 (1992).

208 Jiang X., Paskin M., Weltzien R. and Epstein P.M.: Cell Biochem. Biophys. *28*, 135–160 (1998).

209 Michie A.M., Rena G., Harnett M.M. and Houslay M.D.: Cell Biochem. Biophys. *28*, 161–185 (1998).

210 Savany A., Abriat C., Nemoz G., Lagarde M. and Prigent A.-F.: Cell Signal 8, 511–516 (1996).

211 DiSanto M.E. and Heaslip R.J.: Eur. J. Pharmacol. *290*, 169–172 (1995).

212 DiSanto M.E., Glaser K.B. and Heaslip R.J.: Cell Signal *7*, 827–835 (1995).

213 El Bawab S., Macovschi O., Sette C., Conti M., Lagarde M., Nemoz G. and Prigent A.-F.: Eur J. Biochem. *247*, 1151–1157 (1997).

214 Nemoz G., Sette C. and Conti M.: Mol. Pharmacol. 51, 242–249 (1997).

215 Baroja M.L., Cieslinski L.B., Torphy T.J., Wange R.L. and Madrenas J.: J. Immunol. *162*, 2016–2023 (1999).

216 Seybold J., Newton R., Wright L., Finney P.A., Suttorp N., Barnes P.J., Adcock I.M. and Giembycz M.A.: J. Biol. Chem. *273*, 20575–20588 (1998).

217   Erdogan S. and Housaly M.D.: Biochem J. *324*, 165–175 (1997).

218   Ostlere L.S., Mallett R.B., Kaminski A., Kaminski E.R., Pereira R.S. and Holden C.A.: Br. J. Dermatol. *133*, 1–5 (1995).

219   Gantner F., Gozt C., Gekeler V., Schudt C., Wendel A. and Hatzelmann A.: Br. J. Pharmacol. *123*, 1031–1038 (1998).

220   Marcoz P., Prigent A.-F., Lagarde M. and Nemoz G.: Mol. Pharmacol. *44*, 1027–1035 (1993).

221   Banner K.H., Roberts N.M. and Page C.P.: Br. J. Pharmacol. *116*, 3169–3174 (1995).

222   Crocker I.C., Townely R.G. and Khan M.M.: Immunopharmacology *31*, 223–235 (1996).

223   Foissier L., Lonchampt M., Coge F. and Cante E.: J. Pharmacol. Exp. Ther. *278*, 1484–1490 (1996).

224   Kaminuma O., Mori A., Suko M., Kikkawa H., Ikezawa K. and Okudaira H.: J. Pharmacol. Exp. Ther. *279*, 240–246 (1996).

225   vanWauve J., Aerts F., Walter H. and de Boer M.: Inflamm. Res. *44*, 400–405 (1995).

226   Yoshimura T., Nagao T., Nakao T., Watanabe S., Usami E., Kabayashi J., Yamazaki F., Tanaka H., Inagaki N. and Nagai H.: Gen. Pharmacol. *30*, 175–180 (1998).

227   Essayan D.M., Kagey-Sobotka A., Lichtenstein L.M. and Huang S.-K.: Biochem. Pharmacol. *53*, 1055–1060 (1997).

228   Grunig G., Warnock M., Wakil A.E., Venkayya R., Brombacher F., Rennick D.M., Sheppard D., Mohrs M., Donaldson D.D., Locksley R.M. et al.: Science *282*, 2261–2263 (1998).

229   Li Y., Simons F.E. and HayGlass K.T.: J. Immunol. *161*, 7007–7014 (1998).

230   Lidington E., Nohammer C., Dominguez M., Ferry B. and Rose M.L.: Clin. Exp. Immunol. *104*, 66–71 (1996).

231   Sommer N., Loschmann P.-A., Northoff G.H., Weller M., Steinbrecher A., Steinbach J.P., Lichtenfels R., Meyermann R., Riethmuller A., Fontana A. et al.: Nature Med. *1*, 244–248 (1995).

232   Genain C.P., Roberts T., Davis R.L., Nguyen M.-H., Uccelli A., Faulds D., Li Y., Hedgpeth J. and Hauser S.L.: Proc. Nat. Acad. Sci. *92*, 3601–3605 (1995).

233   Jung S., Zielasek J., Kollner G., Donhauser T., Toyka K. and Hartung H.-P.: J. Neuroimmunol. *68*, 1–11 (1996).

234   Moodley I., Sotsios Y. and Bertin B.: Mediators Inflamm. *4*, 112–116 (1995).

235   Griswold D.E., Webb E.F., Badger A.M., Gorycki P.D., Levandoski P.A., Barnette M.S., Grous M., Christensen S.B. and Torphy T.J.: J. Pharmacol. Exp. Ther. *387*, 705–711 (1998).

236   Webb E.F., Tzimas M.N., Newsholme S.J. and Griswold G.E.: J. Invest Dermatol. *111*, 86–92 (1998).

237   Sekut L., Yarnall D., Stimpson S.A., Noel L.S., Bateman-Fite R., Clark R.L., Brackeen M.F., Menius J.A. and Connolly K.M.: Clin. Exp. Immunol. *100*, 126–132 (1995).

238   Nyman U., Mussener A., Larsson E., Lorentzen J. and Klareskog L.: Clin. Exp. Immunol. *108*, 415–419 (1997).

239   Ross S.E., Williams R.O., Mason L.J., Mauri C., Marinova-Mutafchieva L., Malfait A.-M., Maini R.N. and Feldmann M.: J. Immunol. *159*, 6253–6259 (1997).

240   Liang L., Beshay E. and Prud'homme G.J.: Diabetes *47*, 570–575 (1998).

241   Underwood D.C., Matthew J.K., Osborn R.R., Bochnowicz S. and Torphy T.J.: J. Pharmacol. Exp. Ther. *280*, 21–219 (1997).

242   Fischer W., Schudt C. and Wendel A.: Biochem. Pharmacol. *45*, 2399–2404 (1993).

243   Badger A.M., Olivera D.L. and Esser K.M.: Circulatory Shock *44*, 188–195 (1994).

244   Griswold D.E., Hillegass L.M., O'Leary-Bartus J., Lee J.C., Laydon J.T. and Torphy T.J.: J. Immunol. Methods *195*, 1–5 (1996).

245   Cheng J.B., Watson J.W., Pazoles C.J., Eskra J.D., Griffiths R.J., Cohan V.L., Turner C.R., Showell H.J. and Pettipher E.R.: J. Pharmacol. Exp. Ther. *280*, 621–626 (1997).

246   Pettipher E.R., Labasi J.M., Salter E.D., Stam E.J., Cheng J.B. and Griffiths R.J.: Br. J. Pharmacol. *117*, 1530–1534 (1996).

247   Hadley A.J., Kumari M.K., Cover P.O., Osborne J., Poyser R., Flack J.D. and Buckingham J.C.: Br. J. Pharmacol. *119*, 463–470 (1996).

248   Kumari M., Cover P.O., Poyser R.H. and Buckingham J.C.: Br. J. Pharmacol. *121*, 459–468 (1997).

249   Holbrook M., Gozzard N., James T., Higgs G. and Hughers B.: Br. J. Pharmacol. *118*, 1192–1200 (1996).

250   Uno T., Tanaka H. and Nagai H.: Gen. Pharmac. *30*, 167–173 (1998).

251   Santig R.E., Olymulder C.G., Van der Molen K., Meurs H. and Zaagsma J.: Eur. J. Pharmacol. *275*, 75–82 (1995).

252   Planquois J.M.S., Bonnet S. and Payne A.N.: Am. J. Respir. Crit. Care Med. *157*, A843 (abstract) (1998).

253   Qian Y., Girard V., Martin C.A.E., Molimard M. and Advenier C.: Eur J. Respir *7*, 306–310 (1994).

254   Undem B.J., Meeker S.N. and Chen J.: J. Pharmacol. Exp. Ther. *271*, 811–817 (1994).

255   Imoto A., Yoshida M., Takahashi N. and Ito Y.: J. Auton Nervous System *68*, 1–13 (1998).

256   Ellis J.L. and Conanan D.N.: J. Pharmacol. Exp. Ther. *272*, 997–1004 (1995).

257   Fernandes L.B., Ellis J.L. and Undem B.J.: Am. J. Respir. Crit. Care Med. *150*, 1384–1390 (1994).

258   Palmer D., Tsoi K. and Maurice D.H.: Circ. Res. *82*, 852–861 (1998).

259   Rose R.J., Liu H., Palmer D. and Maurice D.H.: Br. J. Pharmacol. *122*, 233–240 (1997).

260   Tomlinson P.R., Wilson J.W. and Stewart A.G.: Biochem. Pharmacol. *49*, 1809–1819 (1995).

261   Maruno K., Absood A. and Said S.I.: Am. J. Physiol. *268*, L1047–L1051 (1995).

262   Florio C., Martin J.G., Styhler A. and Heisler S.: Am. J. Physiol. *266*, L131–L137 (1994).

263   Noveral J.P. and Grunstein M.M.: Am. J. Physiol. *267*, L291–L299 (1994).

264   Johnson-Mills K., Arauz E., Coffey R.G., Krzanowski J.J. and Polson J.B.: Biochem. Pharmacol. *56*, 1065–1073 (1998).

265   Pan X., Arauz E., Krzanowski J.J., Fitzpatrick D.F. and Polson J.B.: Biochem. Pharmacol. *48*, 827–835 (1994).

266   Souness J.E., Hassall G.A. and Parrott D.P.: Biochem. Pharmacol. *44*, 857–866 (1992).

267   Billington CK, Joseph S.K., Swan C., Scott M.G.H., Jobson T.M. and Hall I.P.: Am. J. Physiol. *276*, L412–L419 (1999).

268   Duttagupta C., Rifas L. and Makman M.H.: Biochim. Biophys. Acta *523*, 385–394 (1978).

269   Saltzman L.E., Moss J., Berg R.A., Hom B. and Crystal R.G.: Biochem. J. *204*, 25–30 (1982).

270   Magnaldo I. and Pouyssegur P.S.: FEBS Lett. *245*, 65–69 (1989).

271   Zitnik R.J., Zheng T. and Elias J.A.: Am. J. Physiol. *264*, L253–L260 (1993).

272   Lindenschmidt R.C. and Witschi H.: Biochem. Pharmacol. *34*, 4269–4273 (1985).

273   Wagner R.S., Smith C.J., Taylor A.M. and Rhoades R.A.: J. Pharmacol. Exp. Ther. *282*, 1650–1657 (1997).

274   Pauwels R.: Clin. Exp. Allergy *26* (Suppl. 2), 55–59 (1996).

275   Spina D., Landells L.J. and Page C.P.: Clin. Exp. Allergy *28* (Suppl. 3), 24–34 (1998).

276 Foster R.W., Rakshi K., Carpenter J.R. and Small R.C.: Br. J. Clin. Pharmac. *34*, 527–534 (1992).

277 Brunnee T., Engelstatter R., Steinijans V.W. and Kunkel G.: Eur. Respir. J. *5*, 982–985 (1992).

278 Ukena D., Rentz K., Reiber C. and Sybrecht G.W.: Respir. Med. *89*, 441–444 (1995).

279 Harbinson P.L., MacLeod D., Hawksworth R., O'Toole S., Sullivan P.J., Heath P., Kilfeather S., Page C.P., Costello J., Holgate S.T. et al.: Eur. Respir. J. *10*, 1008–1014 (1997).

280 Jones T.R., McAuliffe M., McFarlane C.S., Piechuta H., Macdonald D. and Rodger I.W.: Can. J. Physiol. Pharmacol. *76*, 210–217 (1998).

281 Nieman R.B., Fisher B.D., Amit O. and Dockhorn R.J.: Am. J. Respir. Crit. Care Med. *157*, A413 (abstract) (1998).

282 Murdoch R.D., Cowley H., Upward J., Webber D. and Wyld P.: Am. J. Respir. Crit. Care Med. *157*, A409 (abstract) (1998).

283 Compton C., Cedar E., Nieman R.B., Amit O., Langley S.J. and Sapene M.: Am. J. Respir. Crit. Care Med. *159*, A624 (abstract) (1999).

284 Torphy T.J., Barnette M.S., Underwood D.C., Griswold D.E., Christensen S.B., Murdoch R.D., Nieman R.B. and Compton C.H.: Pulmonary Pharmacol. Ther. (in press) (1999).

285 Compton C.H., Gubb, J., Cedar E., Bakst A., Nieman R.B., Amit O., Ayres J. and Brambilla C.: Am. J. Respir. Crit. Care Med. *159*, A522 (abstract) (1999).

286 Compton C.H., Gubb J., Nieman R.B., Amit O., Brambilla A and Ayres J.: Am. J. Respir. Crit. Care Med. *159*, A806 (abstract) (1999).

287 Souness J.E. and Rao S.: Cell Signal *9*, 227–236 (1997).

288 Horowski R., Sastre Y. and Hernandez M.: Curr. Ther. Res. *38*, 23–29 (1985).

289 Carpenter D.O., Briggs D.B., Knox A.P. and Strominger N.: J. Neurophysiol. *59*, 358–369 (1988).

290 Heaslip R.J. and Evans D.Y.: Eur. J. Pharmacol. *286*, 281–290 (1995).

291 Robichaud A., Tattersall F.D., Choudhury I. and Rodger I.W.: Neuropharmacology *38*, 289–297 (1999).

292 Barnette M.S., Grous M., Cieslinski L.B., Burman M., Christensen S.B. and Torphy T.J.: J. Pharmacol. Exp. Ther. *273*, 1396–1402 (1995).

293 Silver P.J., Harris A.L., Buchholz R.A., Miller M.S., Gordon R.J., Dundore R.L. and Pagani E.D., in: K.A. Jacobson, J.W. Daley and V. Manganiello (eds.): *Purines in Cellular Signaling, Targets for New Drugs*, Springer-Verlag, New York 1990, 358–364.

294 Barnette M.S., Manning C.D., Price W.J. and Barone F.C.: J. Pharmacol. Exp. Ther. *264*, 801–812 (1993).

295 Grous M. and Barnette M.S.: Br. J. Pharmacol. *111*, 259–263 (1994).

296 Izzo A.A., Mascolo N. and Capasso F.: Naunyn Schmiedeberg's Arch. Pharmcol. *357*, 677–681 (1998).

297 Schneider H.H., Schmiechen R., Brezinski M. and Seidler J.: Eur. J. Pharmacol. *127*, 105–115 (1986).

298 Jacobitz S., McLaughlin M.M., Livi G.P., Burman M. and Torphy T.J.: Mol. Pharmacol. *50*, 891–899 (1996).

299 Rocque W.J., Tian G., Wiseman J.S., Holmes W.D., Zajac-Thompson I., Willard D.H., Patel I.R., Wisely G.B., Clay W.C., Kadwell S.H. et al.: Biochemistry *36*, 14250–14261 (1997).

300 Kaulen P., Bruning G., Schneider H.H., Sarter M. and Baumgarten H.G.: Brain Res. *503*, 229–245 (1989).

301 Souness J.E., Houghton C., Sardar N. and Withnall M.T.: Br. J. Pharmacol. *121*, 743–750 (1997).

302 Duplantier A.J., Biggers M.S., Chambers R.J., Cheng J.B., Cooper K., Damon D.B., Eggler J.F., Kraus K.G., Marfat A., Masamune H. et al.: J. Med. Chem. *39*, 120–125 (1996).

303 Koe B.K., Lebel L.A., Nielsen J.A., Russo L.L., Saccomano N.A., Vinick F.J. and Williams I.H.: Drug Dev. Res. *21*, 135–142 (1990).

304 Christensen S.B., Guider A., Forster C.J., Gleason J.G., Bender P.E., Karpinski J.M., DeWolf W.E., Barnette M.S., Underwood D.C., Griswold D.E. et al.: J. Med. Chem. *41*, 821–835 (1998).

305 Montana J.G., Buckley G.M., Cooper N., Dyke H.J., Gowers L., Gregory J.P., Hellewell P.G., Kendall H.J., Lowe C., Maxey R. et al.: Bioorganic Med. Chem. Lett. *8*, 2635–2640 (1998).

306 Bolger G.B., Rodgers L. and Riggs M.: Gene *149*, 237–244 (1993).

307 Obernolte R., Bhakta S., Alvarez R., Bach C., Zuppan P., Mulkins M., Jarnagin K. and Shelton E.R.: Gene *129*, 239–247 (1993).

308 Engels P., Abdel'Al S., Hulley P. and Lubbert H.: J. Neuroscience Res. *41*, 169–178 (1995).

309 Iwahashi Y., Furuyama T., Tano Y., Ishimoto I., Shimomura Y. and Inagaki S.: Mol. Brain Res. *38*, 14–24 (1996).

310 Iona S., Cuomo M., Bushnik T., Naro F., Sette C., Hess M., Shelton E.R. and Conti M.: Mol. Pharmacol. *53*, 23–32 (1998).

Index Vol. 53

Index of titles
Vol. 1–53 (1959–1999)

Acetylen-Verbindungen als Arzneistoffe, natürliche und synthetische
14, 387 (1970)

Adenosine receptors: Clinical implications and biochemical mechanisms
32, 195 (1988)

Adipose tissue, the role of in the distribution and storage of drugs
28, 273 (1984)

Adrenal cortex, steroidogenic capacity and its regulation
34, 359 (1976)

β-Adrenergic blocking agents
20, 27 (1976)

β-Adrenergic blocking agents, pharmacology and structure-activity
10, 46 (1966)

β-Adrenergic blocking drugs, pharmacology
15, 103 (1971)

Adrenergic receptor research, recent developments
33, 151 (1989)

Adrenoceptors, subclassification and nomenclature
47, 81 (1996)

Adverse reactions of sugar polymers in animals and man
23, 27 (1979)

Aldose reductase inhibitors: Recent developments
40, 99 (1993)

Allergy, pharmacological approach
3, 409 (1961)

Alternative therapeutic modalities. Alternative medicine
47, 251 (1996)

Alzheimer's disease, implications of immunomodulant therapy
32, 21 (1988)

Alzheimer's disease, neuroimmune axis as a basis of therapy
34, 383 (1990)

Amebic disease, pathogenesis of
18, 225 (1974)

Amidinstruktur in der Arzneistoffforschung
11, 356 (1968)

Amines, biogenic and drug research
28, 9 (1984)

Aminoglycosides and polyamines: Targets and effects in the mammalian organism of two important groups of natural aliphatic polycations
46, 183 (1996)

Amino- und Nitroderivate (aromatische), biologische Oxydation und Reduktion
8, 195 (1965)

Aminonucleosid-Nephrose
7, 341 (1964)

Amoebiasis, chemotherapy
8, 11 (1965)

Amoebiasis, surgical
18, 77 (1974)

Amoebicidal drugs, comparative evaluation
18, 353 (1974)

Anabolic steroids
2, 71 (1960)

Author and paper index
Vol. 1–53 (1959–1999)

Pertussis agglutinins and complement fixing antibodies in whooping cough *19*, 178 (1975)	K. C. Agarwal M. Ray N. L. Chitkara
Pharmacology of clinically useful beta-adrenergic blocking drugs *15*, 103 (1971)	R. P. Ahlquist A. M. Karow, Jr. M. W. Riley
Adrenergic beta blocking agents *20*, 27 (1976)	R. P. Ahlquist
Trial of a new anthelmintic (bitoscanate) in ankylostomiasis in children *19*, 2 (1975)	S. H. Ahmed S. Vaishnava
Development of antibacterial agents of the nalidixic acid type *21*, 9 (1977)	R. Albrecht
The mode of action of anti-rheumatic drugs. Anti-inflammatory and immunosuppressive effects of glucocorticoids *33*, 63 (1989)	Anthony C. Allison Simon W. Lee
Biological activity in the quinazolone series *14*, 218 (1970)	A. H. Amin D. R. Mehta S. S. Samarth
Enhancement and inhibition of microsomal drug metabolism *17*, 11 (1973)	M. W. Anders
Reactivity of rat and man to egg-white *13*, 340 (1969)	S. I. Ankier
Enzyme inhibitors of the renin-angiotensin system *31*, 161 (1987)	Michael J. Antonaccio John J. Wright
Narcotic antagonists *8*, 261 (1965)	S. Archer L. S. Harris

Interbiotype conversion of cholera vibrios by action of mutagens *19*, 466 (1975)	P. Bhattacharya S. Ray
Experience with bitoscanate in hookworm disease and trichuriasis in Mexico *19*, 23 (1975)	F. Biagi
Analysis of symptoms and signs related with intestinal parasitosis in 5,215 cases *19*, 10 (1975)	F. Biagi R. López J. Viso
Untersuchungen zur Biochemie und Pharmacologie der Thymoleptika *11*, 121 (1968) The role of adipose tissue in the distribution and storage of drugs *28*, 273 (1984)	M. H. Bickel
The β-adrenergic-blocking agents, pharmacology, and structure-activity relationships *10*, 46 (1966)	J. H. Biel B. K. B. Lum
Prostaglandins *17*, 410 (1973)	J. S. Bindra R. Bindra
In vitro models for the study of antibiotic activities *31*, 349 (1987)	J. Blaser S. H. Zinner
The red blood cell membrane as a model for targets of drug action *17*, 59 (1973)	L. Bolis
Epidemiology and public health. Importance of intestinal nematode infections in Latin America *19*, 28 (1975)	D. Botero
Clinical importance of cardiovascular drug interactions *25*, 133 (1981) Serum electrolyte abnormalities caused by drugs *30*, 9 (1986)	D. Craig Brater
Update of cardiovascular drug interactions *29*, 9 (1985)	D. Craig Brater Michael R. Vasko
Some practical problems of the epidemiology of leprosy in the Indian context *18*, 25 (1974)	S. G. Browne
Brain neurotransmitters and the development and maintenance of experimental hypertension *30*, 127 (1986)	Jerry J. Buccafusco Henry E. Brezenoff
Die Ionenaustauscher und ihre Anwendung in der Pharmazie und Medizin *1*, 11 (1959)	J. Büchi

Wert und Bewertung der Arzneimittel *10*, 90 (1966)	J. Büchi
Cyclopropane compounds of biological interest *15*, 227 (1971) The state of medicinal science *20*, 9 (1976) Isosterism and bioisosterism in drug design *37*, 287 (1991)	A. Burger
Human and veterinary anthelmintics (1965–1971) *17*, 108 (1973)	R. B. Burrows
The antibody basis of local immunity to experimental cholera infection in the rabbit ileal loop *19*, 471 (1975)	W. Burrows J. Kaur
Les dérivés organiques du fluor d'intérêt pharmacologique *3*, 9 (1961)	N. P. Buu-Hoï
Teaching tropical medicine *18*, 35 (1974)	K. M. Cahill
Anabolic steroids *2*, 71 (1960)	B. Camerino G. Sala
Immunosuppression agents, procedures, speculations and prognosis *16*, 67 (1972)	G. W. Camiener W. J. Wechter
Dopamine agonists: Structure-activity relationships *29*, 303 (1985)	Joseph G. Cannon
Therapeutic applications of cytokines for immunostimulation and immuno- suppression: An update *47*, 211 (1996)	Gaetano Cardi Thomas L. Ciardelli Marc S. Ernstoff
Analgesics and their antagonists: Recent developments *22*, 149 (1978)	A. F. Casy
Chemical nature and pharmacological actions of quaternary ammonium salts *2*, 135 (1960)	C. J. Cavallito A. P. Gray
Contributions of medicinal chemistry to medicine – from 1935 *12*, 11 (1968) Changing influences on goals and incentives in drug research and development *20*, 159 (1976) Quaternary ammonium salts – advances in chemistry and pharmacology since 1960 *24*, 267 (1980)	C. J. Cavallito

Studies on *Vibrio parahaemolyticus* infection in Calcutta as compared to cholera infection *19*, 490 (1975)	B. C. Deb
Biochemical effects of drugs acting on the central nervous system *8*, 53 (1965)	L. Decsi
Some reflections on the chemotherapy of tropical diseases: Past, present and future *26*, 343 (1982)	E. W. J. de Maar
Drug research – whence and whither *10*, 11 (1966)	R. G. Denkewalter M. Tishler
Immunization of a village, a new approach to herd immunity *19*, 252 (1975)	N. S. Deodhar
Profiles of tuberculosis in rural areas of Maharashtra *18*, 91 (1974)	M. D. Deshmukh K. G. Kulkarni S. S. Virdi B. B. Yodh
The interface between drug research, marketing, management, and social, political and regulatory forces *20*, 181 (1976) Medicinal research: Retrospectives and perspectives *29*, 97 (1985) Serendipity and structured research in drug discovery *30*, 189 (1986) Medicinal chemistry: A support or a driving force in drug research? *34*, 343 (1990) Heterocyclic diversity: The road to biological activity *44*, 9 (1995)	G. deStevens
Hypolipidemic agents *13*, 217 (1969)	G. deStevens W. L. Bencze R. Hess
Antihypertensive agents *20*, 197 (1976)	G. deStevens M. Wilhelm
RNA virus evolution and the control of viral disease *33*, 93 (1989)	Esteban Domingo

The use of quantum chemical methods to study molecular mechanisms of drug action *34*, 9 (1990)	H.-D. Höltje M. Hense S. Marrer E. Maurhofer
Relationship of induced antibody titres to resistance to experimental human infection *19*, 542 (1975)	R. B. Hornick R. A. Cash J. P. Libonati
Recent applications of mass spectrometry in pharmaceutical research *18*, 399 (1974)	G. Horváth
Risk assessment problems in chemical oncogenesis *31*, 257 (1987)	G. H. Hottendorf
Bacterial resistence to antibiotics: The role of biofilms *37*, 91 (1991)	Brian D. Hoyle J. William Costerton
Recent developments in disease-modifying antirheumatic-drugs *24*, 101 (1980)	I. M. Hunneyball
The pharmacology of homologous series *7*, 305 (1964)	H. R. Ing
Progress in the experimental chemotherapy of helminth infections. Part. 1. Trematode and cestode diseases *17*, 241 (1973)	P. J. Islip
Pharmacology of the brain: The hippocampus, learning and seizures *16*, 211 (1972)	I. Izquierdo A. G. Nasello
Cholinergic mechanism – monoamines relation in certain brain structures *16*, 334 (1972)	J. A. Izquierdo
The development of antifertility substances *7*, 133 (1964)	H. Jackson
Development of novel anti-inflammatory agents: A pharmacological perspective on leukotrienes and their receptors *46*, 115 (1996)	William T. Jackson Jerome H. Fleisch
Agents acting on central dopamine receptors *21*, 409 (1977)	P. C. Jain N. Kumar
Recent advances in the treatment of parasitic infections in man *18*, 191 (1974) The levamisole story *20*, 347 (1976)	P. A. J. Janssen
Recent developments in cancer chemotherapy *25*, 275 (1981)	K. Jewers

Search for pharmaceutically interesting quinazoline derivatives: Efforts and results (1969–1980) *26*, 259 (1982)	S. Johne
Serotonin in migraine: Theories, animal models and emerging therapies *51*, 219 (1998)	Kirk W. Johnson Lee A. Phebus Marlene L. Cohen
A review of advances in prescribing for teratogenic hazards *29*, 121 (1985)	E. Marshall Johnson
A comparative of bitoscanate, bephenium hydroxynaphthoate and tetrachlor-ethylene in hookworm infection *19*, 70 (1975)	S. Johnson
Polyamines and cerebral ischemia *50*, 193 (1998)	T. David Johnson
Tetanus in Punjab with particular reference to the role of muscle relaxants in its management *19*, 288 (1975)	S. S. Jolly J. Singh S. M. Singh
Virulence-enhancing effect of ferric ammonium citrate on *Vibrio cholerae* *19*, 546 (1975)	I. Joó
Chemical teratogenesis *41*, 9 (1993) Chemical teratogenesis in humans: Biochemical and molecular mechanisms *49*, 25 (1997)	Mont R. Juchau
Drug molecules of marine origin *35*, 521 (1990) Alternative therapeutic modalities. Alternative medicine *47*, 251 (1996) Drug discovery: Past, present and future *50*, 9 (1998)	Pushkar N. Kaul
Toxoplasmosis *18*, 205 (1974)	B. H. Kean
The application of high-throughput screening to novel lead discovery *51*, 245 (1998)	Barry A. Kenny Mark Bushfield David J. Parry-Smith Simon Fogarty Mark Treherne
Tabellarische Zusammenstellung über die Substruktur der Proteine *16*, 364 (1972)	R. Kleine
Bioactive peptide analogs: *In vivo* and *in vitro* production *34*, 287 (1990)	Horst Kleinkauf Hans von Doehren

Die Anwendung von Psychopharmaka in der psychosomatischen Medizin *10*, 530 (1966)	F. Labhardt
The bacterial cell surface and antimicrobial resistance *32*, 149 (1988)	Peter A. Lambert
Therapeutic measurement in tetanus *19*, 323 (1975)	D. R. Laurence
Clinical application of cytokines and immunostimulation and immunosuppression *39*, 167 (1992)	Betty Lee Thomas L. Ciardelli
Physicochemical methods in pharmaceutical chemistry I. Spectrofluorometry *6*, 151 (1963)	H. G. Leemann K. Stich Margrit Thomas
Biochemical acyl hydroxylations 16, 229 (1972)	W. Lenk
Cholinesterase restoring therapy in tetanus *19*, 329 (1975)	G. Leonardi K. G. Nair F. D. Dastur
Perspective and overview of Chinese traditional medicine and contemporary pharmacology *47*, 131 (1996)	E. Leong Way Yong Qing-Liu Chieh-Fu Chen
The histamine H_3-receptor: A targeting for new drugs *39*, 127 (1992)	R. Leurs H. Timmerman
The medicinal chemistry and therapeutic potentials of the histamine H_3 receptor *45*, 107 (1995)	R. Leurs R.C. Vollinga H. Timmerman
Biliary excretion of drugs and other xenobiotics *25*, 361 (1981)	W. G. Levine
Structures, properties and disposition of drugs *29*, 67 (1985) Ribonucleotide reductase inhibitors as anti-cancer and antiviral agents *31*, 101 (1987) Fungal metabolites and Chinese herbal medicine as immunostimulants *34*, 395 (1990) Design and discovery of new drugs by stepping-up and stepping-down approaches *40*, 163 (1993)	Eric J. Lien
Immunopharmacological and biochemical bases of Chinese herbal medicine *46*, 263 (1996)	Eric J. Lien Arima Das Linda J. Lien

Physicochemical basis of the universal genetic codes – quantitative analysis 48, 9 (1997)	Eric J. Lien Arima Das Partha Nandy Shijun Ren
In search of ideal antihypertensive drugs: Progress in five decades 43, 43 (1994)	Eric J. Lien Hua Gao Linda L. Lien
Interactions between androgenic-anabolic steroids and glucocorticoids 14, 139 (1970)	O. Linet
Drug inhibition of mast cell secretion 29, 277 (1985)	R. Ludowyke D. Lagunoff
Reactivity of bentonite flocculation, indirect haemagglutination and Casoni tests in hydatid disease 19, 75 (1975)	R. C. Mahajan N. L. Chitkara
Characteristics of catechol O-methyltransferase (COMT) and properties of selective COMT inhibitors 39, 291 (1992)	P.T. Männistö I. Ulmanen K. Lundström J. Taskinen J. Tenhunen C. Tilgmann S. Kaakkola
Interaction of cancer chemotherapy agents with the mononuclear phagocyte system 35, 487 (1990)	Alberto Mantovani
Mechanisms of fibrinolysis and clinical use of thrombolytic agents 39, 197 (1992)	Maurizio Margaglione Elvira Grandone Giovanni Di Minno
Drugs affecting plasma fibrinogen levels. Implications for new anti-thrombotic strategies 46, 169 (1996)	M. Margaglione E. Grandone F. P. Mancini G. Di Minno
Epidemiology of diphtheria 19, 336 (1975)	L. G. Marquis
Biological activity of the terpenoids and their derivatives 6, 279 (1963)	M. Martin-Smith T. Khatoon
Biological activity of the terpenoids and their derivatives – recent advances 13, 11 (1969)	M. Martin-Smith W. E. Sneader
Antihypertensive agents 1962–1968 13, 101 (1969) Fundamental structures in drug research – Part I 20, 385 (1976)	A. Marxer O. Schier

Fundamental structures in drug research – Part II *22*, 27 (1978) Antihypertensive agents 1969–1980 *25*, 9 (1981)	A. Marxer O. Schier
Relationships between the chemical structure and pharmacological activity in a series of synthetic quinuclidine derivatives *13*, 293 (1969)	M. D. Mashkovsky L. N. Yakhontov
Further developments in research on the chemistry and pharmacology of synthetic quinuclidine derivatives *27*, 9 (1983)	M. D. Mashkovsky L. N. Yakhontov M. E. Kaminka E. E. Mikhlina S. Ordzhonikidze
Role of neutrotransmitters in the central regulation of the cardiovascular system *35*, 25 (1990) Neurotransmitters involved in the central regulation of the cardiovascular system *46*, 43 (1996)	Robert B. McCall
On the understanding of drug potency 13, 123 (1971) The chemotherapy of intestinal nematodes *16*, 157 (1972)	J. W. McFarland
Non-steroidal menses-regulating agents: The present status *44*, 159 (1995)	P.K. Mehrotra Sanjay Batra A.P. Bhaduri
Zur Beeinflussung der Strahlen- empfindlichkeit von Säugetieren durch chemische Substanzen *9*, 11 (1966)	H.-J. Melching C. Streffer
Analgesia and addiction *5*, 155 (1963)	L. B. Mellett L. A. Woods
Comparative drug metabolism 13, 136 (1969)	L. B. Mellett
The oral antiarrhythmic drugs 35, 151 (1990)	Lisa Mendes Scott L. Beau John S. Wilson Philip J. Podrid
Mechanism of action of anxiolytic drugs *31*, 315 (1987)	T. Mennini S. Caccia S. Garattini
Pathogenesis of amebic disease 18, 225 (1974) Protozoan and helminth parasites – a review of current treatment *20*, 433 (1976)	M. J. Miller

Medicinal agents incorporating the 1,2-diamine functionality *33*, 135 (1989)	Erik T. Michalson Jacob Szmuszkovicz
Fluorinated quinolones-new quinolone antimicrobials *38*, 9 (1992)	S. Mitsuhashi (Editor) T. Kojima, N. Nakanishi, T. Fujimoto, S. Goto, S. Miyusaki, T. Uematsu, M. Nakashima, Y. Asahina, T. Ishisaki, S. Susue, K. Hirai, K. Sato, K. Hoshino, J. Shimada, S. Hori
Synopsis der Rheumatherapie *12*, 165 (1968)	W. Moll
On the chemotherapy of cancer *8*, 431 (1965) The relationship of the metabolism of anticancer agents to their activity *17*, 320 (1973) The current status of cancer chemotherapy *20*, 465 (1976)	J. A. Montgomery
Present status of Leishmaniasis *34*, 447 (1990)	Anita Mukherjee Manju Seth A. P. Bhaduri
The significance of DNA technology in medicine *33*, 397 (1989)	Hansjakob Müller
Der Einfluß der Formgebung auf die Wirkung eines Arzneimittels *10*, 204 (1966) Galenische Formgebung und Arznei- mittelwirkung. Neue Erkenntnisse und Feststellungen *14*, 269 (1970)	K. Münzel
Effects of NSAIDs on the kidney *49*, 155 (1997)	M. D. Murray D. Craig Brater
A field trial with bitoscanate in India *19*, 81 (1975)	G. S. Mutalik R. B. Gulati A. K. Iqbal
Comparative study of bitoscanate, bephenium hydroxynaphthoate and tetrachlorethylene in hookworm disease *19*, 86 (1975)	G. S. Mutalik R. B. Gulati
Ganglienblocker *2*, 297 (1960)	K. Nádor
Nitroimidazoles as chemotherapeutic agents *27*, 162 (1983)	M. D. Nair K. Nagarajan
Recent advances in cholera pathophysiology and therapeutics *19*, 563 (1975)	D. R. Nalin

Drug research and human sleep *22*, 355 (1978)	I. Oswald
Effects of drugs on calmodulin-mediated enzymatic actions *33*, 353 (1989)	Judit Ovádi
An extensive community outbreak of acute diarrhoeal diseases in children *19*, 570 (1975)	S. C. Pal C. Koteswar Rao
Drug and its action according to Ayurveda *26*, 55 (1982)	Madhabendra Nath Pal
Oligosaccharide chains of glycoproteins *32*, 163 (1990)	Y. T. Pan Alan D. Elbein
Pharmacology of synthetic organic selenium compounds *36*, 9 (1991)	Michael J. Parnham Erich Graf
Moral challenges in the organisation and management of drug research *42*, 9 (1994)	Michael J. Parnham
3,4-Dihydroxyphenylalanine and related compounds *9*, 223 (1966)	A. R. Patel A. Burger
Mescaline and related compounds *11*, 11 (1968)	A. R. Patel
Experience with bitoscanate in adults *19*, 90 (1975)	A. H. Patricia U. Prabakar Rao R. Subramaniam N. Madanagopalan
The impact of state and society on medical research *35*, 9 (1990)	C. R. Pfaltz
Transfer factor in malignancy *42*, 401 (1994)	Giancarlo Pizza Caterina De Vinci H. Hugh Fudenberg
Monoaminoxydase-Hemmer *2*, 417 (1960)	A. Pletscher K. F. Gey P. Zeller
Antifungal therapy: Are we winning? *37*, 183 (1991)	A. Polak P. G. Hartman
Antifungal therapy, an everlasting battle *49*, 219 (1997)	A. Polak
What makes a good pertussis vaccine? *19*, 341 (1975) Vaccine composition in relation to antigenic variation of the microbe: Is pertussis unique? *19*, 347 (1975) Some unsolved problems with vaccines *23*, 9 (1979)	N. W. Preston

Eradication by vaccination: The memorial to smallpox could be surrounded by others *41*, 151 (1993)	N. W. Preston
Peptide drug delivery into the central nervous system *51*, 95 (1998)	Laszlo Prokai
Antibiotics in the chemotherapy of malaria *26*, 167 (1982)	S. K. Puri G. P. Dutta
Potassium channel openers: Airway pharmacology and clinical possibilities in asthma *37*, 161 (1991)	David Raeburn Jan-Anders Karlsson
Isozyme-selective cyclic nucleotide phosphodiesterase inhibitors: Biochemistry, pharmacology and therapeutic potential in asthma *40*, 9 (1993)	David Raeburn John E. Souness Adrian Tomkinson Jan-Anders Karlsson
Clinical study of diphtheria, tetanus and pertussis *19*, 356 (1975)	V. B. Raju V. R. Parvathi
Epidemiology of cholera in Hyderabad *19*, 578 (1975)	K. Rajyalakshmi P. V. Ramana Rao
Present status of hepatoprotectants *52*, 53 (1999)	Vishnu Ji Ram Atul Goel
Adenosine receptors: Clinical implications and biochemical mechanisms *32*, 195 (1988)	Vickram Ramkumar George Pierson Gary L. Stiles
New synthetic ligands for L-type voltage-gated calcium channels *40*, 191 (1993)	David Rampe David J. Triggle
Problems of malaria eradication in India *18*, 245 (1974)	V. N. Rao
Pharmacology of migraine *34*, 209 (1990)	Neil H. Raskin
The photochemistry of drugs and related substances *11*, 48 (1968)	S. T. Reid
Natural products and their derivatives as cancer chemopreventive agents *48*, 147 (1997) Development of HIV protease inhibitors: A survey *51*, 1 (1998)	Shijun Ren Eric J. Lien
Orale Antikoagulantien *11*, 226 (1968)	E. Renk W. G. Stoll

In search of ideal inotropic steroids: Recent progress *47*, 9 (1996)	Kurt R.H. Repke Kathleen J. Sweadner Jürgen Weiland Rudolf Megges Rudolf Schön
Mechanism-based inhibitors of monoamine oxidase *30*, 205 (1986)	Lauren E. Richards Alfred Burger
Glutamatergic involvement in psychomotor stimulant action *50*, 155 (1998)	Robin W. Rockhold
The hopanoids, bacterial triterpenoids, and the biosynthesis of isoprenic units in prokaryote *37*, 271 (1991)	Michel Rohmer Philippe Bisseret Bertrand Sutter
Isoprenoids biosynthesis via the mevalonate-independent route, a novel target for antibacterial drugs? *50*, 135 (1998)	Michel Rohmer
Tetrahydroisoquinolines and β-carbolines: Putative natural substances in plants and animals *29*, 415 (1985)	H. Rommelspacher R. Susilo
Functional significance of the various components of the influenza virus 18, 253 (1974)	R. Rott
Drug receptors and control of the cardiovascular system: Recent advances *36*, 117 (1991)	Robert R. Ruffolo Jr J. Paul Hieble David P. Brooks Giora Z. Feuerstein Andrew J. Nichols
Behavioral correlates of presynaptic events in the cholinergic neurotransmitter system *32*, 43 (1988)	Roger W. Russell
Epidemiology of pertussis *19*, 257 (1975)	J. A. Sa
Surgical amoebiasis *18*, 77 (1974)	A. E. de Sa
Role of beta-adrenergic blocking drug propranolol in severe tetanus *19*, 361 (1975)	G. S. Sainani K. L. Jain V. R. D. Deshpande A. B. Balsara S. A. Iyer
Studies on *Vibrio parahaemolyticus* in Bombay *19*, 586 (1975)	F. L. Saldanha A. K. Patil M. V. Sant

Immunoregulatory role of neuro-peptides *38*, 149 (1992) Neuropeptides as native immune modulators *45*, 9 (1995) Immunotherapy for brain diseases and mental illnesses *48*, 129 (1997)	Vijendra K. Singh
Natural products as anticancer agents *42*, 53 (1994)	Shradha Sinha Sudha Jain
Biologically active quinazolones *43*, 143 (1994)	Shradha Sinha Mukta Srivastava
Some often neglected factors in the control and prevention of communicable diseases *18*, 277 (1974)	C. E. G. Smith
Tetanus and its prevention *19*, 391 (1975)	J. W. G. Smith
Growth of *Clostridium tetani in vivo* *19*, 384 (1975)	J. W. G. Smith A. G. MacIver
The biliary excretion and enterohepatic circulation of drugs and other organic compounds *9*, 299 (1966)	R. L. Smith
Noninvasive pharmacodynamic and bio-electric methods for elucidating the bio-availability mechanisms of ophthalmic drug preparations *25*, 421 (1981)	V. F. Smolen
On the relation between chemical structure and function in certain tumor promoters and anti-tumor agents *23*, 63 (1979) Relationships between structure and function of convulsant drugs *24*, 57 (1980)	J. R. Smythies
Gram-negative bacterial endotoxin and the pathogenesis of fever *19*, 402 (1975)	E. S. Snell
Benzodiazepine augmentation of the treatment of disruptive psychotic behavior *35*, 139 (1990)	David A. Solomon Edison Miyawaki Carl Salzman
Chemokines as targets for pharma-cological intervention *47*, 53 (1996)	Silvano Sozzani Paola Allavena Paul Proost Jo Van Damme Alberto Mantovani

From genome to drug – optimising the drug discovery process *53*, 157 (1999)	Paul Spence
Emerging concepts towards the development of contraceptive agents *33*, 267 (1989)	Ranjan P. Srivastava A. P. Bhaduri
Strukturelle Betrachtungen der Psychopharmaka: Versuch einer Korrelation von chemischer Konstitution und klinischer Wirkung *9*, 129 (1966)	K. Stach W. Pöldinger
From podophyllotoxin glucoside to etoposide *33*, 169 (1989)	H. Stähelin A. von Wartburg
Chemotherapy of intestinal helminthiasis *19*, 158 (1975)	O. D. Standen
Immunotherapy for leprosy and tuberculosis *33*, 415 (1989)	J. L. Stanford
The leishmaniasis *18*, 289 (1974)	E. A. Steck
The benzodiazepine story *22*, 229 (1978)	L. H. Sternbach
Immunostimulation with peptidoglycan or its synthetic derivatives *32*, 305 (1988)	Duncan E. S. Stewart-Tull
Hypertension: Relating drug therapy to pathogenic mechanisms *32*, 175 (1988)	David H. P. Streeten Gunnar H. Anderson Jr
Progress in sulfonamide research *12*, 389 (1968) Problems of medical practice and of medical-pharmaceutical research *20*, 491 (1976)	Th. Struller
Bacterial resistance to β-lactam antibiotics: Problems and solutions *41*, 95 (1993)	R. Sutherland
Antiviral agents *22*, 267 (1978) Antiviral agents 1978–1983 *28*, 127 (1984)	D. L. Swallow
Ketoconazole, a new step in the management of fungal disease *27*, 63 (1983)	J. Symoens G. Cauwenbergh
Antiarrhythmic compounds *12*, 292 (1968)	L. Szekeres J. G. Papp

U-50,488 and the κ receptor: a personalized account covering the period 1973–1990 *52*, 167 (1999) U-50,488 fand the κ receptor. Part II: 1991–1998 *53*, 1 (1999)	Jacob Szmuszkovicz
Practically applicable results of twenty years of research in endocrinology *12*, 137 (1968)	M. Tausk
Stereoselective drug metabolism and its significance in drug research *32*, 249 (1988)	Bernard Testa Joachim M. Mayer
Age profile of diphtheria in Bombay *19*, 412 (1975)	N. S. Tibrewala R. D. Potdar S. B. Talathi M. A. Ramnathkar A. D. Katdare
On conformation analysis, molecular graphics, fentanyl and its derivatives *30*, 91 (1986)	J. P. Tollenaere H. Moereels M. van Loon
Antibakterielle Chemotherapie der Tuberkulose *7*, 193 (1964)	F. Trendelenburg
Alternative approaches to the discovery of novel antipsychotic agents *38*, 299 (1992)	M. D. Tricklebank L. J. Bristow P. H. Hutson
Insulin resistance, impaired glucose tolerance and non-insulin-dependent diabetes, pathologic mechanisms and treatment: Current status and therapeutic possibilities *51*, 33 (1998)	Nicholas C. Turner John C. Clapham
Diphtheria *19*, 423 (1975)	P. M. Udani M. M. Kumbhat U. S. Bhat M. S. Nadkarni S. K. Bhave S. G. Ezuthachan B. Kamath
Biologische Oxydation und Reduktion am Stickstoff aromatischer Amino- und Nitro- derivate und ihre Folgen für den Organismus *8*, 195 (1965) Stoffwechsel von Arzneimitteln als Ursache von Wirkungen, Nebenwirkungen und Toxizität *15*, 147 (1971)	H. Uehleke
Mode of death in tetanus *19*, 439 (1975)	H. Vaishnava C. Bhawal Y. P. Munjal

Comparative evaluation of amoebicidal drugs *18*, 353 (1974) Comparative efficacy of newer anthelmintics *19*, 166 (1975)	B. J. Vakil N. J. Dalal
Cephalic tetanus 19, 443 (1975)	B. J. Vakil B. S. Singhal S. S. Pandya P. F. Irami
G protein coupled receptors as modules of interacting proteins: A family meeting *49*, 173 (1997)	Olivier Valdenaire Philippe Vernier
The effect and usefulness of early intravenous beta blockade in acute myocardial infarction *30*, 71 (1986)	Anders Vedin Claes Wilhelmsson
Methods of monitoring adverse reactions to drugs *21*, 231 (1977) Aspects of social pharmacology *22*, 9 (1978)	J. Venulet
The current status of cholera toxoid research in the United States *19*, 602 (1975)	W. F. Verwey J. C. Guckian J. Craig N. Pierce J. Peterson H. Williams Jr
Systemic cancer therapy: Four decades of progress and some personal perspectives *34*, 76 (1990)	Charles L. Vogel
Abnormalities of protein kinases in neurodegenerative diseases *51*, 133 (1998)	Ravenska T. E. Wagey Charles Krieger
The problem of diphtheria as seen in Bombay *19*, 452 (1975)	M. M. Wagle R. R. Sanzgiri Y. K. Amdekar
Drug nephrotoxicity – The significance of cellular mechanisms *41*, 51 (1993)	Robert J. Walker J. Paul Fawcett
Protease inhibitors as potential antiviral agents for the treatment of picornaviral infections *52*, 197 (1999)	Q. May Wang
Nicotine: An addictive substance or a therapeutic agent? *33*, 9 (1989)	David M. Warburton
Cell-wall antigens of *Vibrio cholerae* and their implication in cholera immunity *19*, 612 (1975)	Y. Watanabe R. Ganguly

Nonsteroid antiinflammatory agents *10*, 139 (1966)	C. A. Winter
A review of the continuum of drug- induced states of excitation and depression *26*, 225 (1982)	W. D. Winters
Basic research in the US pharmaceutical industry *15*, 204 (1971)	O. Wintersteiner
Light and dark as a "drug" *31*, 383 (1987)	Anna Wirz-Justice
Neuronal prostacyclin receptors *49*, 123 (1997)	Helen Wise
Dioxopiperazines: Chemistry and biology *35*, 249 (1990)	Donald T. Witiak Yong Wey
The chemotherapy of amoebiasis *8*, 11 (1965)	G. Woolfe
Antimetabolites and their revolution in pharmacology *2*, 613 (1960)	D. W. Woolley
Noise analysis and channels and the postsynaptic membrane of skeletal muscle *24*, 9 (1980)	D. Wray
Krebswirksame Antibiotika aus Actinomyceten *3*, 451 (1961)	Kh. Zepf
Developments in histamine H_1-receptor agonists *44*, 49 (1995)	V. Zingel C. Leschke W. Schunack
Fifteen years of structural modifications in the field of antifungal monocyclic 1-substituted 1 H-azoles *27*, 253 (1983)	L. Zirngibl
Lysostaphin: Model for a specific enzymatic approach to infectious disease *16*, 309 (1972)	W. A. Zygmunt P. A. Tavormina

Backlist

Roger M. Freidinger: Toward peptide receptor ligand drugs: Progress on nonpeptides

Reinhard Sarges and Peter J. Oates: Aldose reductase inhibitors: Recent developments

Eric J. Lien: Design and discovery of new drugs by stepping up and stepping-down approaches

David Rampe and David J. Triggle: New synthetic ligands for L-type voltage-gated calcium channels

Indra Dwivedy, Suprabhat Ray and Arvinder Grover: Present status of luteolytic agents in fertility regulation

Vol. 41, 1993, 406 pp. ISBN 3-7643-2925-4

Mont J. Juchau: Chemical teratogenesis

Robert J. Walker and J. Paul Fawcett: Drug nephrotoxicity – The significance of cellular mechanisms

R. Sutherland: Bacterial resistance to β-lactam antibiotics: Problems and solutions

Noel W. Preston: Eradication by vaccination: The memorial to smallpox could be surrounded by others

Sanjay Batra, Manju Seth and A. P. Bhaduri: Chirality and future drug design

Wilhelm Schoner: Endogenous digitalis-like factors

James W. Fisher: Recent advances in erythropoietin research

Hiroshi Ohtaka and Toshio Fujita: Structural modification patterns from agonists to antagonists and their application to drug design – A new serotonin (5HT$_3$)-antagonist series

Vol. 42, 1994, 472 pp. ISBN 3-7643-2995-5

Michael J. Parnham: Moral challenges in the organization and management of drug research

Vera M. Kolb: Luteinizing hormone regulators: Luteinizing hormone releasing hormone analogs, estrogens, opiates, and estrogen-opiate hybrids

Shradha Sinha and Sudha Jain: Natural products as anticancer agents

A. Das, J. H. Wang and E. J. Lien: Carcinogenicity, mutagenicity and cancer preventing activities of flavonoids: A structure-system-activity relationship (SSAR) analysis

Berend Olivier, Jan Mos, Maikel Rayhoebar, Paul de Koning and Marianne Mak: Serenics

H. Hugh Fudenberg and Giancarlo Pizza: Transfer factor 1993: New frontiers

Giancarlo Pizza, Caterina de Vinci and H. Hugh Fudenberg: Transfer factor in malignancy

Vol. 43, 1994, 330 pp. ISBN 3-7643-5042-3

Harold E. Bays and Carlos Dujovne: Drugs for treatment of patients with high cholesterol blood levels and other dyslipidemias

Eric J. Lien, Hua Gao and Linda L. Lien: In search of ideal antihypertensive drugs: Progress in five decades

N. Seiler and C.L. Atanassov: The natural polyamines and the immune system

Shrada Sinha and Mukta Srivastava: Biologically active quinazolones

Mark P. Hayes and Kathryn C. Zoon: Production and action of interferons: New insights into molecular mechanisms of gene regulation and expression

Vol. 44, 1995, 342 pp. ISBN 3-7643-5149-7

George deStevens: Heterocyclic diversity: The road to biological activity

V. Zingel, C. Leschke and W. Schunack: Developments in Histamine H$_1$-receptor agonists

Paul D. Hoeprich: Antifungal chemotherapy

Richard M. Schultz: New antifolates in cancer therapy

P.K. Mehrotra, Sanjay Batra and A.P. Bhaduri: Non-steroidal menses-regulating agents: The present status

Anil K. Saxena and Mridula Saxena: Developments in anticonvulsants

Vol. 45, 1995, 386 pp. ISBN 3-7643-5212-4

Vijendra K. Singh: Neuropeptides as native immune modulators

Shijun Ren and Eric J. Lien: Natural products and their derivatives as cancer chemopreventive agents

Deborah S. Hartman and Olivier Civelli: Dopamine receptor diversity: Molecular and pharmacological perspectives

Vera M. Kolb: Novel and unusual nucleosides as drugs

Vol. 49, 1997, 373 pp. ISBN 3-7643-5672-3

Richard M. Eglen: 5-Hydroxytryptamine (5-HT)4 receptors and central nervous system function: An update

Mont R. Juchau: Chemical teratogenesis in humans: Biochemical and molecular mechanisms

Gillian Edwards and Arthur H. Weston: Recent advances in potassium channel modulation

Helen Wise: Neuronal prostacyclin receptors

M.D. Murray and D. Craig Brater: Effects of NSAIDs on the kidney

Olivier Valdenaire and Philippe Vernier: G protein coupled receptors as modules of interacting proteins: A family meeting

Annemarie Polak: Antifungal therapy, an everlasting battle

Vol. 50, 1998, 373 pp. ISBN 3-7643-5821-1

P.N. Kaul: Drug discovery: Past, present and future

G. Edwards and A.H. Weston: Endothelium-derived hyperpolarizing factor – a critical appraisal

M. Rohmer: Isoprenoid biosynthesis via the mevalonate-independent route, a novel target for antibacterial drugs

R.W. Rockhold: Glutamatergic involvement in psychomotor stimulant action

T.D. Johnson: Polyamines and cerebral ischemia

J.M. Colacino and K.A. Staschke: The identification and development of antiviral agents for the treatment of chronic hepatitis B virus infection

Vol. 51, 1998, 330 pp. ISBN 3-7643-5822-X

Shijun Ren and Eric J. Lien: Development of HIV protease inhibitors: A survey

Nicholas C. Turner and John C. Clapham: Insulin resistance, impaired glucose tolerance and non-insulin-dependent diabetes, pathologic mechanisms and treatment: Current status and therapeutic possibilities

P.N. Kaul: Drug discovery: Past, present and future

G. Edwards and A.H. Weston: Endothelium-derived hyperpolarizing factor – a critical appraisal

M. Rohmer: Isoprenoid biosynthesis via the mevalonate-independent route, a novel target for antibacterial drugs

R.W. Rockhold: Glutamatergic involvement in psychomotor stimulant action

T.D. Johnson: Polyamines and cerebral ischemia

J.M. Colacino and K.A. Staschke: The identification and development of antiviral agents for the treatment of chronic hepatitis B virus infection

Vol. 52, 1999, 280 pp. ISBN 3-7643-5979-X

Bijoy Kundu and Sanjay K. Khare: Recenc advances in immunosuppressants

Vishnu J. Ram and Atul Goel: Present status of hepatoprotectants

Berend Olivier, Willem Soudijn and Ineke van Wijngarden: The 5HT$_{1A}$ receptor and its ligands: structure and function

Jacob Szmuszkovicz: U-50,488 and the κ receptor: A personalized account covering the period of 1973–1990

Q. May Wang: Protease inhibitors as potential antiviral agents for the treatment of picornaviral infections